THE ENDOMETRIUM

THE ENDOMETRIUM

Edited by

Frances A. Kimball, Ph.D.
Research Scientist
Fertility Research
The Upjohn Company
Kalamazoo, MI

Proceedings of the Eighth Brook Lodge Workshop on Problems in Reproductive Physiology

SP MEDICAL & SCIENTIFIC BOOKS

New York • London

Softcover reprint of the hardcover 1st edition 1980

SPECTRUM PUBLICATIONS, INC.
175-20 Wexford Terrace, Jamaica, N.Y. 11432

Library of Congress Cataloging in Publication Data

Brook Lodge Workshop on Problems of Reproductive
Biology, 8th, 1979.
The endometrium.

Includes index.
1. Endometrium—Congresses. I. Kimball, Frances A.
II. Title. [DNLM: 1. Endometrium—Drug effects—
Congresses. 2. Endometrium—Physiology—Congresses.
W3 BR805 8th 1979e / WP400 B871 1979e]
OP265.B76 1979 599.01'6 80-16110
ISBN 978-94-011-7857-0 ISBN 978-94-011-7855-6 (eBook)
DOI 10.1007/978-94-011-7855-6

Contributors

Margaret H. Abel
MRC Reproductive Biology Unit
Dept. of Obstetrics/Gynecology
University of Edinburgh
Edinburgh EH1 2QW, Scotland

G. J. Barbe
Depts. of Obstetrics/Gynaecology
and of Physiology
The University of Western Ontario
London, Ontario, Canada N6A 5A5

Kenneth L. Barker
Department of Biochemistry
Nebraska Medical Center
42nd and Dewey Avenue
Omaha, Nebraska 68105

Donald H. Barron
Dept. of Obstetrics/Gynecology
University of Florida
College of Medicine
Gainesville, Florida 32610

Etienne-Emile Baulieu
Faculté de Médecine de Bicêtre
Lab Hormones
94270 Bicêtre, France

Fuller W. Bazer
Department of Animal Science
Livestock Pavilion - Archer Road
University of Florida
Gainesville, Florida 32611

John D. Biggers
Laboratory of Human Reproduction
and Reproductive Biology
45 Shattuck Street
Boston, Massachusetts 02115

Sam C. Brooks
Department of Biochemistry
Wayne State University
School of Medicine
540 Canfield
Detroit, Michigan 48201

Allen E. Buhl
Fertility Research
The Upjohn Company
Kalamazoo, Michigan 49001

W. R. Butler
Department of Animal Science
Cornell University
Ithaca, New York 14850

John R. Chenault
Animal Health - Reproduction
The Upjohn Company
Kalamazoo, Michigan 49001

E. A. Conner
Department of Pathology
University of Colorado
Health Sciences Center
Denver, Colorado 80262

C. J. Conti
Department of Pathology
University of Colorado
Health Sciences Center
Denver, Colorado 80262

J. R. Depaoli
Department of Pathology
University of Colorado
Health Sciences Center
Denver, Colorado 80262

Eugene R. DeSombre
Ben May Laboratory for Cancer
Research
University of Chicago
Chicago, Illinois 60637

S. K. Dey
Depts. of Obstetrics/Gynecology
and of Physiology
University of Kansas Medical Ctr.
Ralph L. Smith Research Center
Kansas City, Kansas 66103

D. J. Dierschke
Wisconsin Regional Primate Center
Madison, Wisconsin 53701

Richard L. Eckert
Dept. of Physiology & Biophysics
School of Basic Medical Sciences
University of Illinois
Urbana, Illinois 61801

C. A. Evans
Depts. of Obstetrics/Gynecology
and of Physiology
The University of Western Ontario
London, Ontario, Canada N6A 5A5

Colin A. Finn
Dept. of Veterinary Physiology
University of Liverpool
Leahurst, Weston, Wirrol
Merseyside, L647TE, United Kingdom

Larry R. French
732 Animal Science Building
1685 Observatory Drive
University of Wisconsin
Madison, Wisconsin 53706

G. R. Fritz
Department of Physiology
University of Pittsburgh
School of Medicine
Pittsburgh, Pennsylvania 15261

R. Don Gambrell, Jr.
Department of Endocrinology
Medical College of Georgia
Augusta, Georgia 30902

L. E. Gerschenson
Department of Pathology
Univ. of Colorado Medical Center
4200 East Ninth Street
Denver, Colorado 80262

Ernest A. Gilling
Fertility Research
The Upjohn Company
Kalamazoo, Michigan 49001

L. Gimenez-Conti
Department of Pathology
University of Colorado
Health Sciences Center
Denver, Colorado 80262

Stanley R. Glasser
Department of Cell Biology
Baylor College of Medicine
Houston, Texas 77030

Robert B. Greenblatt
Department of Endocrinology
Medical College of Georgia
903 15th Street
Augusta, Georgia 30902

Harold C. Halvorson
International - Medical
The Upjohn Company
Kalamazoo, Michigan 49001

J. William Hendrix
Medical Endocrinology
The Upjohn Company
Kalamazoo, Michigan 49001

E. Keith Inskeep
Division of Animal Science
West Virginia University
Morgantown, West Virginia 26506

D. C. Johnson
Depts. of Obstetrics/Gynecology
and of Physiology
University of Kansas Medical Ctr.
Ralph L. Smith Research Center
Kansas City, Kansas 66103

Benita S. Katzenellenbogen
Dept. of Physiology & Biophysics
School of Basic Medical Sciences
Unitersity of Illinois
Urbana, Illinois 61801

Thomas G. Kennedy
Depts. of Obstetrics/Gynecology
and of Physiology
The Univ. of Western Ontario
London, Ontario, Canada N6A 5A5

Frances A. Kimball
Fertility Research
The Upjohn Company
Kalamazoo, Michigan 49001

Kenneth T. Kirton
Fertility Research
The Upjohn Company
Kalamazoo, Michigan 49001

E. Knobil
Department of Physiology
University of Pittsburgh
School of Medicine
Pittsburgh, Pennsylvania 15261

Nancy C. Lan
Dept. of Physiology & Biophysics
School of Basic Medical Sciences
University of Illinois
Urbana, Illinois 61801

James W. Lauderdale
Experimental Agricultural Biology
The Upjohn Company
Kalamazoo, Michigan 49001

Thomas J. Lobl
Fertility Research
The Upjohn Company
Kalamazoo, Michigan 49001

Frederique Logeat
Groupe de Recherches sur la Biochimie
Endocrinienne et le Reproduction
(INSERM U 135), Faculté de Médecine
Paris-Sud, 94270 Bicêtre, France

C. Richard Lyttle
Ben May Laboratory for Cancer Research
The University of Chicago
Chicago, Illinois 60637

James Mazella
Dept. of Obstetrics/Gynecology
School of Medicine
Health Sciences
State University of New York at Stony Brook
Stony Brook, New York 11794

Shirley A. McCormack
Department of Cell Biology
Baylor College of Medicine
Houston, Texas 77030

Edwin Milgrom
Groupe de Recherches sur la Biochimie
Endocrinienne et le Reproduction
(INSERM U 135), Faculté de Médecine
Paris-Sud, 94270 Bicêtre, France

William L. Miller
Fertility Research
The Upjohn Company
Kalamazoo, Michigan 49001

Rodrigue Mortel
Hershey University Medical Center
Hershey, Pennsylvania 17033

Harland W. Mossman
Department of Anatomy
University of Wisconsin
Madison, Wisconsin 53706

Bruce C. Moulton
University of Cincinnati
College of Medicine
Dept. of Obstetrics/Gynecology
Cincinnati, Ohio 45267

J. T. Murai
Department of Pathology
University of Colorado
Health Sciences Center
Denver, Colorado 80262

Helen A. Padykula
Department of Anatomy
University of Massachusetts
Medical School
55 Lake Avenue, N.
Worcester, Massachusetts 01605

Edward J. Pavlik
Dept. of Physiology & Biophysics
School of Basic Medical Sciences
University of Illinois
Urbana, Illinois 61801

Paul Robel
Faculté de Médecine de Bicêtre
Lab Hormones
94270 Bicêtre, France

Pierre Sartor
Laboratoire des Interactions Cellulaires
Université de Bordeaux II
33076 Bordeaux, France

Paul C. Schwallie
Fertility Research
The Upjohn Company
Kalamazoo, Michigan 49001

S. S. Shapiro
Dept. of Obstetrics/Gynecology
University of Wisconsin
Center for Health Sciences
Madison, Wisconsin 53706

Edward M. Southern
Fertility Research
The Upjohn Company
Kalamazoo, Michigan 49001

Charles H. Spilman
Fertility Research
The Upjohn Company
Kalamazoo, Michigan 49001

Linda Tseng
Dept. of Obstetrics/Gynecology
School of Medicine
Health Sciences Center
State University of New York
at Stony Brook
Stony Brook, New York 11794

Mai T. Vu Hai
Groupe de Recherches sur la
Biochimie
Endocrinienne et le Reproduction
(INSERM U 135), Faculté de Médecine
Paris-Sud, 94270 Bicêtre, France

John W. Wilks
Fertility Research
The Upjohn Company
Kalamazoo, Michigan 49001

Laird Wilson, Jr.
Dept. of Obstetrics/Gynecology
University of Illinois
Medical Center
Chicago, Illinois 60612

Yang-Dar Yuan
Pathology & Toxicology Research
The Upjohn Company
Kalamazoo, Michigan 49001

Preface

The Eighth Brook Lodge Conference on Problems of Reproductive Physiology is the latest in a series of small meetings held over 18 years. The topics for these meetings have reflected the changing interests and backgrounds of the organizers. The recent rapidly increasing quantity of information on the uterine endometrium and its continuing relevance to fertility control stimulated the organizers to focus the 1979 workshop on this topic. The first four speakers provided a histological background for the molecular and biochemical studies described subsequently. The interaction of biochemist, physiologist, pathologist and physician as they focus their thoughts and talents on this limited area of the body is apparent in the discussions of presentations. This workshop was planned to provide insight and a sense of proportion for the participants. For the reader, the record of the proceedings should serve as a useful reference to the state of the art in this area of research.

The uterine endometrium is central in the successful implantation and development of the embryo. Examination of the physical relationships, biochemical interactions and hormonal influences in this tissue could further advance the understanding of this pivotal tissue in the reproductive process. The depth of the understanding of endometrial physiology should be reflected in our ability to better control this reproductive endpoint and to treat its dysfunction.

The efforts of many individuals made these Proceedings possible. Members of Fertility Research at The Upjohn Company planned and organized the program. We appreciate the contributions of the workshop participants who prepared manuscripts and participated in the discussions. We also wish to thank Doctors F. W. Bazer, L. E. Gerschenson, B. S. Katzenellenbogen and B. C. Moulton for serving as session chairpersons. The hospitality provided by the staff of Brook Lodge was an important feature in providing the atmosphere for this workshop. The editorial assistance of Suzanne K. Moyer and the efforts of Edna Bronson, Ruth Ann Connors, Marty Klerk and Lois VandeGiessen in the preparation of the discussions are appreciated.

Frances A. Kimball, Ph.D.

January 1980

Contents

PART I
ENDOMETRIAL MORPHOLOGY

1

Comparative Morphology of the Endometrium

Harland W. Massman

To my knowledge, no one has ever written a comprehensive treatise on the comparative morphology of the mammalian endometrium. There is a fair amount of information available, but it has to be gleaned from the literature on other subjects, such as estrous cycles, pseudopregnancy, etc. Thus I have had to rely to a large extent on my own experience in examining microscopic sections made in my study of placentation. What I am able to present is therefore not a well-rounded finished thesis, but rather a somewhat fragmentary and tentative sketch of the field.

The sole purpose of the uterus of a placental mammal is to furnish a conduit through which spermatozoa reach the eggs, and to contain and sustain the developing conceptus from the morula or early blastocyst period until parturition. A major part of these functions is borne by the endometrium, which is the mucous membrane lining that part of the uterus in which the conceptus is housed. The mucosa of the cervical region is not endometrium proper and usually differs structurally from the true endometrium.

Before proceeding further, it may be that some are thinking of the uterine luteolytic factor as a separate uterine function. This feature is, I believe, best regarded as part of the complex preparation of a uterus for a subsequent pregnancy. The inactivity and regressed state of the uterus of a monestrous mammal during a long anestrous period is good evidence of its uselessness in the animal's day-to-day existence when not involved in reproduction.

The uterus of mammals has, no doubt, evolved from part of the oviduct of their presumed egg-laying ancestors, but its function has changed dramatically. The ancestral reptiles and probably even the early ancestral mammals had large-yolked (megalecithal) eggs into which the ovary had deposited enough yolk to sustain the embryos until hatching time. If the oviduct or its so-called uterine segment contributed anything other than shell membranes and shell, it must have been principally albumin and water. Most modern reptile eggs have relatively little albumin compared to those of birds, and most of their need for additional water seems to be satisfied by absorption through the egg shell and shell membranes from the external environment in which the eggs are deposited. Both marsupials and placental mammals (Eutheria) have minimal-yolked (miolecithal) eggs, consequently their embryos must be nourished until birth by the uterus, i.e. directly by the endometrium.

Nutritive substances presented to the embryos by the endometrium vary in different mammalian groups both in type and in relative importance. All endometria supply nutrition by direct transfer through the interhemal membrane (placental barrier) of the zona intima from the maternal to the fetal bloodstream. Probably all, in one way or another, supply endometrial epithelial and glandular secretions to absorptive areas of the fetal membranes. Many also supply the breakdown products from dead endometrial surface and gland epithelial cells (Prasad et al., 1979), and from dead stroma and decidua. These are absorbed or phagocytosed by the adjacent fetal membrane. Carnivores (Creed and Biggers, 1963; Sinha and Mossman, 1966) and a few others (certain bats and insectivores, and at least the sheep (Steven, 1975) among bovoids) also provide extravasated maternal blood. Of course, the direct transfer from maternal to fetal bloodstreams is the most important of these mechanisms as is indicated by the large and elaborate choriovitelline and chorioallantoic placentas of marsupials and eutherians respectively. It certainly accounts for most of the transmission of electrolytes, other small molecules, and respiratory gases. However, the other mechanisms have an importance only now beginning to be fully recognized, and they are the most directly related to endometrial structure and type. Thus, for purposes of this discussion, endometrial epithelium, glands, and stroma will be emphasized; and endometrial blood vascular and lymph vascular systems and innervation will be largely ignored. Likewise slight reference will be made to electron microscopy of the endometrium, as too little has been published to have much significance from a comparative viewpoint. The following references may be useful to anyone wishing to enter the relatively recent literature on these aspects of endometrial morphology. Innervation: Kuhnel and Beier, 1976. Capillary supply: MacDonald, 1976. Transmission electron microscopy: Wynn, 1977. Scanning EM: Hafez and Ludwig, 1977. Delayed implantation: Enders and Given, 1977.

The uterus of viviparous mammals probably evolved from the glandular portion of the oviduct of oviparous ancestors. Although its glands no longer secrete massive amounts of albumin or the fibrous shell membranes and calcareous shell, they are always present and are known to secrete at least mucoproteins and glycogen (Spilman and Wilks, 1978). They probably have far more important functions in some mammals than these two products suggest. Many species, especially those with epitheliochorial and endotheliochorial placentation, usually have numerous and well-developed phagocytic and absorptive areas on the chorioallantois apposed to the gland mouths (Figs. 1-4). These range from simple absorptive and phagocytic plaques, through so-called areolae, to large often somewhat villous folds such as those surrounding the placentomes of most ruminants (Fig. 4).

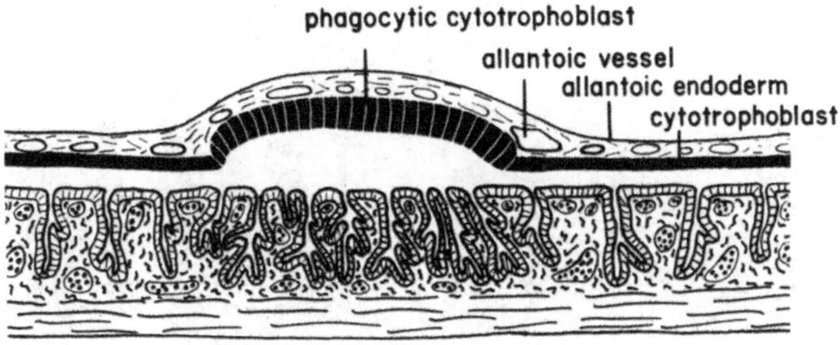

Fig. 1. Diagram of the simplest form of areola as described on the smooth chorioallantois of carnivores. The areolar dome often covers only one gland mouth.

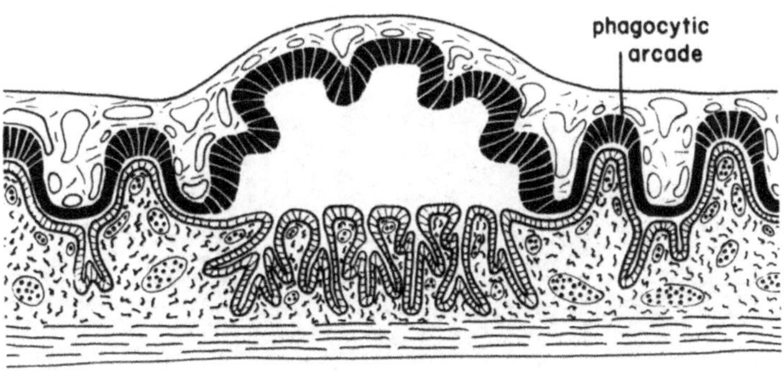

Fig. 2. Diagram of an areola and the arcade system as seen in the chorioallantoic placenta of swine. The dome lining of the areola may be heavily rugose and may cover only one gland mouth.

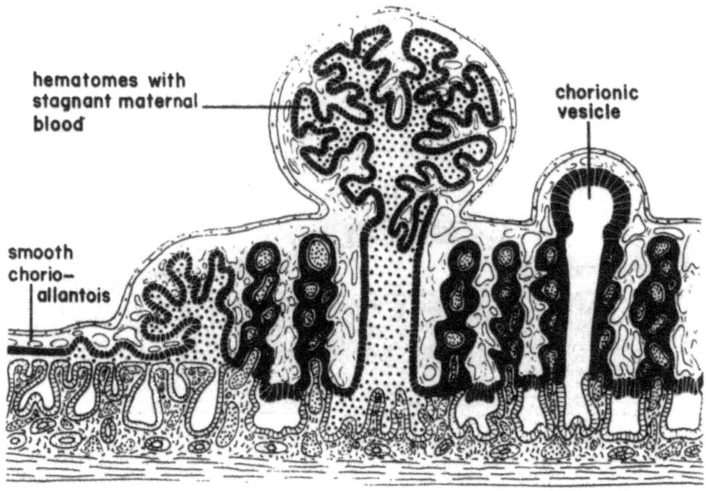

Fig. 3. Diagram of a carnivore placenta showing at the left a marginal hematome such as that of canids, a central hematome common in mustelids and the raccoons, chorionic vesicle or areola, and the absorptive tips of villi covering the gland mouths.

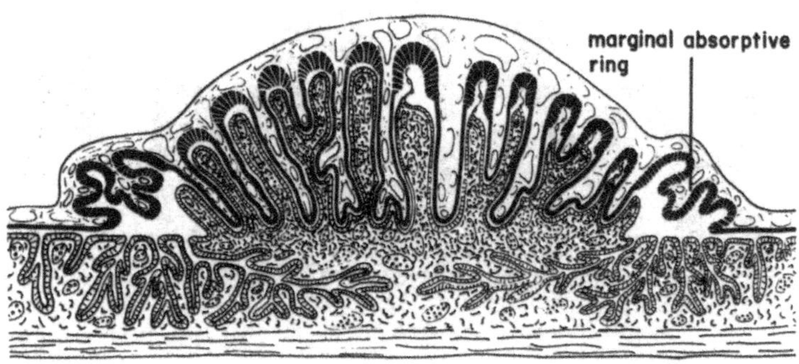

Fig. 4. Diagram of a placentome (cotyledon) of a ruminant showing the marginal absorptive ring and the arcade system. The left half shows the crypt septa before atrophy of their edges; the right half shows them atrophied, a condition especially prominent in deer.

The endometrium of all viviparous mammals has the same general type of tubular somewhat coiled, and usually unbranched glands, but they vary greatly in number. Rats and mice tend to have relatively few and irregularly scattered glands. In many other rodents and in most mammals they are relatively numerous, and usually quite uniform in distribution. Typically the mammalian endometrium is lined by a simple cuboidal epithelium which also lines the mouths and a fairly distinct neck region of each gland. The gland body is usually somewhat coiled and may be slightly branched (Fig. 5). The endometrial stroma is

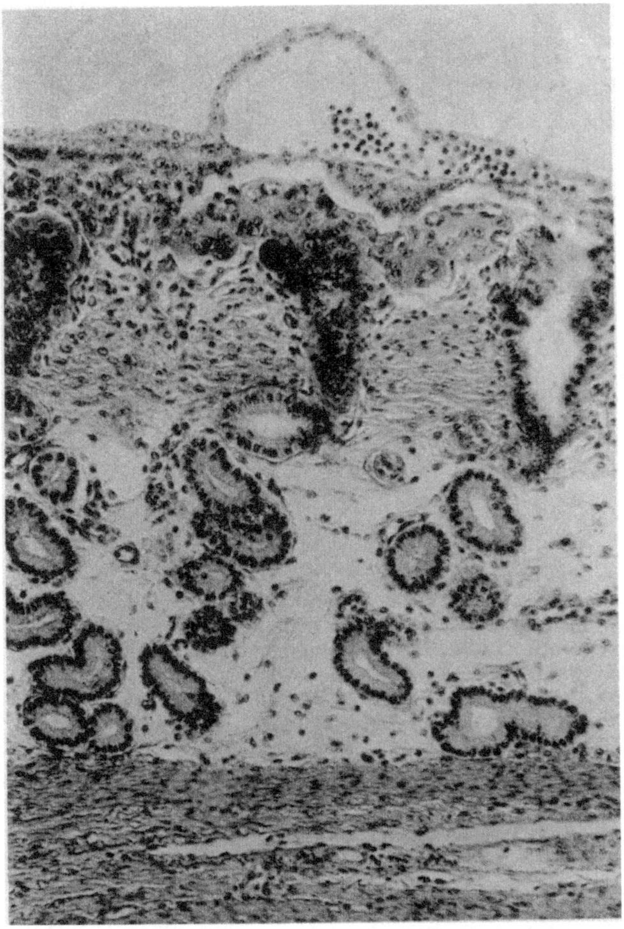

Fig. 5. Mole (Scalopus aquaticus) uterine wall with early attaching choriovitelline membrane showing beginning modification of gland mouth and neck epithelium. Note that the gland body epithelium is in the same state of development throughout. In deciduate placentas the gland tips tend to remain functionally inactive.

usually quite dense between the gland necks (stratum compactum), relatively loose and often edematous between the bodies (stratum spongiosum), and more dense where it connects to the myometrium (stratum basale). In larger, and especially in simplex uteri, the junction with the myometrium is irregular, for the latter is made up of interwoven trabeculae of smooth muscle forming a so-called inner circular and an outer longitudinal coat.

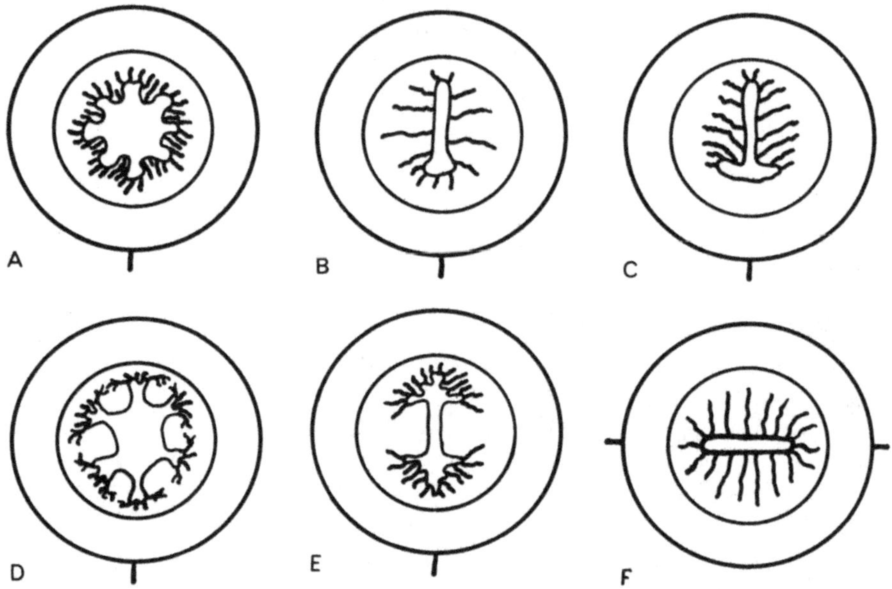

Fig. 6. Diagrams of different thicknesses and patterns of gland distribuions characteristic of endometria of certain eutherian groups. A. Uniform (carnivores, swine). B. Varying thickness and gland distribution along the mesometrial to antimesometrial wall (rabbits, rodents). C. Same (shrews, moles). D. Numerous aglandular caruncles (most ruminants). E. Paired aglandular ridges (tree shrews). F. Relatively uniform distribution of glands and relatively minor differences in thickness as in most simplex uteri (monkeys, apes, man).

These muscle coats are usually not the clear-cut circular and longitudinal layers seen in such organs as the small intestine; rather they consist of more or less interwoven trabeculae that are longitudinal on the outer uterine surface but gradually become more circular as they spiral deeper and deeper into the uterine wall. Thus it is common in larger mammals to find endometrial projections among the inner muscular trabeculae, and in women, even portions of the villous placenta may be gripped and held in these pockets at parturition. Unlike many other mucosae the endometrium has no muscularis mucosae.

There is commonly at least one difference in the glands between the endometria of mammals having deciduate and nondeciduate placentas. In the deciduate forms the basal ends of the gland bodies tend to remain embryonic and nonfunctional during pregnancy as in man. At parturition these basal portions are not deciduated, and it is from them that the new glands and at least some of the new surface epithelium are regenerated. In nondeciduate species (Fig. 5) the tips of the gland bodies function like the rest of the body and after parturition the whole gland becomes functionally inactive until stimulated by the next estral and gestational activity. In other words, extensive proliferation of new glands and endometrial tissue after each menstruation or pregnancy does not occur in mammals which do not shed uterine tissue at parturition or during a reproductive cycle.

It is through the contact of the endometrium with the conceptus or its secretions that the mother learns physiologically that she is pregnant, and that the complicated reactions appropriate to pregnancy are initiated and carried out. Yet, when a pregnancy fails, it is unlikely to be the fault of the endometrium. It seems probable that an endometrial abnormality must be rather extreme to result in pregnancy interruption, and also that most such endometrial pathology is secondary to some endocrine disturbance. The well-known ability of the mother and embryo of man and a few other species to adjust to completely extra-uterine pregnancy, even to the production of a normal full-term fetus, indicates a remarkable capacity for feto-maternal anatomical adjustment, provided the basic physiological systems of both are normal. This ability of the blastocyst to attach and establish a functional placentation on the peritoneal lining of the abdominal cavity does not necessarily argue that the endometrium normally has little importance, but rather that the feto-maternal partnership at least in some mammals, has remarkable adaptive capacity in emergency situations.

Since the endometrium relates the mother to the conceptus structurally and functionally by virtue of close anatomical contact or actual intermingling of tissue elements in the form of various types of placentation, it would be almost meaningless to discuss the comparative aspects of the endometrium without also considering the types of placentation with which each endometrial type is involved. However, we shall see that the endometrium is, or at least appears to be, anatomically much alike among many species that have very different forms of placentation. However, we shall also find that in a few cases very obvious anatomical correlations do exist between the two.

It is almost impossible to make a logical, completely inclusive and at the same time exclusive yet simple classification of any large biological system, for nature has no need to classify and has made no effort to have her features conveniently classifiable. Hence, the outline and organization of the following presentation and of Table I are by no means perfect. They could probably be made more logical by basing them on a classification of fetal membranes; but since comparative fetal membranology seems to be terra incognita to most biologists, I have devised a relatively artificial system based on easily observed gross and histological characteristics of the endometrium

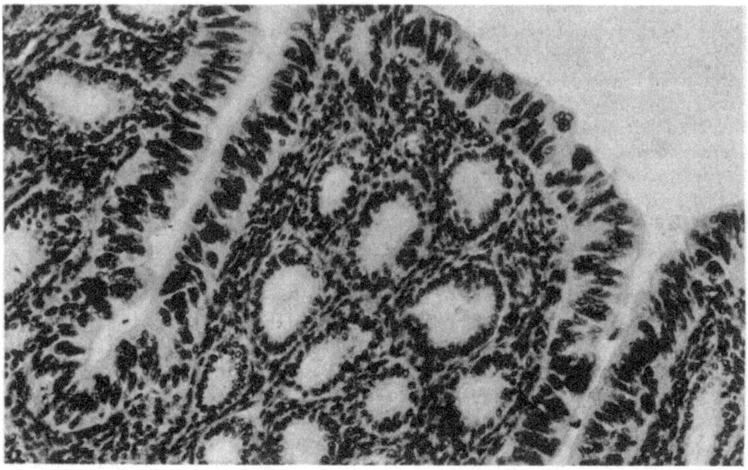

Fig. 7. Endometrium of an intergestation sac area of a snowshoe hare (Lepus americanus) in mid-gestation. Note that the simple columnar surface epithelium has been greatly modified by the formation of numerous multinucleate cells and syncytial masses while the gland epithelium has retained its simple columnar forms. Klein (1933) showed and illustrated well this same condition in the domestic rabbit. It also occurs in the nonpregnant horn of a unilaterally pregnant doe.

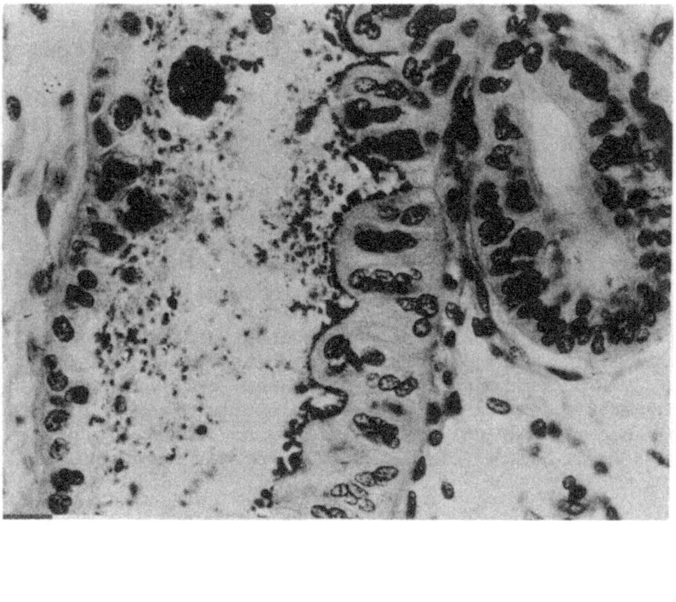

Fig. 8. Higher magnification of snowshoe hare endometrium at the end of a gestation sac, showing chorion at the left with multinucleate trophoblastic masses and cellular debris in the uterine lumen.

(Fig. 6). However, the fetal membrane types involved with each have been mentioned along with examples of some of the better-known mammalian groups possessing each type. This should give an experimentalist some help is selecting suitable species for use as experimental subjects for specific problems. For example, absorption of uterine gland secretions is clearly an important part of fetal nutrition throughout gestation in carnivores and hoofed animals, but the behavior of the glands in animals having a decidua, such as anthropoids and man, suggests that their function, whatever it may be, except during the nidation period, is carried out chiefly by decidual cells, and surface epithelium (Figs. 7, 8, 9).

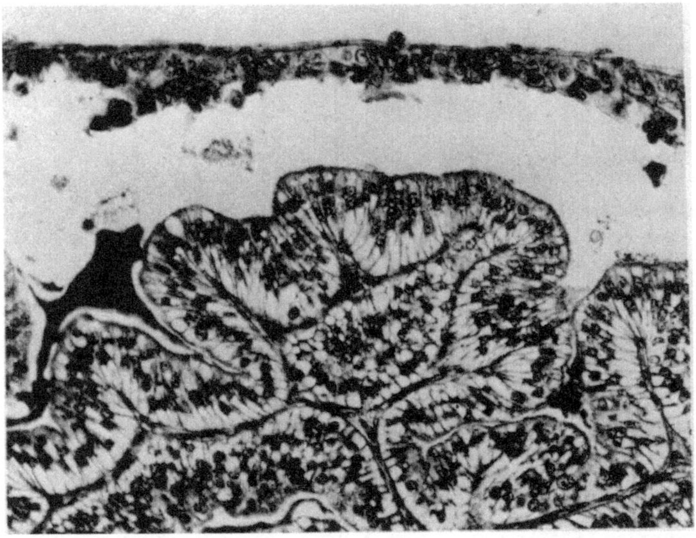

Fig. 9. Uterine epithelium at the end of a gestation sac of a flying squirrel (Glaucomys volans) in mid-pregnancy. This extreme reaction occurs throughout the intergestation sac areas and in both uterine horns even though embryos may be present in only one.

The range and quality of placental interchange is known to be somewhat related to the morphology of the interhemal membrane (placental barrier), and this is generally believed to depend upon the aggressiveness of the trophoblast in penetrating the endometrium. It could as well depend upon endometrial defense against trophoblastic penetration. At present, I at least, can see nothing in the morphology of an endometrium to explain why it thwarts or why it succumbs to trophoblastic invasion. More cytological studies comparing the endometria of mammals with noninvasive epitheliochorial placentation to those with invasive endotheliochorial or hemochorial types may someday reveal at least some of the reasons why these different degrees of endometrial invasion occur.

Pertinent to our classification and discussion of endometrial type is the gross anatomy of mammalian uteri. All arise from the paired female ducts (mullerian ducts) of the embryo (Fig. 10, 11). During development, these fuse in varying degrees in different species. Fusion always begins at their caudal ends. No fusion or only superficial fusion, not involving the lumina, results in duplex uteri. Complete fusion at the caudal ends, including the lumina, produces long, medium, or short bicornuate uteri, depending upon how much of the lumina of the original ducts is involved. Complete fusion the entire length of the uterine portions of the ducts, i.e., forward as far as the attachment of the proper ligament (gubernaculum) of the ovary, produces a simplex uterus, although many of these, as in anthropoids and man, retain short internal remnants of the lumina of the two cornua.

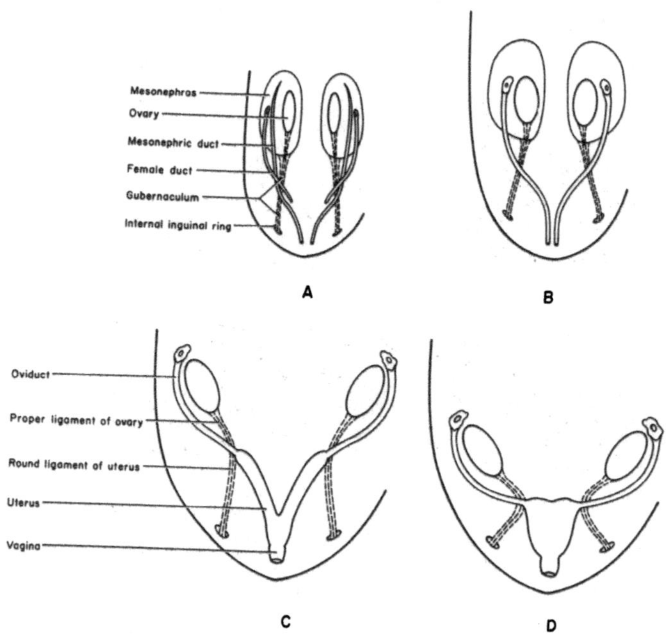

Fig. 10. Ventral view diagrams to show the relations of the gubernaculum to the female duct, and the relations of the derivatives of each to one another. Most other urogenital organs are omitted. A. - early fetal stage. B. - later fetal stage. C.- definitive stage in the case of a long bicornuate uterus with minimal caudal migration of the internal genital organs. D. - definitive stage in the case of a simplex uterus with maximal caudal migration. (From: Biology of the Uterus, Ralph M. Wynn, ed., Plenum Pr., 1977).

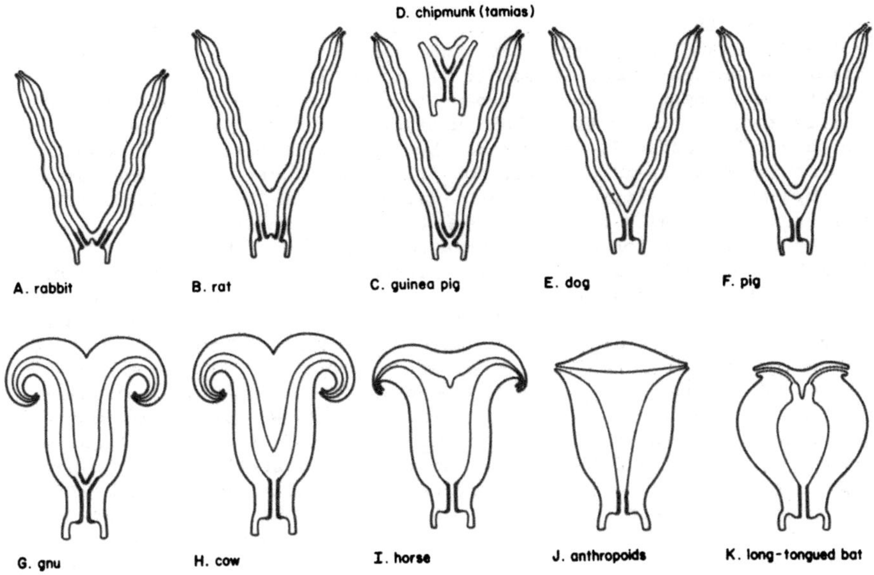

Fig. 11. Diagrammatic frontal sections of the types of uteri found among Eutheria. One known possessor of each is given. Oviducts are indicated cut near their uterotubal junctions and the vaginae just caudal to the cervices. Heaviest line = cervical mucosa; lightest line = endometrial surface epithelium; dashed line = oviduct epithelium. A to D long duplex: A. most primitive; B. caudal ends fused externally, simulating a corpus uteri; C., D. V-shaped and Y-shaped cervical canals, respectively. E., F. long bicornuate: E. very short corpus, rarely permitting a conceptus to extend from one cornu to the other; F corpus large enough to permit a conceptus with its placenta in one cornu to extend into the other cornu. G. medium length duplex: Y-shaped cervical canal. H. medium length bicornuate: corpus permits fetal membranes, but usually not the fetus, to extend into opposite cornu. I. short bicornuate: very short septum, which is essentially obliterated during pregnancy, permitting fetal membranes and sometimes the fetus to extend into the opposite cornu. J. simplex: cornua represented only by the lateral angles of the lumen and their surrounding tissues: K. cornua represented by small tubular pits (with surrounding tissues) connecting with the intramural portions of the oviducts. The blastocyst implants in one of these pits (modified from Rasweller, 1974). (From: Biology of the Uterus, Ralph M. Wynn, ed., Plenum Pr., 1977).

The importance of the gross differences between the simplex and the others is that while many duplex and bicornuate uteri have rather marked differences between the endometrium on the mesometrial side compared to that of the antimesometrial area (Fig. 12), simplex uteri, so far as I am aware, have only a moderate variation in thickness or other characters from one side to the other (Fig. 6). In all uterine types the endometrium usually does become noticeably thinner near the cervix and near the utero-tubal junction. However, there seems to be an occult but effective difference between the lateral and midsagittal regions in some simplex uteri, for it is known that in anthropoids and man by far the greater number of nidations occur in the midsagittal plane, not laterally near the mesometrial attachments.

The classification of endometria that follows (Table I) relates them to adeciduate and deciduate placentation and to the presence or absence of true decidual tissue. True is emphasized because more or less isolated cells, presumed to be of maternal origin but of unknown function, have been described as decidual cells in carnivores where no typical decidual cell tissue exists. Carnivores do shed a fair amount of the highly glandular endometrium at the base of their placentas at parturition and are therefore considered to have deciduate placentas, although they have no true decidual cell tissue. As a matter of fact, the full function of decidua is still unknown; hence we can recognize no specific characteristics that will identify with certainty an isolated cell as one of true decidua. Until we can do this, it only causes confusion to designate such a cell as decidua simply because it appears to be maternal and superficially resembles the cells of decidual tissue.

There are several gestational phenomena among mammals that indicate physiological differences in the endometrium between species, and also local physiological differences within the same female. For most of these, no clearly correlated morphological features have been recognized. Some of these unexplained phenomena are: 1. The relatively uniform spacing of nidation sites in mammals with multiple embryos. 2. The apparent lack of spacing and consequent crowding of embryos in certain species, especially those with excessively large litters such as the multimammate mouse, *Mastomys erythroleucus* (Brambell and Davis, 1941). 3. The ovulation and fertilization at one estrus of two hundred or more eggs, but the nidation and gestation of only one per uterine horn in the plains viscasha, *Lagostomus maximus* (Weir, 1971). 4. The death of all but two embryos in the pronghorn antelope, *Antilocapra americana*, presumably because only one in each horn is able to attach to the specific nidation area (O'Gara, 1969). 5. The usual midsagittal plane line of the simplex uteri of anthropoids and man in which most nidations occur. 6. The specific nidation area in the central segment of the uterine horn in ruminants (Lee, Mossman and Mossman, 1977). 7. The high percentage of right horn nidation in some bats (Wimsatt, 1944), in the muntjac deer (Chapman and Dansie, 1969; Chaplin and Harrison, 1971), and in several African antelope (Kellas, 1955; Buechner, 1961; Mossman and Mossman, 1965; Robinette and Child, 1964; Child and Mossman, 1965; Spinage, 1969; Symington and Paterson, 1970). 9. The obligate antimesometrial nidation site of rodents.

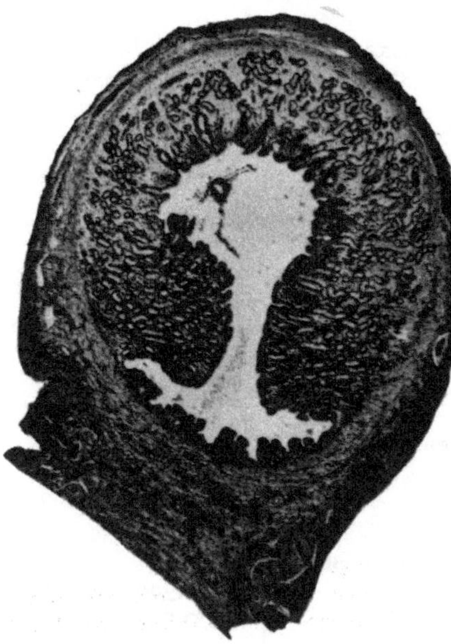

Fig. 12. Cross section of mole (Scalopsus aquaticus) uterus in early pregnancy to show the variation in endometrial thickness and gland distribution along the mesometrial to antimesometrial wall.

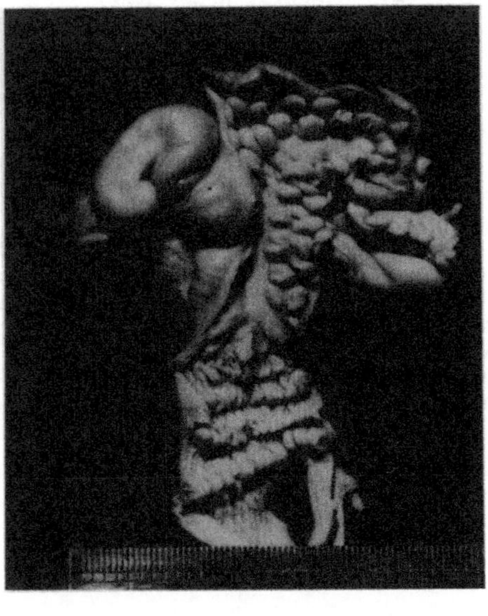

Fig. 13. Reproductive tract of 54 cm (tip of nose to root of tail) cow fetus. Vagina, cervix, uterine body, and right uterine horn opened. Note the numerous endometrial caruncles already differentiated in the body and horn.

TABLE I

I. Thickness and number of glands relatively uniform (Fig. 6a, 6f).

A. No true decidual tissue.

1. Adeciduate placentation.

PIGS, CAMELS, HORSES, LEMURS
Suoidea (pigs, hippos), Camelidae (camels, llamas), Perissodactyla (horses, tapirs, rhinos), Lemuridae, Lorisidae, Daubentonidae (galagos), Manidae (pangolins), Tragulidae (chevrotains).
Duplex or bicornuate uteri.
Epitheliochorial placentation.
Areolae and arcade systems.

2. Deciduate placentation.

*DOG, CATS, FERRETS
Carnivora
Bicornuate uteri.
Endotheliochorial placentation, except hyena which is hemochorial.
Areolae, absorptive areas at tips of villi, hematomes.

B. True decidual tissue.

1. Deciduate placentation.

a. SOME INSECTIVORES AND BATS, DASSIES
Tenrecidae(tenrecs), Chiroptera (bats), Chrysochloridae (gold moles), Hracoidea (dassies), Orycteropus (aardvark), Tarsius (tarsiers).
Duplex or bicornuate uteri.
Endotheliochorial or hemochorial placentation.
Yolk sac inversion in some bats.

b. MONKEYS, APES, MAN
Anthropoidea, Phyllostomatidae (Am. leaf-nosed bats), Bradypodidae (sloths), Dasypodidae (armadillos).
Simplex Uteri.
Endotheliochorial or hemochorial placentation.

* Carnivores are considered to have deciduate placentas because a small amount of glandular endometrium is shed at parturition. However, they have no true decidual cell tissue, although scattered, isolated, presumably maternal cells in their placental labyrinths have been described as decidua, because they bear a general resemblance to decidual cells of other groups. They are not located in the usual position of true decidual tissue, which is at the base of the placental labyrinth.

TABLE I, continued

II. Thickness and number of glands change from the mesometrial to the antimesometrial side of the uterus (Figs. 6b, 6c; 12).

A. No true decidual tissue.

1. Adeciduate placentation.

PRARIE MOLE
(Scalopus aquaticus).
Bicornuate uterus.
Epitheliochorial placentation (Prasad et al., 1979).
Numerous areolae (Fig. 15).

B. True decidual tissue.

1. Deciduate placentation.

RABBITS, RODENTS
Lagomorpha (rabbits), Rodentia, Erinaceidae (hedge-hogs).
Soricidae (shrews), Vespertilionidae (many common bats).
Duplex or bicornuate uteri.
Endotheliochorial or hemochorial placentation.
Inversion of the yolk sac.

III. Localized aglandular ridges or caruncles (Figs. 6d, 6e; 13, 14).

A. No true decidual tissue.

1. Adeciduate placentation.

CATTLE, GOATS, SHEEP, ANTELOPE, DEER
Bovidae, Cervidae (deer), Giraffidae, Antilocapridae (pronghorns).
Duplex or bicornuate uteri.
Epitheliochorial placentation.
Areolae, arcade systems, and marginal absorptive rings around cotyledons.
(Some breeds of sheep have melanin pigmentation of the caruncles).

B. True decidual tissue.

1. Deciduate placentation.

TREE SHREWS
Tupaiidae.
Bicornuate uteri.
Endotheliochorial placentation.

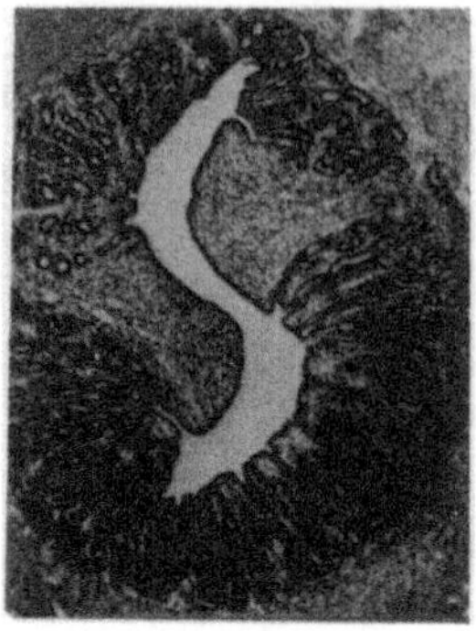

Fig. 14. Cross section of the uterus of an immature tree shrew (Tupaiia minor) showing the paired aglandular ridges on which the paired placental discs develop. (From Luckett, 1968).

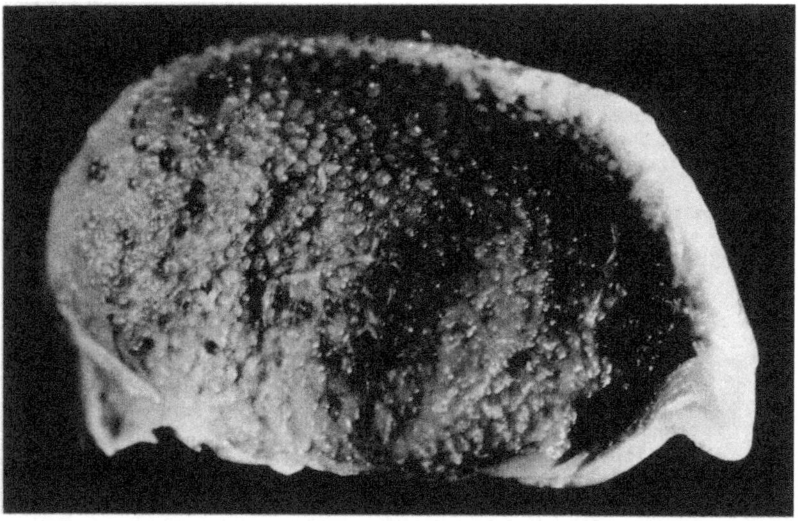

Fig. 15. Photograph of the inner surface of the epitheliochorial placenta of a mole (Scalopus aquaticus) to show the numerous absorptive areolae covering the endometrial gland mouths. X3. The villi occupy the net-like space between the areolae. Glandular products must be a major item in the nutrition of the embryos of these moles (see Prasad et al., 1979 for more details, including EM studies).

What morphological clues should one look for to help explain these phenomena? There could be peculiarities of nerve or blood supply, muscular arrangement, ciliation, epithelial cell type, or gland type. Casual observations have shown no definite evidence of this sort, but no intensive studies have been made. However, there is good evidence that in some species the blastocysts produce secretions that trigger physiological reactions in the mother (Spilman and Wilks, 1978), but there is no indication, of which I am aware, that the message must be received at a specific attachment area in order to be effective. It is somewhat discouraging to contemplate a thorough search for any of these possible morphological factors, for they all would seem to require long and tedious procedures and to promise little likelihood of success. Nevertheless, if one knew the mechanisms involved in the natural transport of blastocysts to a favorable attachment site, and what there is about these sites that allows the blastocysts to recognize them and attach, the applications of such information obviously would be substantial.

A completely comparative morphological approach to these problems has little chance of solving any of them, but it can and has given some information as to what species would make favorable experimental subjects, and as to the areas of their uteri and endometria in which to probe for clues.

The following tabular outline gives the distribution of the three somewhat arbitrarily defined types of endometrium among eutherian mammals (see also Fig. 6). Heading each list are the common names of some of the more familiar and easily available species. Following this are scientific names, including the common animals mentioned and others. Several important groups of mammals are omitted because of lack of information. These include Elephantidae, Cetacea (whales), and several groups of bats and insectivores. It should be mentioned that many subgroups of the major groups listed have never been examined, so exceptions to this tentative classification no doubt exist. Uterine and placental types are mentioned, as are the various absorptive and phagocytic areas of the chorioallantois, since the latter are directly related to the glandular pattern of the endometrium.

ACKNOWLEDGEMENTS

I am indebted to the following: for typing - Donna Leonard and Julie Michels; for photography - Don Chandler and Cheryl Adams; and for drawing of figures 10 and 11 - Lucy Taylor; for providing work space - the Department of Zoology and the Zoology Museum of the University of Wisconsin. NIH Grants HE-03331 and HD-00277, and NSF Grants GB 19732 have contributed to this work.

REFERENCES

Brambell, F.W.R. and D.H.S. Davis (1941) Reproduction in the multimammate mouse (Mastomys erythroleucus Temm.) of Sierra Leone. Proc. Zool. Soc. London B, 111:1-11.

Buechner, H.K. (1961) Unilateral implantation in the Uganda kob. Nature, 190:738.

Chapman, D.I. and O. Dansie (1969) Unilateral implantation in the muntjac deer (Muntiacus muntjak Zimmerman and M. reevesi Ogilby). J. Zool., 159:534-436.

Chaplin, R.E. and R.J. Harrison (1971) Uterus, ovaries and placenta of Chinese muntjac deer (Muntiacus reevesi). J. Anat., 110:147.

Child, G. and A.S. Mossman (1965) Right horn implantation in the common duiker. Science, 149:1265-1266.

Creed, R.F.S. and J.D. Biggers (1963) Development of the raccoon placenta. Am. J. Anat., 113:417-445.

Enders, A.C. and R.L. Given (1977) The endometrium of delayed and early implantation. In: Biology of the Uterus, R.M. Wynn, ed., Plenum Pr., NY and London.

Grant, R. (1933) The pigmentation of the uterine mucosa in the ewe. Vet. J., 89:271-274.

Hafez, E.S.E. and H. Ludwig (1977) Scanning electron microscopy of the endometrium. In: Biology of the Uterus, R.W. Wynn, ed., Plenum Pr. NY and London.

Kellas, L.M. (1955) Observations on the reproductive activities, measurements, and growth rate of the dik-dik (Rhyncotragus kirkii thomasi Neumann). Proc. Zool. Soc. London, 124:751-784.

Klein, M. (1933) La muqueuse utérine de la lapin. Contribution à l' histophysiologie des muqneuses. Bull. D'Histologie Appliquée, 10:327-354.

Kuhnel, W. and H.M. Beier (1976) Studies on the innervation of the endometrium. Cell and Tissue Res., 167:527-536.

Lee, Sue Y., H.W. Mossman, A.S. Mossman and Guido del Pino (1977) Evidence of a specific nidation site in ruminants. Am. J. Anat., 150:631-640.

Luckett, W.P. (1968) Morphogenesis of the placenta and fetal membranes of the tree shrews (Family - Tupaiidae). Am. J. Anat., 123: 385-428.

MacDonald, A.A. (1976) Uterine vasculature of the pregnant pig: a scanning electron microscope study. Anat. Rec., 184:689-698.

Mossman, A.S. and H.W. Mossman (1962) Ovulation, implantation and fetal sex ration in impala. Science, 137:869.

O'Gara, B.W. (1969) Unique aspects of reproduction in the female pronghorn (Antilocapra americana). Am. J. Anat., 125:217-232.

Prasad, M.R.N., H.W. Mossman and G.L. Scott (1979) Morphogenesis of the fetal membranes of an American mole, Scalopus aquaticus. Am. J. Anat., 155:31-68.

Robinette, W.L. and G.F.T. Child (1964) Notes on the biology of the lechwe (Kobus leche). The Puku, The occasional papers of the Dept. of Game and Fisheries (Northern Rhodesia), 2:84-117.

Sinha, A.A. and H.W. Mossman (1966) Placentation of the sea otter. Am. J. Anat., 119:521-554.

Spilman, C.H. and J.W. Wilks, eds. (1978) Novel Aspects of Reproductive Biology. Brook Lodge Workshop on Problems of Reproductive Biology. SP Medical and Scientific Books, Spectrum Publications Inc., NY and London.

Spinage, C.A. (1969) Reproduction in the Uganda Defassa waterbuck, Kobus defassa ugandae Neumann. J. Reprod. Fert., 18:445-457.

Steven, D.H., ed. (1975) Comparative Placentation. Essays in Structure and Function. Academic Pr., London.

Symington, R.B. and N.J. Paterson (1970) Preliminary report on the phenomenon of unilateral implantation in the right uterine horn of the common duiker, Sylvicapra grimmea. Arnoldia, 4:1-5.

Weir, B.K. (1971) The reproductive organs of the female plains viscacha, Lagostomus maximus. J. Reprod. Fert., 25:365-373.

Wimsatt, W.A. (1979) Reproductive asymmetry and unilateral pregnancy in Chiroptera. J. Reprod. Fert., 56:345-357.

Wynn, R.M. (1977) Histology and ultrastructure of the human endometrium. In: Biology of the Uterus. R.M. Wynn, ed., Plenum Pr., NY and London.

DISCUSSION

GLASSER: I have just been entertaining myself with the idea of what NIH would do with a budget item statement asking for per diem support for six black bears. In 1975, in one of their papers on rabbit implantation, Alan Enders and Sandra Schlafkey presented a unique figure that suggested that the transfer of materials between trophectoderm and endometrium may not follow the usual synthesis/secretion pattern but fusion and eventual dissolution of the interfacing membranes between the two cells may occur instead. Recently, at the implantation conference in Houston, Enders presented a similar one for the rat (Enders et al, 1980). This in-situ somatic hybridization was very attractive in biochemical terms, but I have never seen other figures like these. Have you, in your comparative studies of placentation ever seen an arrangement between trophectoderm and the stroma or epithelium which suggests that fusion and mixing of cell contents rather than exocytosis transfers materials between the two cells?

MOSSMAN: No, because I haven't done electronmicroscopy of trophectoderm and endometrium.

GLASSER: Are you aware of anybody else who has ever reported it?

MOSSMAN: Well, I don't think reports of fusion and dissolution are too uncommon. As I understand it, the fusion of cells results in the ultimate destruction of the maternal cell.

GLASSER: The process is more than absorption of a dead cell. It involves two different but viable cells, one from the trophectoderm and one from the endoderm.

MOSSMAN: Yes, I know. It is first a fusion, but it is actually a way of incorporating the maternal cells. Perhaps we shouldn't call it phagocytosis, but it has the same results.

PADYKULA: My wildest adventure in placentation was to go to Australia to study the Australian bandycoot because of evidence of cell fusion in the chorioallantoic placenta in that marsupial family. Only they form a chorioallantois; all other marsupials have only a yolksac placenta. Hill and then Flynn had demonstrated that when the bandycoot trophoblast disappears at the chorioallantoic site the maternal epithelium is formed of multinucleate cells that are homokaryons, and all the nuclei are alike and euchromatic. Before the trophoblast disappearance, it is a simple columnar epithelium with lots of free ribosomes. When this trophoblastic layer disappears, homokaryons become heterokaryons, and they have the big heterochromatic nuclei characteristic of the trophoblast. It looked like an implantation process which stopped at the stage when Schlafkey and Enders (1975) had seen the fusion in the rabbit. There would be a transient formation of a heterokaryon with maternal and fetal nuclei, and then in the Eutheria heterokaryon developed into the stroma. I think that fusion may, with formation of a transient heterokaryon with maternal and fetal nuclei, happen in many mammals that form hemochorial placenta. Intracellular mixing has an immunologic effect.

GLASSER: The strategic importance of such immunoparalysis is quite short and wouldn't require cell surface antigens.

PADYKULA: Larsen (1970) suggested that cell fusion occurs in primate implantation. There may be heterokaryon formation in the early human implantation sites. Dr. Mossman, is epithelial shedding fairly common among the different orders of mammals? You mentioned epithelial shedding a number of times, and I was wondering about its prevalence among the mammalian orders.

MOSSMAN: Shedding of surface epithelium occurs to some extent in the nonpregnant uterus, but is far more common and extensive during pregnancy, especially in ruminents and rodents. It also occurs in the moles and carnivores.

GERSCHENSON: In the rabbit, which is in estrus all the time except during pregnancy or pseudopregnancy, epithelial cells have to be shed or eliminated some other way. If one perfuses rabbits with ^{3}H-thymidine for several days, labeled nuclei appear in about 60% of the cells in the glandular epithelium and about 11% of the luminal cells. Without shedding, the endometrium would keep growing and the uterus would eventually become bigger than the rabbit.

In the beginning, cell proliferation and progesterone treatment induce shedding and then the cells stop dividing becoming probably terminally differentiated. However, we checked for shedding following therapy and found none. Progesterone may increase the anchorage of epithelial cells to the basement membrane. Since epithelial cells are anchored, the only solution is for the epithelium to fold and form what I used to call glands. I am not sure they are glands; maybe some Ob/Gyn people are right when they call them crypts.

BAULIEU: Could you describe for us the differences among implantation in the human, chimps, the very highest apes, and baboons, rhesus and other monkeys.

MOSSMAN: Implantation is very much alike in all the anthropoids and humans.

BAULIEU: Do you think that the findings in baboons can be extrapolated to humans?

MOSSMAN: Well, the chimps and the humans have essentially the same type of implantation.

BAULIEU: What is the basic difference between humans and baboons?

MOSSMAN: The baboons have a more superficial implantation.

References:

Enders, AC, Chavez, DJ and Schlafke, S (1980). Comparison of implantation in utero and in vitro. In: Cellular and Molecular Aspects of Implantation (SR Glasser and DW Bullock, eds.) Plenum Publishing Co., New York (in press).

Larsen, JF (1970). In: Ovo-implantation, Human Gonadotropins and Prolactin. Karger, Basel.

Padykula, HA and Taylor, JM (1976). Cellular mechanisms involved in cyclic stromal renewal of the uterus. I. The opossum, Didelphis virginiana. Anat Rec 184:5.

Schlafke, S and Enders, AC (1975). Cellular basis of interaction between trophoblast and uterus at implantation. Biol Reprod 12:41-65.

The Endometrium

2

Uterine Cell Biology and Phylogenetic Considerations: An Interpretation

Helen A. Padykula

INTRODUCTION

The strong evolutionary imprint on mammalian reproductive systems creates an impressive barrier to interpretation of uterine cellular differentiation among different species. Especially during placental involvement, the uterus displays striking species variation which is considerably greater than occurs in other organs (e.g., liver, kidney, lung). During implantation, in most orders of mammals the uterine mucosa is eroded to varying degree during the formation of several principal types of chorio-allantoic placental associations characterized by differences in the number and types of cellular and tissue layers intervening between the maternal (uterine) and the fetal (allantoic) bloodstreams (Mossman, 1937; Amoroso, 1952; Enders, 1965; Steven, 1975). In rodents, rabbits, Old World monkeys, and human beings, the uterine luminal epithelium, stroma, and microvasculature are progressively destroyed as the formation of the hemochorial placenta places the maternal blood into direct contact with the fetal trophoblast. Ultrastructural analysis has reduced Grosser's original classification of the chorioallantoic placental barriers into three major categories: (1) epitheliochorial (Artiodactyla, Perissodactyla, Cetacea, Lemuroidae), (2) endotheliochorial (most Carnivora, Pinnipedia), and hemochorial (Insectivora, Rodentia, Lagomorpha, Sirenia, most Primates) (Steven, 1975). Within the hemochorial type, the number (1 to 3) of trophoblastic layers intervening between the maternal and fetal bloodstreams varies (Enders, 1965).

Evolutionary imprint is somewhat less conspicuous during cyclic uterine differentiation than during pregnancy, except for features such as the number of glands, degree of endometrial storage of glycogen, etc. (see Finn and Porter, 1975). During the anabolic phase of the uterine cycle, considerable similarity exists in the sequential differentiation of endometrial cells and tissues as they respond to increasing estrogenic stimulation through hyperplasia and hypertrophy and then to the superposition of rising progesterone during ovulation and the early luteal phase, particularly by secretory activity.

In the final stages of the catabolic phase a drastic difference exists between menstruating primates and all other mammals. Cyclic uterine renewal in these primates involves menstrual shedding of the superficial region (functionalis) of the endometrium with distinct external signs of bleeding. In New World monkeys the external bleeding has been described as being "microscopic in dimensions" (Kaiser, 1947). In most mammals, however, uterine regression at the close of the estrous cycle is accomplished without endometrial shedding. Instead, a "bloodless" intrauterine catabolism involving cellular atrophy and death, and degradation of the extracellular matrix effects reduction of uterine mass. This remodeling occurs without destruction of mucosal integrity. Thus, menstruation is a drastic mechanism for cyclic endometrial renewal which is a highly restricted biologic phenomenon. It is part of human biology and analysis of the menstrual cycle should include this terminal event.

Investigators have thus far concentrated effort on the anabolism of uterine differentiation to gain understanding of the action of estrogen and progesterone. This effort has provided considerable definition of steroidal mitogenic action as well as identified the role of the steroid-receptor complex in regulation of DNA, RNA, and protein synthesis in uterine target cells (O'Malley and Birnbaumer, 1978). Much less attention has been given to the obvious point that uterine catabolism is as necessary as anabolism for cyclic activity. Modern investigations of regression have been performed on the rodent uterus (see bibliographies in Tansey and Padykula, 1978 and Padykula and Tansey, 1979). Increased study is necessary not only for biological interpretation of cyclicity but particularly because of current widespread control of human uterine differentiation by oral contraceptives which includes artificial scheduling of regression. Moreover, irregularities and abnormalities of the human menstrual cycle and pregnancy may include unexpected regression. Thus, it is surprising that present knowledge of cyclic uterine differentiation at the tissue level rests largely on the early classic studies on the human and rhesus monkey which originated largely in relation to the activities of the Department of Embryology at the Carnegie Institution between 1930 to 1958 (e.g., Hartman, 1932; Bartelmez, 1933; Wislocki and Dempsey, 1939; Markee, 1940; Daron, 1936, 1937; Bartelmez, Corner, and Hartman, 1951; Bartelmez, 1957). An ultrastructural literature on human uterine cyclic changes is growing steadily (Lawn, 1973; Ferenczy and Richart, 1974) but informational and interpretive discontinuities exist because of limitations inherent in studying a specimen isolated at only a point in an individual's cycle as well as the difficulty of performing close sequential analyses of serum estrogen and progesterone.

Here an attempt will be made to demonstrate the degree to which cyclic and postpartum regression-renewal centers on differentiative changes in the cells and extracellular matrix of the stromal compartment of the uterus. Secondly, the possibility that a fundamental unity may exist between non-menstruating and menstruating mammals in terms of uterine stromal cell populations will be explored.

STROMAL CELL POPULATIONS OF THE UTERINE ENDOMETRIUM

The uncomplicated histologic design of the uterine endometrium belies the everchanging nature of this dynamic mucosa with its remarkable regenerative potential as well as its tolerance of allografts. Its structural components enlarge or diminish in relation to the steadily changing hormonal levels of the cycle or pregnancy. A simple columnar luminal epithelium is associated with a lamina propria which is generally referred to as the "uterine stroma" (Figure 1). Tubular glands lined by simple cuboidal-columnar epithelium may branch or coil. Stromal vascularity, as with all other structural features,

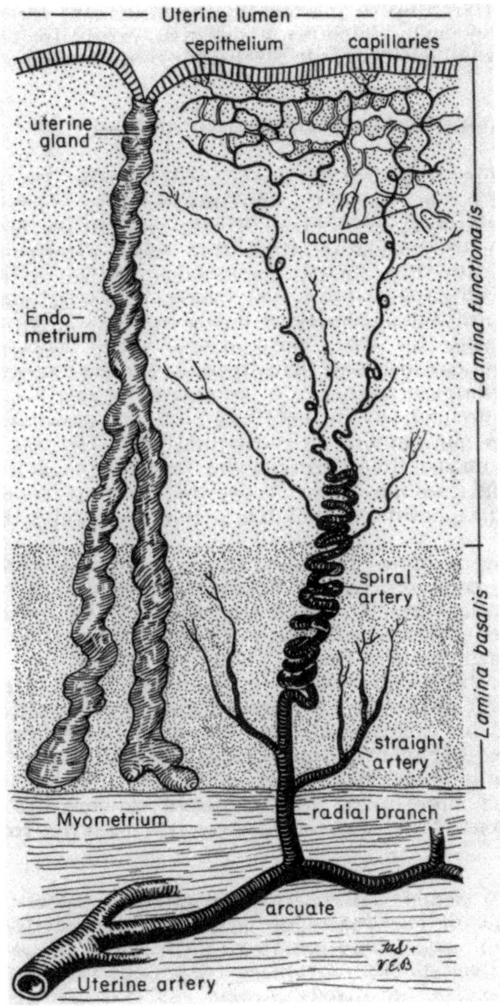

Figure 1. Diagram of the histologic organization of the human endometrium. (Taken from Blandau, R.J., page 911 in the Weiss-Greep Histology, 4th edition, McGraw-Hill Company.

varies with reproductive stage. In mammals with hemochorial placentae, lymphatic vessels are absent from the endometrium, except near the junction with the myometrium (Hoggan and Hoggan, 1881; Wislocki and Dempsey, 1939; McLean and Scothorne, 1970). This anatomic feature may be a major factor in immunologic tolerance of the fetal allograft. Discussion here will be limited to differentiative changes in the stroma of three mammals, the North American opossum, albino rat, and human, except for brief comment on the primate epithelial component in relation to endometrial zonation.

The Basoluminal (proximo-distal) Endometrial Gradient

Sequential stimulation by ovarian hormones during the cycle and early pregnancy creates an elaborate microvasculature (arteriole-capillaries-venule) in the superficial endometrial stroma beneath the luminal epithelium (Figure 1). This microvasculature arises from radial arteries that carry blood in a centripedal direction toward the uterine luminal surface from large circumferentially directed arteries that course between myometrial layers. This concentration of microvasculature in the superficial stroma establishes a basoluminal polarity in the endometrium with important functional implications, since an abundant subepithelial vascular supply characterizes the specialized transport surfaces of absorptive organs, such as the small intestine, renal proximal tubule, and lung. This microvasculature with the luminal epithelium may provide the structural basis for transport processes that modify the uterine fluid during sperm transport-capacitation and later for reception of the free blastocyst. It lays the maternal foundation for early establishment of the placental association with the implanting blastocyst.

In menstruating primates the coiled (spiral) artery is comparable to the radial artery of non-menstruating mammals. However, a second type of artery, the basal or straight artery, serves only the basal endometrium (basalis) and is less obviously involved in cyclic differentiation than the upper endometrium ("functionalis") (Daron, 1936 and Figure 1). It is generally assumed that only the basalis remains in the human uterus after menstruation and is the source of stem cells for regeneration of the functionalis; however, the exact extent of endometrial loss among primates has not yet been adequately defined (Bartelmez, Corner and Hartman, 1951). The stroma of the basalis is usually described as "more cellular and fibrous" than that of the functionalis. Much more study will be needed to elucidate the structure, function, and extent of the endometrial layer that persists from one cycle to the next.

The concept of endometrial zonation presented by Bartelmez, Corner and Hartman (1951) was derived from close histologic study of the rhesus uterus. This useful concept assists interpretation of the thick primate endometrium with its abundant long glands. Bartelmez recognized four histologic zones on the basis of differences in glands, stroma, and vascular supply (Figure 2). Zone 1 is composed of the luminal epithelium and the highly vascular superficial stroma; it is equipped for transport functions as well as the initiation of placentogenesis. Zone 2 contains the uppermost portions of the glands that are straight and widely separated by stroma whereas in the deeper zone 3 the glandular segments are more coiled and closely packed. Besides reflecting cyclic epithelial responses related to secretion, zones 2 and 3 are mitotic centers for the glandular epithelium and stroma. Zone 4, presumably the counterpart of the basalis, possesses the potential inherently for total regeneration of the endometrium because, after physical removal of all visible traces of rhesus endometrium, it is entirely reconstituted from

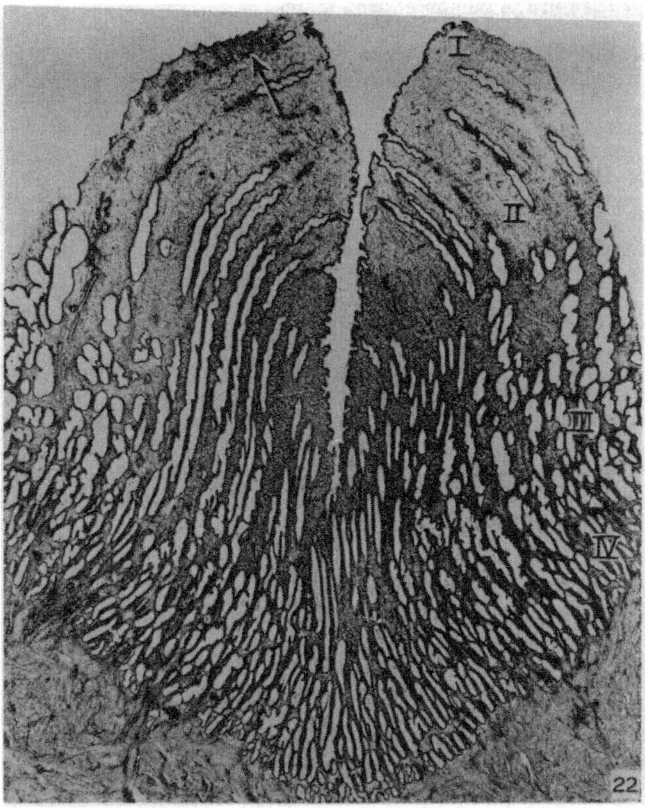

Figure 2. Histologic zonation in the late secretory endometrium of the rhesus monkey. Note the regional (indicated as I, II, III, and IV) differences in the glandular shape as well as in stromal cellular in the four zones. (Taken from Bartelmez, Corner, and Hartman, 1951. Contributions to Embryology, Carnegie Institution, 34:99.)

remaining glandular segments that extend into the myometrium (Hartman, 1944). Thus, stem cells capable of producing all endometrial tissue components may exist in zone 4.

Zonation in the primate endometrium is also evident in the cleavage plane of menstrual sloughing in the rhesus monkey. Bartelmez, Corner and Hartman (1951) provided strong histologic evidence that only zone 1 and the upper part of zone 2 are eliminated and that the sloughed tissue separates in an uneven manner. From this, it seems that there is less menstrual reduction in the rhesus than in the human endometrium.

The Bartelmez zonation was recently applied to ultrastructural interpretation of the normal human endometrium on days 16 and 19 of the menstrual cycle (Statz, Padykula, and Driscoll, 1979, unpublished). Our experience indicates that the human endometrium exhibits comparable quadruple zonation and that recognition of this regional variation as a sampling problem is obligatory, particularly in ultrastrauctural analyses. Additional support for a basoluminal gradient comes from recent proliferation kinetics of normal human uterus (Ferenczy, Bertrand, and Gelfand, 1979). Highest mitotic rates were observed in the upper third of the human endometrium on days 8-10 of the cycle, an observation that is in general agreement with earlier mitotic counts and localizations in the rhesus endometrium (Bensley, 1951; Bartelmez, Corner and Hartman, 1951).

In the rat endometrium with its sparse glands, only bipartite histologic zonation is evident. The superficial stroma is more densely cellular and less collagenous than the deeper stroma (Tansey and Padykula, 1978). During late pregnancy and early postpartum regression, monocytes, neutrophils, and lymphocytes are more concentrated in the superficial stroma whereas tissue eosinophils and mast cells reside primarily in the deepest stroma (Padykula and Tansey, 1979, Figure 3).

COMMON FEATURES OF MAMMALIAN UTERINE STROMAL DIFFERENTIATION

The cell populations of the uterine stroma (endometrial and myometrial) may be divided into two categories, the <u>resident cells</u> that are regularly present in the adult uterus and will persist after ovariectomy and the <u>transient cells</u> that appear intermittently in relation to changing ovarian hormonal stimulation. Most of the transient cells are leucocytes that emigrate from the blood to the stromal and epithelial tissue compartments. The following 11 cell types occur in the uterine stroma of three mammals that are phylogenetically quite distinct, the North American opossum (marsupial with only a yolk sac placenta in epithelio-chorial association without endometrial erosion), the albino rat (non-menstruating rodent with a hemotrichorial placenta with endometrial erosion and an inverted yolk sac placenta without erosion), and the human being (menstruating primate with only a hemomonochorial placenta with endometrial erosion):

RESIDENT CELLS	TRANSIENT CELLS
Fibroblasts	Decidual cells
Mast cells	Monocyte-macrophages
T & B lymphocytes	T & B lymphocytes
Stem cells	Eosinophils
	Heterophils (neutrophils)
	Plasma cells
	Endometrial granular cells

All of these cell types occur in rat and human uteri. The opossum uterus does not have decidual cells, and so far the counterpart to the endometrial granular cell has not been observed (Padykula and Taylor, 1976 and Figure 4; Padykula and Campbell, 1976; Padykula, 1976; Padykula, Driscoll, and Cardasis, 1978; Tansey and Padykula, 1978; Padykula and Tansey, 1979; for earlier studies consult reviews in Finn and Porter, 1975 and Schmidt-Mathiessen, 1963). The presence of B lymphocytes is indicated indirectly by the transient occurrence of plasma cells (Padykula, 1976) as well as by the recent immunocytochemical demonstration of the presence of B immunoblasts in the mouse uterus (McDermott and Bienenstock, 1979). In the above list, the presence of T lymphocytes is also inferred because of their known involvement with the other cells of the immune response.

Resident Cells of the Normal Uterine Stroma

As in all connective tissues, the uterine fibroblast is the fundamental cell in that it produces the macromolecular precursors of the collagen and elastic fibers as well as the proteoglycans and glycoproteins of the extracellular matrix. In addition to this role as the producer of the matrix, the fibroblast participates also in its degradation, as the synthesizer of collagenase and proteoglycan-degrading enzymes (Werb and Burleigh, 1974; Werb et al., 1977). The sensitive responsiveness of the uterine fibroblast to ovarian hormones, as reflected in well known ultrastructural modulations (Brinsfield and Hawk, 1974) as well as biochemical changes, sets it apart from fibroblasts on non-target organs. The extracellular matrix changes steadily in relation to fibrous and proteoglycan content as a consequence of fibroblastic differentiation.

A small population of mast cells occurs normally, and their number appears to be hormonally regulated (see Finn and Porter, 1975). The mast cells are involved local histamine release. In the rat uterus they occur primarily in the basal region of the endometrium near the origin of the radial arteries. Lymphocytes are regularly present in variable numbers in the epithelial and stromal compartments. Their presence may reflect, in part, a role in the common mucosal immunologic system which has recently been recognized as occurring in the mucosae of the female reproductive system as well as in the respiratory and gastrointestinal system (McDermott and Bienenstock, 1979). Stem cells for epithelial, stromal, and vascular cells are regularly present, as evident from radioautographic studies, (e.g., Martin and Finn, 1968; Marcus, 1974) but their morphologic identity remains largely unknown.

Transient Cells of the Normal Uterine Stroma

Relatively little investigative attention has been directed toward cell types, other than the fibroblast and decidual cell, that inhabit the uterine stroma. Leucocytic invasion may occur at certain points during the cycle and pregnancy. It has long been realized that the premenstrual period in the human (Bartelmez, 1933; Noyes, Hertig, and Rock, 1950; Noyes, 1973) and rhesus endometria (Markee, 1940; Bartelmez, Corner, and Hartman, 1951) is characterized by the onset of decidualization as well as immigration of blood leucocytes into the uterine tissue compartments. Detailed characterization of this cellular invasion in the primate uterus remains to be done, but progress has been made with the rodent and opossum uteri.

Our studies of normal postpartum regression in the North American opossum (Padykula and Taylor, 1976) (Figure 4) and albino rat (Padykula and Campbell, 1976) (Figure 3) have demonstrated that uterine involution is marked by the immigration of monocytes, heterophils, eosinophils, and lymphocytes as well as by intratissue conversion of monocytes to macrophages and the appearance of plasma cells (Figures 3 and 4). From this enumeration of transient cell types, it is evident that an inflammatory and/or humoral immune response occurs during regression. This leucocytic invasion coincides with rapid and massive reduction in uterine mass. The possibility of the interrelationship of these two events has been suggested (Padykula, 1976; 1980). Overall, these observations suggest that cellular mechanisms usually associated with pathologic response may participate in normal remodeling of the uterus.

Factors Associated with the Appearance of Leucocytes in Normal Uterine Stroma

Declining serum and tissue levels of progesterone may represent the negative hormonal signal that leads to uterine regression in the postpartum rat and to menstruation in primates. Discussion here will be limited to factors that have been studied in the albino rat.

Rat uterine progesterone nuclear receptors exist in maximal tissue concentrations between days 9 to 15 of pregnancy and decline to a low or undetectable level at parturition (VuHai et al., 1978). During days 16 to birth as serum and tissue levels of progesterone are declining, heterophils, monocytes, and eosinophils appear in the gestational stroma and epithelia in increasing numbers (Padykula and Tansey, 1979). Heterophilic and monocytic infiltration might be related to the postulated function of progesterone as an anti-inflammatory (or immunosuppressive) agent, when present in high local concentrations, as in a target organ (Siiteri et al., 1977). On the other hand, it is likely that rising serum estrogen levels during late pregnancy (Yoshinaga, 1976) may lead to emigration of blood eosinophils into the peripartum uterus (Ross and Klebanoff, 1966).

The onset of massive reduction of the uterus proceeds during a steadily changing inverse relationship between declining progesterone and rising estrogen serum levels (Yoshinaga, 1976). This is manifested at the cellular level in the endometrium as a mixture of simultaneous catabolic and anabolic events over a period that extends at least from day 16 of pregnancy through day 4 postpartum (Figure 3). Besides this leucocytic invasion, neutral collagenase is activated at birth and results in an unusually rapid destruction of collagen fibrils within 72 hours (see review by Gross, 1974). Concomitant

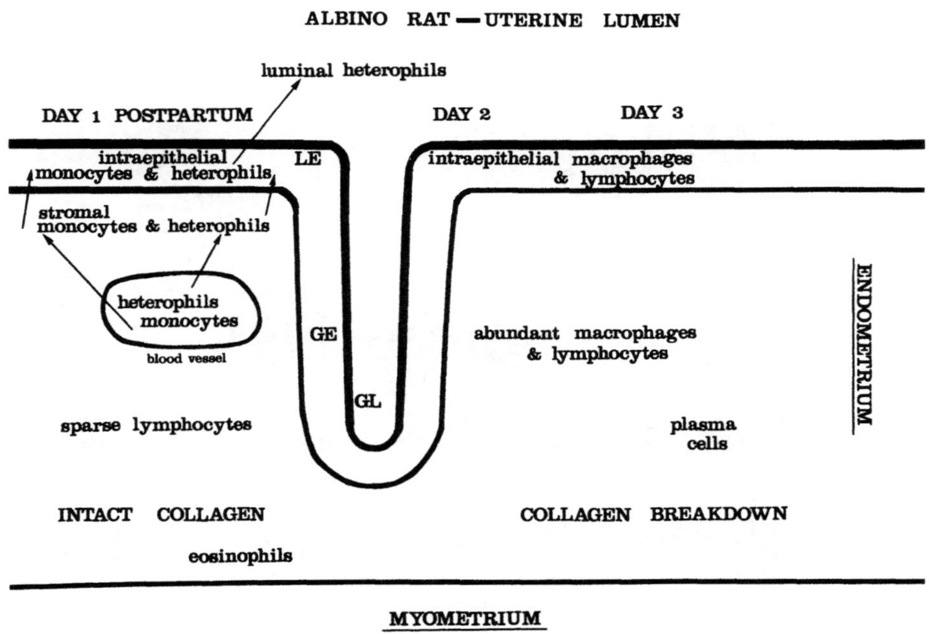

Figure 3. Diagram illustrating sequential changes in stromal cell populations in the rat uterus during the first three postpartum days. (Taken from Padykula, 1980.)

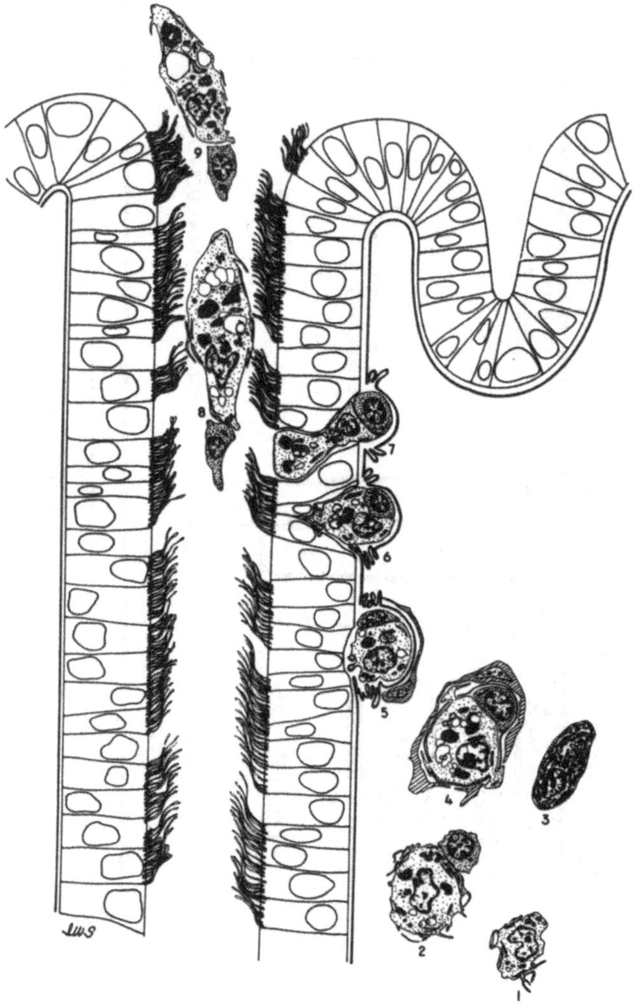

Figure 4. Hypothetical representation of the occurrence of a humoral immune response and a pathway of macrophagic and lymphocytic migration during regression in the early postpartum opossum uterus. 1, tissue monocyte; 2, macrophagic-lymphocytic interaction; 3, plasma cell; 4, segregation of macrophage and lymphocyte; 5-9, transepithelial and intraglandular emigration of lymphocytes and macrophages toward the uterine lumen. (Taken from Padykula, 1976.)

with rapid degradation of the extracellular matrix, tissue monocytes convert steadily into macrophages that are involved in phagocytosis of luminal epithelial cells (Sandow, West and Brenner, 1978) and possibly in removal of the remains of the matrix (Padykula, 1976; 1980). Uterine lymphocytic populations increase during the first three postpartum days. Near the close of stromal catabolism, plasma cells are present (Figure 3). During the first three postpartum days, anabolism is manifested by features such as division of luminal epithelial cells and expansion of the cytoplasmic membranes of fibroblasts, presumably for initiation of synthesis of a new extracellular matrix.

The regulation of collagenase activity is fundamental to control of the stability of the extracellular matrix, since latent collagenase is widely distributed in the uterus (Wirl, 1975; Woessner, 1977). This regulation may be linked to the invasion of uterine leucocytes, since macrophages in cell culture produce collagenase as well as plasminogen activator, a known activator of collagenase (Werb et al., 1977). Collagenase activity is strongly inhibited in vitro and in vivo by progesterone (Jeffrey and Koob, 1973). As described above, uterine leucocytes increase in number steadily in relation to the declining prepartum progesterone and increasing estrogen serum and tissue levels. When exogenous progesterone is administered in vivo daily from day 19 of pregnancy through day 3 postpartum, parturition is delayed and the postpartum stromal changes illustrated in Figure 3 are largely blocked (Tansey and Padykula, 1978). That is, the endometrium retains its late gestational differentiation. When the administration of exogenous progesterone is commenced at birth, stromal differentiation is delayed but not blocked during the first 48 hours postpartum. Endometrial zonation was striking at this time because macrophages and other infiltrating cells occurred in the superficial stroma but were sparse in the deep stroma where collagen was retained (see Figures 8 and 9 in Tansey and Padykula, 1978). Plasma cells were not observed in the progesterone-treated uteri in both experiments. Thus progesterone given in vivo prevented or delayed collagen breakdown and concomitantly leucocytic immigration into the stroma was delayed or blocked. Overall, this cellular evidence links the declining serum and tissue progesterone levels just before birth with the translocation of blood leucocytes into the uterine stromal and epithelial compartments; the activation of collagen degradation at birth is temporally correlated with the cellular array associated with an inflammatory and/or humoral immune response.

The occurrence of cellular manifestations of a humoral immune response was a surprising observation. Possible explanations for this phenomenon may be derived from other kinds of evidence. Wira and Sandoe (1977) have reported that the uterus secretes immunoglobulins into the uterine fluid and that this process is regulated by estrogen and progesterone, i.e., estrogen stimulates while progesterone suppresses. Thus the uterine local immune system may be functioning here as component of the postpartum estrus. On the other hand, we have demonstrated that monocytes and granulocytes infiltrate the uterus as early as day 16 of gestation. Such a widespread monocytic infiltration under normal circumstances is unusual; the monocytes assume locations that will be occupied by macrophages after degradation of the extracellular matrix has commenced at birth (Figure 3). An hypothesis has been suggested that monocytic-macrophagic differentiation might be stimulated by rapid production of antigenic sites from fragments of collagen molecules arising from enzymic cleavage of the triple helix by collagenase (Padykula, 1976). Moreover, these peptide fragments undergo subsequent denaturation (Gross, 1974). A transient powerful local antigenic stimulus to the maternal organism would occur and produce an inflammatory response. This inflammation would be novel in that its expression depends directly on levels of estrogen and progesterone.

In the early primate pregnancy (human and rhesus monkey), a transient drop in serum progesterone occurs during the period of switchover from ovarian to placental production of progesterone. In the human, this event occurs between 4 to 11 weeks of pregnancy with its nadir at 9 weeks (Mishell et al., 1973). We have observed between 5 to 11 weeks that a lymphoid infiltration occurs throughout the decidua parietalis which is heavier in paraglandular and paravascular locations (Padykula, Driscoll, and Cardasis, 1978). Clinical pathologists have been aware of this normal phenomenon and designated it as a "mononuclear infiltration." Our ultrastructural evidence indicates that this infiltration consists of numerous endometrial granular cells at various stages of development as well as of lymphocytes, monocytes, macrophages, and plasma cells. This differs from the peripartum phenomenon in the rat uterus by the absence of tissue neutrophils and eosinophils. Since this period corresponds to a high frequency of spontaneous abortion, this stromal event may represent a period of endometrial instability.

The so-called period of the "placental sign" in the rhesus monkey (Hartman, 1932) coincides with a transient period of low serum progesterone. The placental sign is manifested by the appearance of vaginal blood which probably originates from the implantation sites. In relation to this matter, it is relevant to note that during implantation in the mouse, maternal immunoglobulins are widely distributed in the uterine extracellular matrix as well as along the surface of the trophoblast and within the embryo (Bernard, Ripoche, and Bennett, 1977). These investigators offer the tentative interpretation that these tissue maternal immunoglobulins may be "enhancing antibodies", i.e., immunoglobulins with immunosuppresive properties and/or simply "nutritive proteins".

GENERAL CONCLUSION

Our studies on the organization of the uterine stroma at the cellular level indicate considerable unity exists among diverse mammals (opossum, rat, human, rhesus monkey). Also they highlight a long ignored stromal differentiation, i.e., that leucocytic populations appear within the uterine extracellular matrix and epithelia under normal circumstances. Consideration is given to the existence of a structural-functional basoluminal (proximo-distal) gradient in the mammalian uterus which reaches considerable complexity in the primate (human and rhesus) uterus. The interpretation presented here may seem to be, in part, a simplification; however, it is hoped that description and analysis of basic cellular differentiations will provide a common background for interpretation of specialized features related to species differences.

ACKNOWLEDGMENT

This study was supported by funds from USPH Research Grant HD 13941-01.

BIBLIOGRAPHY

Amoroso, E.C. 1952 Placentation. Chapter 15 in Marshall's Physiology of Reproduction, Vol. 2, Longmans, Cambridge, England.

Bartelmez, G.W. 1933 Histological studies on the menstruating mucous membrane of the human uterus. Contrib. Embryol. Carnegie Inst., 24:143-187.

Bartelmez, G.W. 1957 The form and the functions of the uterine blood vessels in the rhesus monkey. Contrib. Embryol. Carnegie Inst., 36:153-182.

Bartelmez, G.W., G.W. Corner and C.G. Hartman 1951 Cyclic changes in the endometrium of the rhesus monkey (Macaca mulatta). Contrib. Embryol. Carnegie Inst., 34:99-146.

Bensley, C.M. 1951 Cyclic fluctuations in the rate of epithelial mitoses in the endometrium of the rhesus monkey. Contrib. Embryol. Carnegie Inst., 34:87-98.

Bernard, O., M.A. Ripoche and D. Bennett 1977 Distribution of the maternal immunoglobulin in the mouse uterus and embryo in the days after implantation. J. Exp. Med., 145:58.

Brinsfield, T.H. and H.W. Hawk 1974 Ultrastructure of sheep endometrial stromal cells after ovariectomy and hormone treatment. Biol. Reprod. 10:98.

Daron, G.H. 1936 The arterial pattern of the tunica mucosa of the uterus of Macacus rhesus. Am. J. Anat., 58:349-419.

Daron, G.H. 1937 The veins of the endometrium (Macaca rhesus) as a source of the menstrual blood. Anat. Rec. 67, Suppl. 13.

Enders, A.C. 1965 A comparative study of the fine structure of the trophoblast in several hemochorial placentas. Am. J. Anat. 116:29.

Ferenczy A., G. Bertrand, and M.M. Gelfand 1979 Proliferation kinetics of human endometrium during the normal menstrual cycle. Am. J. Obstet. Gynecol., 133:859-867.

Ferenczy, A. and R.M. Richart 1974 Female Reproductive System: Dynamics of Scan and Transmission Electron Microscopy. John Wiley & Sons, N.Y.

Finn, C.A. and D.G. Porter 1975 The Uterus. Reprod. Biol. Handbook, Vol. 1, Publishing Sciences Group, Inc. Acton, Ma.

Gross, J. 1974 Collagen biology: structure, degradation and disease. In: The Harvey Lectures, 1972-1973. Academic Press, N.Y., pp. 351-432.

Hartman, C.G. 1932 Studies in the reproduction of the monkey, Macacus (Pithecus) rhesus, with special reference to menstruation and pregnancy. Contrib. Embryol. Carnegie Inst., 23:1.

Hartman, C.G. 1944 Regeneration of the monkey uterus after surgical removal of the endometrium and accidental endometriosis. West. J. Surg. Obst. Gynec., 52:87-102.

Hoggan, G. and F.E. Hoggan 1881 On the comparative anatomy of the lymphatic of the uterus. J. Anat., 16:50-89.

Jeffrey, J.J. and T.J. Koob 1973 Hormonal regulation of collagen catabolism in the uterus. Endocrinology: Excerpta Med. Intl. Congr. Series 273:1115.

Kaiser, I.H. 1947 Histological appearance of coiled arterioles in the endometrium of rhesus monkey, baboon, chimpanzee and gibbon. Anat. Rec., 99:199.

Lawn, A.M. 1973 Ultrastructure of the endometrium during the sexual cycle. In: Advances Reprod. Physiol., 1:61.

Marcus, G.J. 1974 Mitosis in the rat uterus during the estrous cycle, early pregnancy, and early pseudopregnancy. Biol. Reprod. 10:447.

Markee, J.E. 1940 Menstruation in intraocular endometrial transplants in the rhesus monkey. Contrib. Embryol. Carnegie Inst., 28:219-308.

Martin, L. and C.A. Finn 1968 Hormonal regulation of cell division in epithelial and connective tissues of the mouse. J. Endocrinol. 41:363.

McDermott, M.R. and J. Bienenstock 1979 Evidence for a common mucosal immunologic system. I. Migration of B immunoblasts into intestinal, respiratory, and genital tissues. J. Immunology, 122(5):1892.

McLean, J.M. and R.J. Scothorne 1970 The lymphatics of the endometrium in the rabbit. J. Anat., 107:39-48.

Mishell, D.R., I.H. Thorneycroft, Y. Nagata, T. Murata and R.M. Nakamura 1973 Serum gonadotropin and steroid patterns in early human gestation. Am. J. Obst. Gynec., 117:631-639.

Mossman, H.W. 1937 Comparative morphogenesis of the fetal membranes and accessory uterine structures. Contrib. Embryol. Carnegie Inst., 26:129.

Noyes, R.W., A.T. Hertig and J. Rock 1950 Dating the endometrial biopsy. Fert. Steril., 1:3.

Noyes, R.W. 1973 Normal phases of the endometrium, Chapter 7. In: The Uterus. Eds.: H.J. Norris, A.T. Hertig and M.R. Abell. The Williams & Wilkins Co., Baltimore, Md.

O'Malley, B.W. and L. Birnbaumer (eds.) 1978 Receptors and Hormone Action, Vol. 11, Academic Press.

Padykula, H.A. 1976 Cellular mechanisms involved in cyclic stromal renewal of the uterus. III. Cells of the immune response. Anat. Rec., 184:49.

Padykula, H.A. 1980 Shifts in uterine stromal cell populations during pregnancy and regression. Conference on Cellular and Molecular Aspects of Implantation, eds. S. Glasser and D. Bullock.

Padykula, H.A. and A. Campbell 1976 Cellular mechanisms involved in cyclic stromal renewal of the uterus. II. The albino rat. Anat. Rec., 184:27.

Padykula, H.A., S.G. Driscoll, and C.A. Cardasis 1978 Decidual cell differentiation in the normal early gestational human uterus includes lymphoid infiltration. Anat. Rec., 190:500.

Padykula, H.A. and T.R. Tansey 1979 The occurrence of uterine stromal and intraepithelial monocytes and heterophils during normal late pregnancy in the rat. Anat. Rec., 193:329.

Padykula, H.A. and J.M. Taylor 1976 Cellular mechanisms involved in cyclic stromal renewal of the uterus. I. The opossum, Didelphis virginiana. Anat. Rec., 184:5.

Ross, R. and S. Klebanoff 1966 The eosinophilic leukocyte. Fine structure studies of changes in the uterus during the estrous cycle. J. Exp. Med., 124:653-660.

Sandow, B.A., N.B. West, and R.M. Brenner 1978 Hormonal regulation of an unusual form of cellular degeneration in hamster uterine luminal epithelium. Anat. Rec., 190:529.

Schmidt-Mathiessen, H. 1963 The Normal Human Endometrium. Ed. H. Schmidt-Mattheissen. The Blakiston Division, McGraw-Hill Co., N.Y.

Siiteri, P., F. Febres, L.E. Clemens, R.J. Chang, B. Gondos and D.P. Slites 1977 Progesterone and maintenance of pregnancy. Is progesterone nature's immunosuppressant? Ann. N.Y. Acad. Sci., 286:384.

Statz, E.M. H.A. Padykula, and S.G. Driscoll 1979 Unpublished.

Steven, D.H. (ed.) 1975 Comparative Placentation. Essays in Structure and Function. Academic Press.

Tansey, T.R. and H.A. Padykula 1978 Cellular responses to experimental inhibition of collagen degradation in the postpartum rat uterus. Anat. Rec., 191(3):287.

VuHai, M.T., F. Logeat, and E. Milgrom 1978 Progesterone receptors in the rat uterus: Variations in cytosol and nuclei during the oestrous cycle and pregnancy. J. Endocr., 76:43.

Werb, Z., C.L. Mainardi, C.A. Vater, and E.D. Harris, Jr. 1977 Endogenous activation of latent collagenase by rheumatoid synovial cells. Evidence for a role of plasminogen activator. New Eng. J. Med., 296:1017.

Werb, Z. and M.C. Burleigh 1974 A specific collagenase from rabbit fibroblasts in monolayer culture. Biochem. J., 137:373.

Wira, C.P. and C.P. Sandoe 1977 Sex steroid hormone regulation of IgA and IgG in rat uterine secretions. Nature., 268:534.

Wirl, G. 1975 Extraction of collagenase from the 6000 x 8 sediment of uterine and skin tissues of mice. A comparative study. Hoppe-Seyler's Z. Physiol. Chem. 356:1289.

Wislocki, G.B. and E.W. Dempsey 1939 Remarks on the lymphatics of the reproductive tract of the female rhesus monkey (Macaca mulatta). Anat. Rec., 75:341.

Woessner, J.F., Jr. 1977 A latent form of collagenase in the involuting rat uterus and its activation by a serine proteinase. Biochem. J. 161:535.

Yoshinaga, K. 1976 Ovarian hormone secretion and ovum implantation. In: Implantation of the Ovum. Eds: K. Yoshinaga, R.K. Meyer and R.O. Greep, pp. 3-17. Harvard University Press, Cambridge, Ma.

DISCUSSION

DEY: One of the early events in implantation is an inflammatory type of reaction and, secondly, for the maintenance of pregnancy, the immunological responses of the mother directed towards the embryo should be suppressed. You mentioned that during the parturition process an inflammatory type of reaction and a simultaneous immuno-rejection occur. That's why you get the parturition process.

PADYKULA: I didn't say it was immuno-rejection. It is an immunologic response.

DEY: It should be an immuno-rejection.

PADYKULA: No, it might be part of the local immune system, because postpartum in the opposum and the rat there is an estrus, and it could be that synthesis of antibodies at that time could be a hormonally regulated, local immune response also. That is another possibility. So, I wouldn't say immuno-rejection.

DEY: What functions do you ascribe to those immunological responses?

PADYKULA: One was that this could potentially, at least theoretically, arise from degradation of the uterine extracellular matrix. It is quite unusual in a normal body to have such rapid matrix degradation, but all the collagen diseases have a similar morphology. Another possibility is suggested in the paper by Bernard, Ripoche and Bennett (1977), dealing with implantation in the mouse, in which they demonstated maternal antibodies present at implantation in the matrix of the uterus covering the decidual cells. They interpreted these tissue maternal immunoglobulins as possibly "enhancing antibodies" that would mask antigen sites on the trophoblast. This would be kind of a protective role for the immune system. They also commented, that another possibility is that the antibodies are nutritive proteins. But they saw plasma cells present. You raised your question about implantation in the human, I think. However, in the rat, and in the mouse, plasma cells are present at implantation, but no one has made a leukocytic study, as far as I know.

GLASSER: You've described the action of the cells that migrate in and out of the uterine stroma during the remodeling in the peri-parturition period, what happens to the resident cells? Is this a fixed population that is being cleaned out, or is there preparation for the next parturient cycle by the appearance of a new fibroblast population?

PADYKULA: Well, in terms of the fibroblast, the lysosomal system is activated, but not for very long because of the onset of postpartum estrus. The fibroblasts soon acquire big cytoplasmic membranes. My impression is that those fibroblasts survive by reducing their volume and then building it up again.

GLASSER: But there isn't a new generation of fibroblasts?

PADYKULA: Well, that I can't comment on. Dr. Finn can. I don't know if anyone has looked at that, but it would be comparable to during a postpartum estrus or during estrus, when you would have a fibroblastic burst of mitosis.

FINN: Well, my guess would be that you wouldn't get very much mitosis in the fibroblasts unless the rat mated at the postpartum estrus, when you would get corpora lutea formed and progesterone secreted.

GERSCHENSON: You showed an illustration showing a decrease in the number of nuclear progesterone receptors postpartum, or was it pregnancy?

PADYKULA: No, that was pregnancy.

GERSCHENSON: There is a decrease of receptors at the end of pregnancy?

PADYKULA: The nuclear progesterone receptor concentration started to decline during the last week of pregnancy when the monocytes are invading.

GERSCHENSON: It would seem that you get addition of another cell of population into the tissue. If you express your data by the number of receptors per amount of DNA, you have an invasion basically by cells that probably do not have progesterone receptors. Maybe it is a relative decrease. Maybe it is not a real decrease.

MILGROM: I am going to talk about this problem in my presentation. At the end of pregnancy the concentration of nuclear receptors decreases and in some animals is undetectable.

FINN: Have you any quantitative data on what proportion of cells in the stroma will be fibroblasts at the time of implantation? I ask this with some conscience because we tend to assume in our work in the mouse that the great majority are fibroblasts and although we see others, we tend to ignore them.

PADYKULA: Well, I've decided I must simply sit down and study that period in detail as I have done for the postpartum period. But I imagine that this infiltration, which presumably occurs, will be occurring mostly in the superficial stroma near the implantation area. I'd like to comment that I have been studying early human gestation, where there is a mononuclear infiltration at implantation, and fibroblast infiltration occurring at the time when the ovarian progesterone production declines and the placental progesterone production increases. There is a small drop in serum progesterone levels at that time, coinciding with fibroblast infiltration. The rhesus monkey, in that same switch over from ovarian to placental progesterone production, has something Hartman called the placental sign, which is a period of endometrial instability. This occurs at a time when spontaneous abortion is apt to occur in women. This whole infiltration story might relate to that period also.

Reference:

Bernard, O, Ripoche, MA and Bennett, D (1977). Distribution of the maternal immunoglobulin in the mouse uterus and embryo in the days after implantation. J Exp Med 145:58.

Padykula, HA, Driscoll, SG, and Cardasis, CA (1978). Decidual cell differentiation in the normal early gestational human uterus includes lymphoid infiltration. Anat Rec 190:500.

Tansey, TR and Padykula, HA (1978). Cellular responses to experimental inhibition of collagen degradation in the postpartum rat uterus. Anat Rec 191(3):287.

3

The Endometrium During Implantation

Colin A. Finn

The principal function of the uterus is the sustenance of the developing embryo, and in mammals this involves the attachment of the blastocyst to the wall of the endometrium. Most of the cellular changes taking place in the tissues of the uterus are concerned with preparation for this event or with regression if it does not occur. As implantation is a very late evolutionary occurrence and was presumably brought about by adaptation of existing structures, it is not surprising that different species of mammals have evolved different solutions to the problem of bringing the embryo into close contact with the mother. Thus when considering the endometrium during implantation we are concerned with a series of cellular changes culminating in the formation of the placenta, and, as would be expected, there is considerable variation between different species.

Implantation of the blastocyst is normally the central event of the fertile oestrous cycle, and the sequence of cellular changes in the endometrium during the cycle are adaptations to allow it to take place. In the absence of a blastocyst the preparation of the endometrium is reversed with regression and maybe sloughing of tissue. It is a fascinating fact of the endometrium that it has to undergo a whole series of changes in preparation for implantation, but having developed to this stage it cannot be maintained in a fully prepared state for an extended period. In the event of implantation not taking place, the endometrium must undergo regression before being prepared again for the next blastocyst. In the interim, of course, the uterine lumen has to provide a suitable environment for the sperm during their transport to the oviduct. This requires very different conditions from those required for implantation. Viewed from this angle the build up and breakdown of the endometrium during every cycle seems more understandable. Some animals, those exhibiting delayed implantation, can hold the uterus in a partially prepared state for an extended period, but even in these, once full sensitivity has been achieved, implantation must be consummated within a short period or regression will ensue. Outside the short period of sensitivity the uterus is actively hostile to the blastocyst.

For convenience we can discuss the cellular changes in the endometrium associated with implantation under three headings; proliferation, differentiation and death. All the main cell types in the endometrium; (luminal epithelium, glandular epithelium and stroma) go through this cycle of changes. Each has its own special role to play in implantation so that although proliferation and death are similar processes in all the cells, differentiation involves a completely different set of parameters. The processes appear to be largely controlled by the ovarian hormones (oestrogens and progesterone). It is in fact remarkable how two simple steroids can bring about such a precise sequence of differing changes in the three main tissues of the endometrium.

As this paper is concerned with the endometrium during implantation, I shall discuss mainly the differentiation of the endometrium at the time of implantation; however, it may be of interest first to summarise the findings regarding cell proliferation. The observable stages of mitosis take place over a very short time period, so that unless special measures are taken, one will not see many cells undergoing division in histological sections and thus will get a very distorted view of the extent of cell proliferation. Equally, cells which have died are rapidly removed from the tissues thus again precluding a true picture of cell turnover. It is however, fairly easy to get an assessment of the extent of mitosis, either by blocking cells in metaphase and counting the number going into mitosis over a predetermined time period in histological sections or by administering labelled thymidine and assessing the number of cells in the S phase of cell division after autoradiography. The S phase of the cell cycle is a fairly lengthy stage compared with mitosis.

Fig. 1 shows the changing levels of mitosis in the various tissues of the mouse uterus, assessed by counting the mitotic figures (two hours after a colchicine injection) taken from uteri on various days of early pregnancy (Finn and Martin, 1967). Guinea pigs show a similar pattern although the glandular mitosis is more prominent (Mehrotra and Finn, 1974; Marcus, 1974).

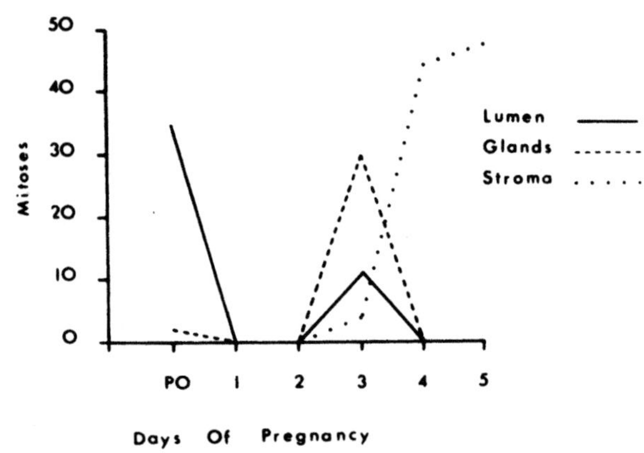

FIGURE 1. Pattern of cell division assessed by counting mitotic figures in histological sections of mouse endometrium 2 hours after the injection of colchicine (from Finn and Martin, 1967).

It will be seen that the luminal epithelium undergoes proliferation chiefly during prooestrus with a small secondary peak on day 3, when the main peak of glandular mitosis takes place. Stromal mitosis takes place on days 4 and 5. In ovariectomised animals there is little mitosis in any tissue. However, if the mice are treated with hormones on the schedule shown in Fig. 2 mitosis can be induced in a pattern very similar to that found in pregnancy. The two doses of 100 ng oestradiol stimulate mitosis mostly in the luminal epithelium on the two days following injection and at the same time cornification of the vagina two days later. As this is equivalent to the day of mating, it is designated as day 1. Subsequently a peak of glandular mitosis occurs on day 3 as in pregnancy with a small secondary peak in the lumen. The administration of progesterone on day 3 initiates stromal mitosis which is increased by giving small doses of 10 ng oestradiol on days 4 and 5. At the same time the uterus becomes sensitive to implantation or to a decidual stimulus on day 5. Thus by using this pattern of hormone injections we can mimic, in ovariectomised mice, the pattern of cell division occurring during pregnancy. As we shall see later, we can also get cell differentiation with this hormone schedule, which not surprisingly follows the pattern of hormone secretion during pregnancy.

Schedule of Hormone Injections

d-2	d-1	d0	d1	d2	d3	d4	d5
E	E	-	-	-	P	Pe	Pe

E = 100ng Estradiol P = 500µg Progesterone

e = 20ng estradiol

FIGURE 2. Schedule of hormone injections.

As mentioned earlier, differentiation varies according to the cell type. Luminal epithelial cells, having divided at the beginning of the cycle in response to the prooestrous oestrogen, differentiate later in the cycle in response to progesterone. However we have shown recently, in the mouse, that between oestrus and day 3, or in the schedule shown,

2 days after the injection of oestradiol, a very large number of luminal epithelial cells die. It is difficult to assess cell death accurately in tissues but we have recently devised a method which we think gives a rough guide to the number of cells dying. This involves labelling the luminal epithelial cells with H^3 thymidine when they are in the S phase of mitosis, that is, after the oestrogen injection or during the dioestrus preceding mating, and then, using scintillation counting of the whole uteri at intervals to follow the amount of radioactivity in the tissues. We assume that the majority of the label will be in the nuclei of the luminal epithelial cells and if they die there will be a reduction in labelling.

As will be seen in Fig. 3, radioactivity drops very sharply over the two days following the cessation of oestrogen injections, whereas after this there is very little loss regardless of treatment. We have also shown that there is a similar drop between prooestrus and day 3 of pregnancy. We assume that the loss of label is due mainly to cell death in the epithelium. In fact if one looks at sections of the uterus at oestrus and on day 4, it is apparent that the lumen has contracted very much in size, so that although one may not get much impression of cell proliferation and death (turnover) from fixed sections, this is probably the dominant activity in the epithelium at this time. During oestrus, the uterus is ballooned out with fluid presumably to allow the passage of spermatozoa to the oviduct. After oestrus, the fluid is dispelled, and the lumen takes on a slit-like shape (Finn and Porter, 1975). Presumably the proliferation and death are part of the cellular differentiation in preparation for these two different events.

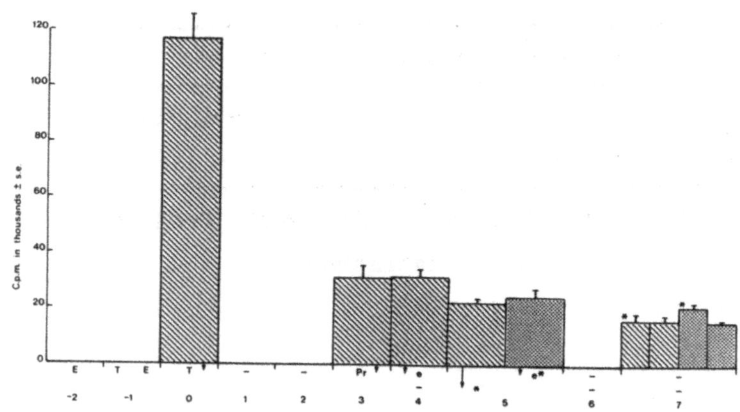

FIGURE 3. Radioactivity in uterus of animals killed on various days of hormone treatment as indicated. All the mice were given 30 μ C ^{3}H thymidine (T) on day 0 and the first group was killed 1 hour later. Subsequent groups were killed on days 3-7. Cross hatched groups did not receive oestradiol on days 4 and 5. Asterisk indicates that oil was injected into one uterine horn to stimulate a decidual reaction.

After progesterone treatment or on day 4 of pregnancy, the luminal cells that do not die prepare for the attachment of the blastocyst. In the mouse there is a well defined closure reaction in which the lumen is more or less obliterated and forms a slit-shaped structure in the mesometrial-antimesometrial direction. The luminal surface of the epithelial cells undergoes a characteristic change. On day 4 of pregnancy the two surfaces are closely opposed with interdigitation of microvilli; whilst on day 5, at the time of implantation, the microvilli flatten so that opposing surfaces run parallel in a very complex pattern. Similar changes occur on days 4 and 5 in ovariectomised mice on the schedule shown earlier. This change in the cell surface is to allow attachment of the trophoblast (Fig. 4). In many species implantation consists of little more than this close apposition of surfaces, which, due to the very large area of attachment, will allow sufficient exchange of materials with the embryo. However, other species have evolved beyond this stage. Basically the aim of implantation in these species is to get the blood vessels of the embryo into closer apposition to the maternal vessels, which at the same time become more permeable (Psychoyos, 1961). This involves the blastocyst penetrating deep into the stromal tissue. There appear to be two main methods for achieving this. In the mouse and rat the luminal epithelial cells surrounding the blastocyst die and are removed by the phagocytic activity of the trophoblast so that the blastocyst comes to lie in a chamber within the stroma and the epithelium re-forms above it. There is good evidence to suggest that this cell death is controlled from within the nucleus of the luminal epithelial cells,

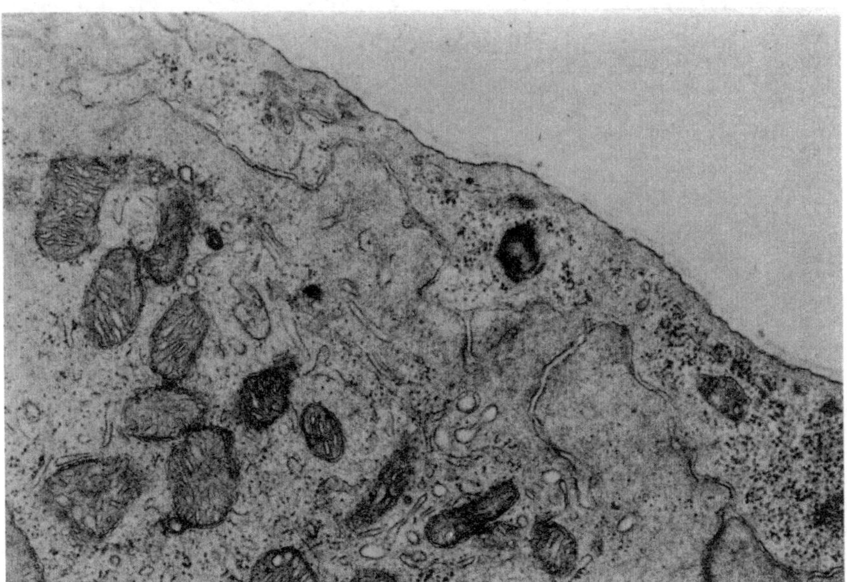

FIGURE 4. Electronmicrograph showing attachment of trophoblast (T) to luminal epithelial surface.

that is, by programmed cell death. The trophblast provides the stimulus for the initiation of the implantation reaction, probably by contact with the surface of the epithelial cells, but once initiated the subsequent chain of events including the breakdown of the epithelial cells surrounding the blastocyst is controlled from within the cells of the endometrium. Thus if one injects a small droplet of oil into the lumen of pseudopregnant or hormonally prepared mice at the time when the endometrium is sensitive to the stimulus of implantation, it will stimulate the uterine side of the implantation reaction including degeneration of the epithelial cells of the anti-mesometrial side of the uterus where implantation would normally take place suggesting that these cells are programmed to die once appropriately prepared and stimulated (Finn and Hinchliffe, 1964). Further evidence for nuclear control comes from experiments using actinomycin D. If this drug is injected systemically into mated mice before implantation, the early stages of implantation, such as the pontamine sky blue reaction and attachment take place, whereas breakdown of the epithelium does not (Finn and Martin, 1972; Finn and Bredl, 1973). However the activation of the blastocyst which in mice is another consequence of the implantation reaction is not stopped. So we have a situation, as depicted in Fig 5, where the blastocyst grows but remains surrounded by epithelial cells, which instead of degenerating appear to actually increase in number. A fairly consistent finding in these cases is that at one point the trophoblast appears to be attempting to penetrate the epithelial cells.

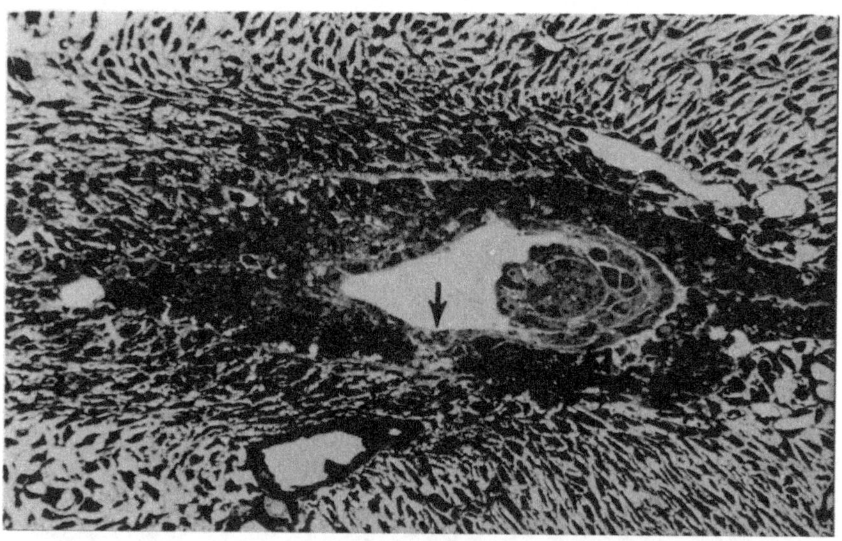

FIGURE 5. Cross section of mouse uterus showing implantating blastocyst 48 hours after initiation of implantation. The trophoblast appears to be penetrating the epithelium at one point (arrowed). (From Finn and Bredl, 1973, by permission of the Editor, J. Reprod. Fertil.)

This is particularly interesting as it appears to be similar to the second method of getting the blastocyst within the stroma, as found in the guinea pig and probably the human. In this method the uterine epithelium appears to be largely passive whereas the trophoblast becomes very active and penetrates between the epithelial cells and actively invades the stroma.

In collaboration with Carol Green, I have recently been looking at this process in guinea pigs with the electron microscope. We first wished to see whether the attachment reaction of the uterine epithelium occurred in this species, either during the infertile cycle or during implantation. We followed changes in the epithelium throughout the cycle. We found that there were changes on the surface of the epithelial cells on days 6 and 7 when implantation would be expected but these were much less obvious than those found in the mouse. There appeared to be closure of the lumen with interdigitation of microvilli but the very distinct contact of opposing membranes was not seen. When uteri of day 6 pregnant guinea pigs were examined, occasional tongue-like protrusions from the trophoblast were seen passing through the zona pellucida to touch the surface of the luminal epithelium; but the contact between trophoblast and epithelium seen in the mouse was not found. On day 7 of pregnancy a few blastocysts were found with the trophoblast, penetrating between the luminal epithelial cells. We looked carefully at the epithelial cells in contact with the trophoblast and they appeared to be healthy. We never found any signs of degenerating cells in the luminal epithelium or of phagocytosis by trophoblast cells. Once the blastocyst had passed into the stroma, the epithelium joined together above it with the formation of gap junctions between cells to reestablish the lumen. One interesting finding was the rarity with which we found specimens at this stage. Altogether we found 25 blastocysts between days $6\frac{1}{2}$ and 7 but found only 4 actually passing through the epithelium. This suggests that the process of passing through must be very rapid. A noticeable feature of this stage was the sudden change in the appearance of the trophoblast. At the time of passage, the polar trophoblast becomes syncytial and takes on the appearance of an actively secreting tissue with a massively developed and dilated endoplasmic reticulum.

Thus the role of the luminal epithelium appears to be different in the guinea pig and mouse: a very active role in the former whilst a passive one in the latter.

The degree of differentiation of the stroma also varies between species. In those species in which the trophoblast does not penetrate through the epithelium there appears to be little differentiation of the stromal cells, although one must not be too dogmatic about this in view of the paucity of information on most non-rodent species. As mentioned earlier women and some other primates are unique in that differentiation of stromal cells starts during the cycle regardless of whether mating occurs or not. Differentiation, however, does not progress very far unless pregnancy ensues, although if exogenous ovarian hormones are administered considerable decidualization can be induced.

Most rodents appear to undergo decidual differentiation of the stroma. Although artificial decidualization appears to have been first demonstrated in the guinea pig, later work has concentrated on the rat and mouse. We have recently been looking at decidual development during implantation in the guinea pig with the electron microscope. In view of the similarity between the mechanism of trophoblast invasion in this species and the human we were interested to see whether decidual development was similar. We wished first to see whether differentiation started during the cycle in the absence of implantation and then to see whether we could cause further development by administering ovarian hormones. In the mouse decidual cells are characterised by their large size and increased numbers of inclusions and the fact that neighbouring cells are joined by gap junctions (Finn and Lawn, 1968). With special staining they can be shown to synthesise alkaline phosphatase (Finn and Hinchliffe, 1964). The predecidual cells in women have also been shown to be joined by gap junctions (Lawn, Wilson and Finn, 1971) and to synthesise alkaline phosphatase (Wilson, 1969). In the guinea pig Deenesley (1971) has shown that alkaline phosphatase is present in small quantities in the stroma before implantation, but this increases dramatically at sites of an implanting blastocyst. It would probably be wrong to interpret this single feature as evidence of preimplantation differentiation of stromal cells in the absence of further evidence, so we have looked at stromal cells throughout the oestrous cycle with the electron microscope.

In the guinea pig, unlike the mouse (Finn and Lawn, 1968), we were able to find a few gap junctions between decidual cells throughout the cycle, but they were most abundant on day 7, that is, when implantation would be expected. However, the stromal cells do not enlarge very much so that the degree of differentiation is probably considerably less than in women. We next administered progesterone or progesterone plus oestrogen to animals during the luteal phase to see if we could get further decidual development. In fact the reverse happened; the cells becoming smaller with fewer junctions. Thus the guinea pig unlike the human appears to need the stimulus of the blastocyst to get further decidual development.

In mice and rats one of the first signs of differentiation of the stroma is increased permeability of the blood vessels supplying the implantation site. This can be demonstrated by injecting pontamine blue into the blood stream, when areas containing a blastocyst will stain blue (Psychoyos, 1961). It has been reported that a similar reaction occurs in guinea pigs (Orsini and Donovan, 1971). However in our experience, in the early stages of implantation in the guinea pig increased vascular permeability is a very irregular occurrence.

Once the blastocyst has started penetrating through the epithelium in the guinea pig the polar trophoblast becomes syncitial and extremely invasive. This is shown in electron micrographs by an immense proliferation of organelles, especially the endoplasmic reticulum. The stromal cells immediately in the area of invasion appear to differentiate little before degenerating and being phagocytosed by the trophoblast, which sends out masses of syncitium in a fan like manner. Around this immediate area there is a layer of larger, more typical looking decidual cells, which have numerous junctions, as in the mouse. However, they never appear to be binucleate. Very soon the syncitiotrophoblast itself degenerates leaving the embryo in a cavity surrounded by decidual cells. This is different from the early stages of implantation in the mouse and rat in which the trophoblast does not become syncitial, but the individual cells grow into giant cells which invade the surrounding decidual tissue. Furthermore the stroma decidualizes well before the trophoblast makes contact with it.

Thus the early stromal response in the guinea pig comes somewhere between that seen in the mouse and the human. In all three species full decidual development only occurs after implantation although in the human it can be artificially stimulated by exogenous ovarian hormones.

In the absence of the stimulus of implantation, the corpus luteum dies and stops secreting progesterone, and the endometrium regresses. In view of the great amount of cell proliferation before implantation, one would expect considerable cell death to occur later in the cycle. In women of course this is obvious at menstruation; however, it appears to have been little studied in other animals. We have attempted to get some quantitative estimate of cell death in the stroma using the same technique as with the epithelium, by labelling a population of stromal cells when they are undergoing their peak of division and then following their fate. In order to label the stromal cells we injected tritiated thymidine one day after the first progesterone injection of the standard schedule that is at the time when the stromal cells would be undergoing synthesis of DNA. In autoradiographic sections we showed that this labelled almost entirely stromal cells. We then followed the amount of radioactivity in the tissues after various treatments (Table 1). We found that if progesterone treatment was

Table 1. Radioactivity (mean counts per horn) in uterine horns following injection of ^{3}H thymidine on day 4 and various treatments as indicated.

d3	d4	d5	d8	n	mean	se
P	TK			10	31,095	± 3,046
P	TPre	K		10	28,073	1,862
P	TPre	e*	K	10	(L)34,100 (R)11,481	5,004 699
P	T		K	10	6,279	606

P = 500 μg progesterone. T = 30 μC ^{3}H thymidine
Pr = 1 mg medroxyprogesterone acetate. e = 10 ng oestradiol
K = autopsy. The mice all received 100 ng oestradiol on days -2 and -1 as in Fig. 2. * Oil injected into left horn (L).

discontinued, the amount of label dropped off dramatically. If progesterone and oestradiol were administered, the drop off was still quite considerable; but if the uterus was stimulated to undergo decidualization by the injection of oil then the level of radioactivity remained high, indicating that few cells had died. Thus it appears that the population of cells which was proliferated just before implantation cannot be maintained unless the cells decidualize. The stromal cells seem to have a choice of two pathways, one leading to death and the other to differentiation.

The nature of the stimulus given to the stromal cells and how it is transmitted from cell to cell is not known. Administration of actinomycin D (AMD) to pregnant mice before decidualization does not prevent the early stages of the implantation reaction; the increased vascular permeability and stromal oedema, indicates that the stimulus has reached the stroma, but it does prevent the onset of decidualization for about 30 hours. Interestingly enough during this time, stromal cells labelled with tritiated thymidine remain, awaiting decidualization (Finn and Bredl, 1977) so that whatever change has been induced in the cells is checked by the AMD with the result that differentiation does not proceed but equally neither does cell death. Once the effect of the drug wears off, decidualization proceeds.

I have left the glands to last as the evidence regarding their role in implantation is weakest. They form a continuous tissue with the luminal epithelium and appear to develop from it; and conversely, at least in the human, the luminal epithelium appears to reestablish itself from the mouths of the glands. Yet as shown earlier their peak of division occurs at a different time from the luminal division. Furthermore their differentiation is completely different. Not surprisingly differentiation involves the synthesis of a secretion. This can clearly be seen in histological sections especially if they are stained with the PAS technique. In the electron microscope it appears as an electron dense material in the gland lumen. It is generally assumed that this secretion is taken up by the blastocyst and provides nutrient material during the critical phase before close vascular apposition. However, it is difficult to get proof of this. An interesting finding in the mouse is that the glands contain little secretion until day 6 of pregnancy by which time the blastocyst is well encased in the deciduum. At this time the yolk sac is at the height of its development so that it is possible that the glands are involved in a short phase of yolk sac placentation.

Studying the secretions from the uterus is a very difficult procedure. As discussed earlier there are extensive changes in the uterine lumen during the cycle and early pregnancy; so that although it is quite feasible to collect fluid from the oestrous uterus, it is a very different problem after closure of the lumen. Len Martin has shown that the instillation of small quantities of fluid into the uterus causes extensive damage to the epithelium so that substances which may appear to have been washed out of the uterus may in fact have been leached out of the cells. The glands are, of course, too small and numerous to canulate so that the only techniques available involve histological sectioning of the uterus. With this limited technique all that one can say with certainty is that the secretion is mucopolysaccharide, and changes in composition with the cycle have been reported in the human.

I hope in this paper to have shown something of the complexity of the cellular events in the endometrium during implantation and of the problems presented by the variation among species.

REFERENCES

Deansley, R. (1971). The differentiation of the decidua at ovo-implantation in the guinea pig contrasted with that of the traumatic deciduoma. J. Reprod. Fertil. 26, 91-97.

Finn, C.A. and Bredl, J.C.S. (1973). Studies on the development of the implantation reaction in the mouse uterus: influence of actinomycin D. J. Reprod. Fertil. 34, 247-253.

Finn, C.A. and Bredl, J.C.S. (1977). Autoradiographic study of the effect of actinomycin D on decidual differentiation of stromal cells in the mouse uterus. J. Reprod. Fertil. 50, 109-111.

Finn, C.A. and Hinchliffe, J.R. (1964). The reaction of the mouse uterus during implantation and deciduoma formation as demonstrated by changes in the distribution of alkaline phosphatase. J. Reprod. Fertil. 8, 331-338.

Finn, C.A. and Lawn, A.M. (1968). Specialized junctions between decidual cells in the uterus of the pregnant mouse. J. Ultrastruct. Res. 20, 321-327.
Finn, C.A. and Martin, L. (1967). Patterns of cell division in the mouse uterus during early pregnancy. J. Endocrinol. 39, 593-597.
Finn, C.A. and Martin, L. (1972). Temporary interruption of the morphogenesis of deciduomota in the mouse uterus by actinomycin D. J. Reprod. Fertil. 31, 353-358.
Finn, C.A. and Porter, D.G. (1975). The Uterus. Elek Science, London.
Lawn, A.M., Wilson, E.W. and Finn, C.A. (1971). The ultrastructure of the human decidual and predecidual cells. J. Reprod. Fertil. 26, 85-90.
Marcus, G.J. (1974). Hormonal control of proliferation in the guinea pig uterus. J. Endocrinol. 63, 89-97.
Mehrotra, S. and Finn, C.A. (1974). Cell proliferation in the uterus of the guinea pig. J. Reprod. Fertil. 37, 405-409.
Orsini, M.W. and Donovan, B.T. (1971). Implantation and induced decidualization of the uterus in the guinea pig, as indicated by Pontamine Blue. Biol. Reprod. 5, 270-281.
Psychoyos, A. (1961). Permeabilile capillaire et decidualisation uterine. C.R. Hebd. Seanc. Acad. Sc. Paris, 252, 1515.
Wilson, E.W. (1969). Alkaline phosphatase in pre-decidual cells of the human endometrium. J. Reprod. Fertil. 19, 567-568.

DISCUSSION:

GREENBLATT: I do not wish to subtract anything from your excellent exposition, but I question the importance of the glands in the implantation process. I have seen decidual cell reaction of the serosa of the appendix during pregnancy and a similar reaction of serosal surface of the ovary following gonadotropin medication. These observations indicate that the mesenchyma can form decidua. The blastocyst can and does implant itself in the abdominal cavity which has no endometrial glands. Several live births have been reported following such instances.

FINN: Yes, I think whether the glands play an important part in implantation in all species is very doubtful. Certainly, in the mouse and guinea pig, the animals I have studied, I would guess that the glands play very little part; I don't know about the human. That the ovum will implant outside the uterus demonstrates, I think, the fact that the ovum can't implant in the uterus except when the uterus allows. The uterus seems to be the only organ which can actually control implantation, that is, the only place where a controlled series of reactions form an implantation chamber and placenta.

GERSCHENSON: Are they really glands or crypts? I have been asking myself this question for years. The so-called endothelial glands are not very well defined functionally.

FINN: Whether they are glands depends on your definition of a gland. In their reaction to hormones and their differentiation, what we call glandular epithelial cells do appear to be different from the luminal cells. They do appear to be secreting something you can see in the lumen.

DEY: During blastocyst attachment, luminal cell death occurs at the site of attachment and can be prevented by injecting actinomycin-D. You saw a similar reaction in pseudopregnant animals injected with oils. Can that be prevented by actinomycin-D?

FINN: Yes, we have done that. The cell breakdown is inhibited as during implantation.

BAULIEU: I must thank you for your very good paper. I find it ter ribly interesting, especially because the three animal species seem to have similar changes, but they occur to different degrees and under different circumstances. Do you mean that in all species, some stromal cells are committed to differentiate to decidual cells in such a way that hormones and implantation or both could extend decidualization and make it more or less invasive according to the stimulus?

FINN: Well, the human is the only animal we know in which some differentiation of stromal cells occurs under the influence of ovarian hormones only. I wouldn't say we know for certain about the guinea pig. There are a few gap junctions between stromal cells, and we have always thought of these as a sign of decidualization because in the mouse and the rat cells don't connect unless they have decidualized. Gap junctions between stromal cells certainly develop in the human before blastocyst attachment, which might be evidence for decidualization. If you administer progesterone/estrogen to a woman you can get quite good decidualization; the whole uterus can become a mass of decidual cells. But in the guinea pig that doesn't happen at all.

BAULIEU: And I assume it is even worse in the rat or the mouse.

FINN: In the rat and the mouse you can give as much hormone as you like but without the stimulus of the blastocyst, oil or trauma, you can't get decidualization. In these species and any other species that have been studied, you must stimulate the endometrium as well as administer hormones.

BAULIEU: Does decidualization start around vessels in the human?

FINN: Yes.

BAULIEU: Does something similar happen in the guinea pig or rat?

FINN: In the guinea pig we didn't notice any relationship topographically between the decidual cells and the blood vessels. As far as I know, the human is the only species in which that connection has been shown.

SOUTHERN: My question is about endometriosis in the human. Whatever everyone believes about the histogenesis of endometriosis, sometimes endometrium develops in the absence of glandular tissue. .Implantation occurs occasionally in ectopic endometrium. That would seem to suggest that glands are not necessary for implantation.

FINN: I would tend to agree. In experiments in animals blastocysts transplanted outside the uterus attached and the trophoblast grew. But in the experimental animals the embryo does not grow. It dies off very rapidly. In the human, the whole embryo will grow. Perhaps the uterus is adapted to prevent implantation at most times and only to allow it when the animal is fully prepared so that implantation takes place under properly controlled conditions. Perhaps the uterus is the place where implantation of the embryo can be controlled. Ectopic implantations can be very dangerous to the animal. If they are not removed they can cause death. So, I think of the uterus as being adapted for the safe sojourn of the embryo.

MOULTON: Did the autophagic or lysosomal activity differ at implantation sites of the rat and the guinea pig?

FINN: We could not see anything. We didn't do anything quantitative so I could not be sure there wasn't any difference.

ABEL: Just two points. The first, the human, as far as I am aware needs just progesterone for the change from predecidual cells to decidual cells. My second point is that in primates including the human you don't seem to get the restriction in time for implantation as you do in the mouse, rat and rabbit. A fertilized ovum was removed from the oviduct of a rhesus monkey, immediately transferred to the uterus, and implantation resulted (Marston et al, 1977). This suggests that the uterine environment is not hostile to the developing primate blastocyst as it is in the mouse and rat.

FINN: This actually is quite the opposite of what I had understood. I thought that Marston did find that he needed synchrony. Certainly Edwards and Steptoe have concluded that putting the fertilized egg into the human uterus at the proper time is very important and that many of their failures have been from improper timing. What was your first point?

ABLE: That the change from predecidual to full decidual cells is progesterone dependent.

FINN: Oh, yes. The work I had in mind referred to women taking a contraceptive tablet which I think did contain estrogen in addition to a progestin. But you are probably quite right, the estrogen would not be essential.

ABLE: Edwards and Steptoe cultured the fertilized ova in vitro for 72 hours before returning them to the uterus. Could the embryo have arrived too late to rescue the corpus luteum and could the pregnancies have failed, in part, for this reason? This differs from the problem of whether or not a sensitive period for implantation exists in the primate.

In addition tubal pregnancies appear to be peculiar to the primate. Thus, if ovum transport through the Fallopian tube is delayed or prevented, the embryo will implant in the epithelial lining of the tube. This does not occur in the mouse, rat, rabbit or guinea pig.

FINN: Isn't this going back to what we were saying earlier about ectopic pregnancies generally? The uterus is the only place where attachment of the blastocyst can be properly controlled. When a blastocyst gets outside the uterus, problems follow.

BIGGERS: Fifteen preimplantation stages of the human have now been recovered. From these limited data we can say that the embryo enters the uterus on about the third day at the 16-cell stage. It then floats in the uterine fluid for three more days before implanting. Therefore, the uterus is not hostile to the embryo during this period. Marston and his colleagues at Birmingham transferred a 2-cell monkey embryo from the oviduct to the uterus in the same animal. This shows that the uterine milieu is not hostile to early development in this species.

Because of the pattern of development of the uterus simplex in the human, the lower part of the oviduct, the isthmus region, has the same type of cellular lining as the uterus. In other words, the uterus extends into the lower part of the oviduct. Therefore it is not surprising that ectopic pregnancies occur frequently in this site.

BAZER: I just had a comment about the uterine glands. From our work with large domestic animals, we feel that the animals that have actual implantation do not need uterine glands because they form an implantation site that allows the direct exchange of feed to the conceptus. Dr. Barron and I have talked about this. The mother seems to benefit during the development of the conceptus. On the other hand, in the pig and the sheep and cow which have a central implantation or placentation, the uterine glands seem to be important for a major portion of pregnancy. So, as Dr. Mossman pointed out, it is almost like going in an evolutionary sense, from the chicken where you have the liver and glands of the reproductive tract secreting everything to the uterine endometrium alone under the hormonal control of the ovary and the placenta secreting material involved in nutrition of the developing conceptus.

FINN: That was just the thought that struck me as I listened to Dr. Mossman this morning and saw his pictures.

GLASSER: In mammals the uterus is as important in the evolutionary strategy as the mammary glands because the uterus restricts the development of the progeny. With respect to John Marston's work, which I think is being much more broadly interpreted than John would care to have it interpreted, you have to differentiate between hostility and synchrony, particularly in those animals with a long preimplantation period and a long period of uterine hospitality during which the blastocyst orients somewhat towards the endometrium. One of the differences that we find between epithelium taken from nonreproductive sites and cast down as monolayers and epithelium taken from the uterus cast down as monolayers is that epithelium from nonreproductive sites does not discriminate about implantation. You can culture the blastocyst and it will attach. However, epithelium from reproductive sites imposes time and rate restrictions on the blastocyst attachment and perhaps penetration.

Reference:

Marston, JH, Penn, R and Sivelle, PC (1977). Successful autotransfer of tubal eggs in the Rhesus monkey (Macacca mulatta). J Reprod Fertil 49:175-176.

4

Endometrial Changes in the Infertile Woman with Particular Reference to Atypism and Its Management

Robert B. Greenblatt
R. Don Gambrell, Jr.

Endometrial changes in infertile women depend on their hormonal status, i.e., ovulatory, anovulatory, or ovarian (follicular) failure. If an endocrinologic or psychophysical disorder cannot be detected and secretory changes are in phase, then "no reason infertility" may be suspected. However, ovulatory women may be infertile if the luteal phase is inadequate.

Luteal phase defects are associated with less than normal progesterone production because of poor corpus luteum function. The diagnosis is made by comparing the secretory changes of the endometrium to the cycle date following the post-ovulatory rise in basal body temperature (Noyes et al, 1950). A luteal phase defect is associated with stromal-glandular disparity. Secretory glandular maturation is delayed and the histologic picture is out of phase (Fig. 1). Unequal ripening, resulting in a mixed follicular and secretory endometrium, occurs occasionally (Fig. 2). Such changes arise from disturbed estrogen-progesterone production or unequal tissue response. G.S. Jones found luteal phase defects in 3-7% of patients with primary infertility and in 35% with secondary infertility related to early, repeated abortions (Jones, 1979).

Three other types of ovulatory women may be infertile. In one type, uterine synechiae more or less obliterate the uterine cavity (Asherman's syndrome). This usually follows post-abortal infection and at times a too rigorous curettage. The diagnosis is made by uterosalpingography and inability to obtain any or only very little endometrial tissue on curettage. A second type is due to chronic inflammation like that caused by an acid-fast infection (tubercular endometritis). Uterosalpingography may resemble that in Asherman's syndrome, but endometrial biopsy usually reveals the characteristic histopathology. A third type occurs in the woman with an endocrinopathy. For instance, women with Cushing's disease or an adrenogenital syndrome are usually amenorrheic; a few may have regular ovulatory periods but rarely conceive until the endocrinopathy is corrected (Greenblatt and Roy, 1963).

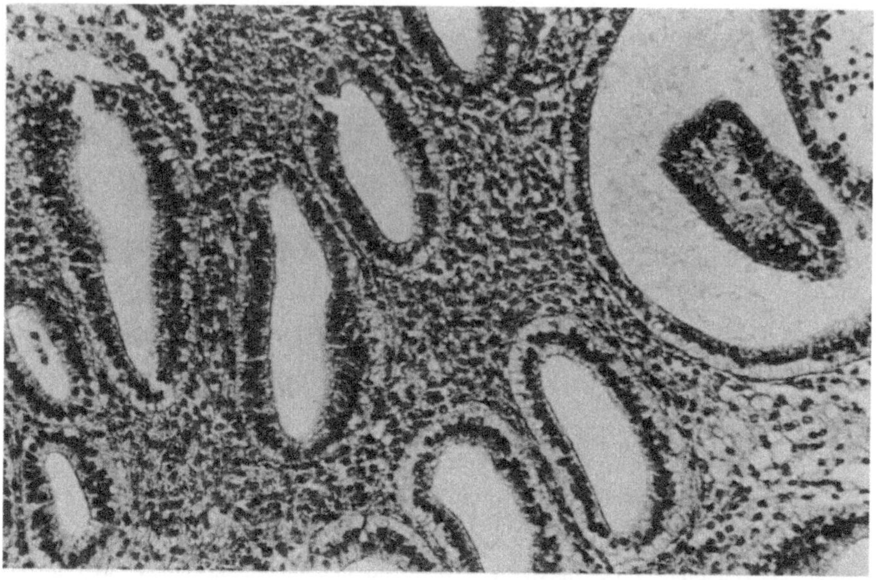

Fig. 1. Luteal phase defect: secretory changes of endometrium are out of phase. Biopsy taken on 11th day of basal body temperature rise, but maturation is comparable to third post-ovulatory day.

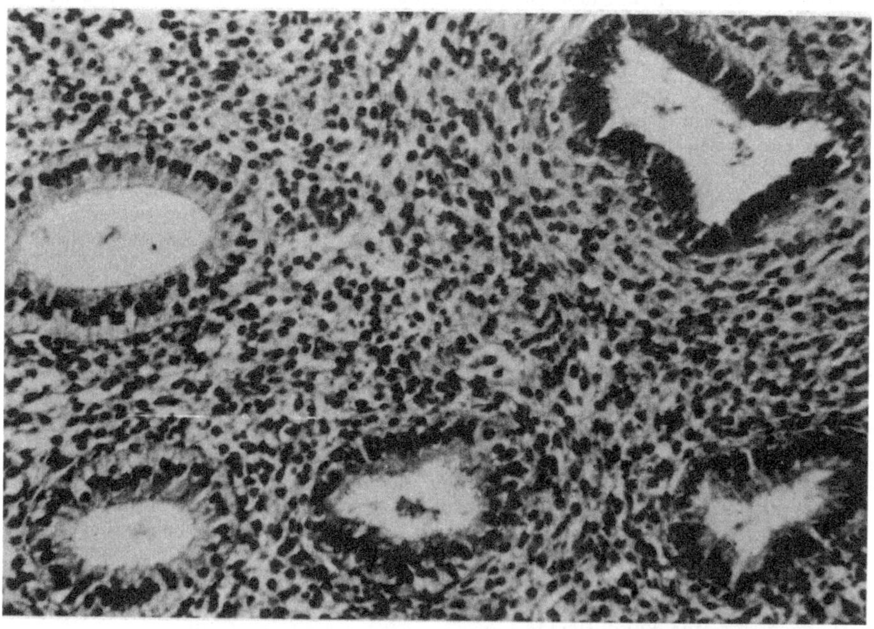

Fig. 2. Unequal estrogen-progestogen response: mixed endometrium. Note secretory glands on left, proliferative glands on right.

Infertility due to primary follicular failure, as in gonadal dysgenesis, resistant ovaries (Savage syndrome), and premature menopause are irremediable although in a few cases massive doses of Pergonal® have overcome the resistance (Rabinovitz et al, 1979). Hypothalamic-pituitary disorders may cause secondary follicular failure, as in patients with pituitary and parapituitary tumors, Sheehan's disease, panhypopituitarism, and in isolated gonadotropin deficiency often associated with anosmia (Kallman's syndrome). The endometrium in patients with these diseases is atrophic with a few sparse tubular glands.

In another group of amenorrheic women, those with hypothalamic-pituitary disorder, estrogen stimulation is usually minimal as in amenorrhea-galactorrhea syndromes, psychogenic amenorrhea, and in post-pill amenorrhea. The results of endometrial studies in this group are, as a rule, not unusual. The histologic picture varies from atrophic to a resting-type of follicular endometrium (Fig. 3).

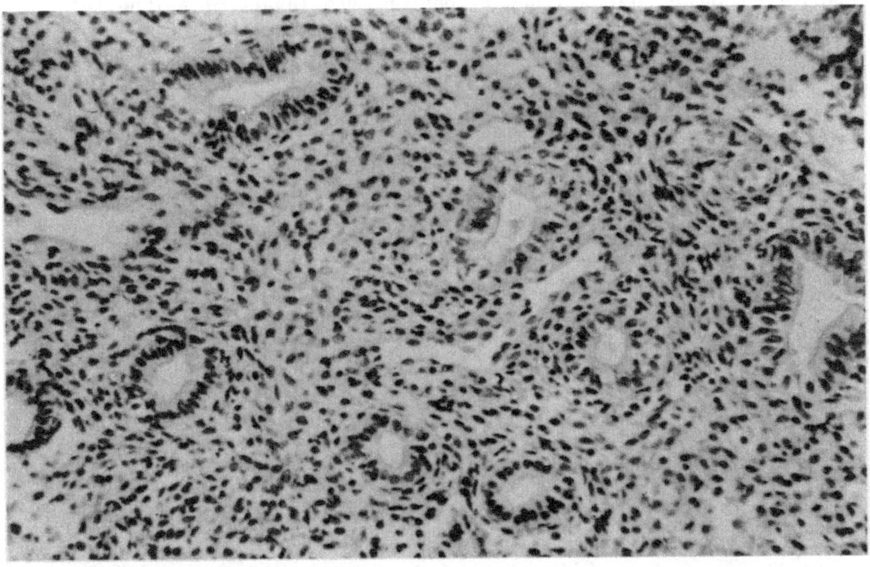

Fig. 3. Resting follicular endometrium in a 21-year-old female complaining of oligomenorrhea and infertility. Patient conceived after first trial of Clomid® therapy.

The most common female factor in infertility is ovulatory failure resulting from hypothalamic-pituitary dysfunction. The varied endometrial changes depend not only on duration and intensity of estrogen stimulation but also on individual tissue responsiveness. The resultant endometrial proliferation may be focal or diffuse and occurs in women with polycystic ovarian disease, dysfunctional uterine bleeding, incretory tumors of the ovary, and various forms of amenorrhea, and oligomenorrhea. Persistent estrogen stimulation may cause complex glandular patterns which simulate neoplastic processes. The pathologist is often taxed to differentiate severe atypical hyperplasia from adenocarcinoma. In fact, many severe hyperplasias are diagnosed as malignancies to protect both the pathologist and the patient. Realizing this dilemma, Halban admitted, "nicht Karzinom aber besser heraus (not carcinoma but better out)" (Halban, 1952).

The histopathologic characteristics of endometrial atypism have been catalogued and described by Ng and Richart (1979), Hertig et al (1949), Kistner (1959), Ng et al (1973), and Novak (1952) and the following review is perfunctory. The spectrum of endometrial changes in anovulatory women with hypothalamic-pituitary dysfunction ranges from simple follicular (proliferative) endometrium (Fig. 4) to adenocarcinoma (Fig. 11). Some typical examples follow.

FOLLICULAR (PROLIFERATIVE) ENDOMETRIUM

A proliferative endometrium is usually composed of more or less uniform tubular glands lined by one or more layers of epithelial cells. The stroma is cellular but not too dense (Fig. 4).

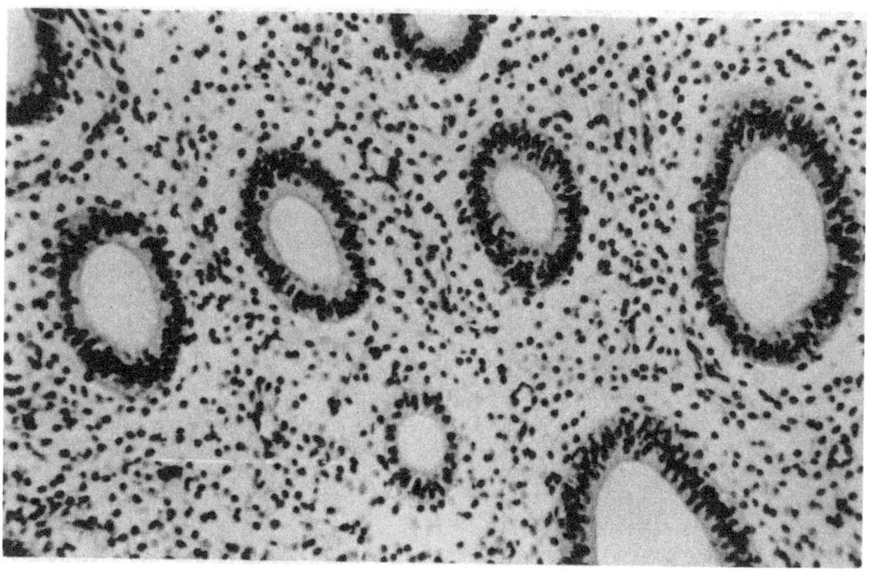

Fig. 4. Proliferative endometrium.

ENDOMETRIAL HYPERPLASIA

When the response to estrogen stimulation is somewhat greater than normal, the number of glands increases and an increased disparity in their size and shape occurs. The glands are lined by pseudostratified, well stained epithelial cells. Such a histologic picture is labelled simple hyperplasia. The stroma is abundant, and mitoses are usually found in both the epithelial and stromal elements (Fig. 5).

CYSTIC GLANDULAR HYPERPLASIA

At times the glands enlarge considerably and appear cystic, giving a Swiss-cheese appearance. The cells lining the glands are usually reduced to a single layer. This type of glandular reaction may or may not accompany hyperplasia in adjacent areas. Cystic glandular hyperplasia is believed due to slow and prolonged estrogen stimulation; the cystic hyperplasia may be an expression of exhaustion or of regression (Fig. 6).

ADENOMATOUS HYPERPLASIA

Adenomatous hyperplasia differs grossly from the pattern of simple hyperplasia; the glands are well formed, lined by mature cells, and greatly increased in number (Fig. 7).

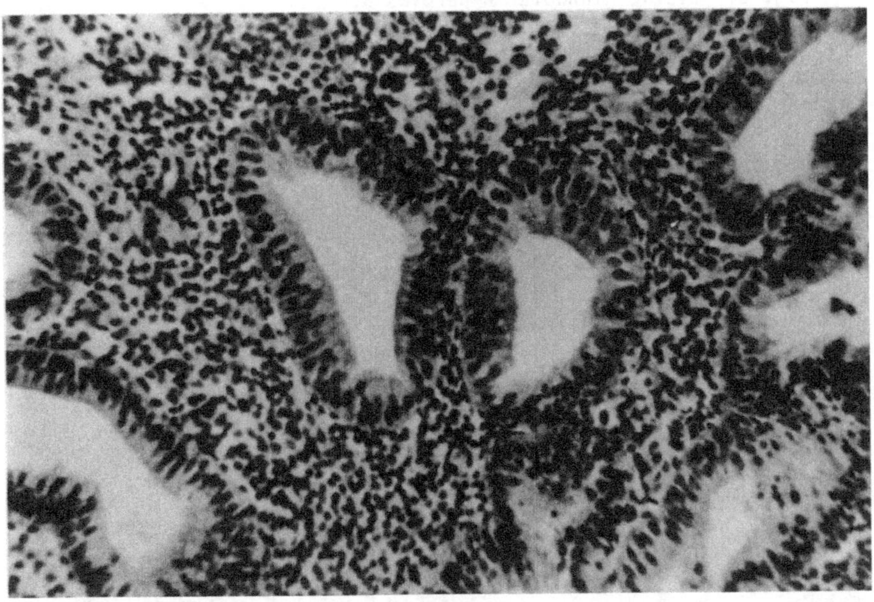

Fig. 5. Endometrial hyperplasia.

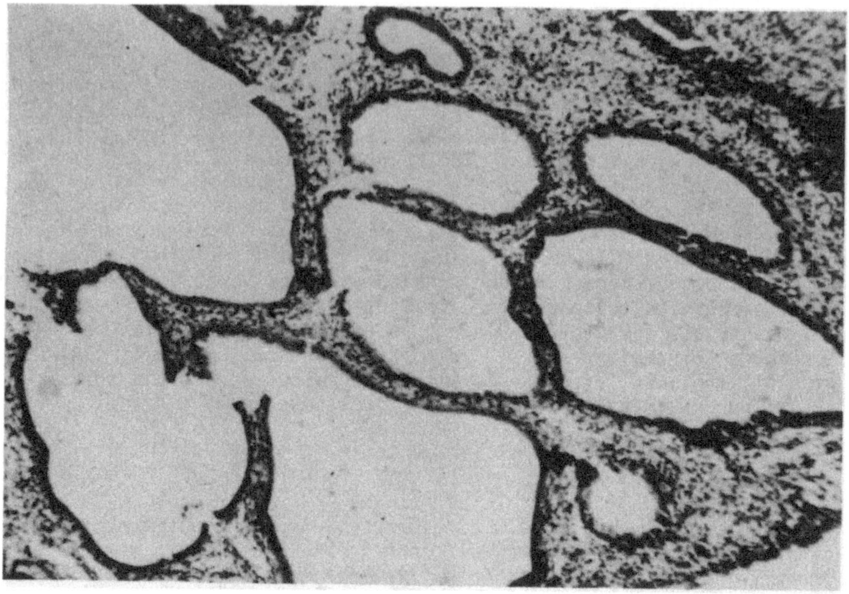

Fig. 6. Cystic glandular hyperplasia.

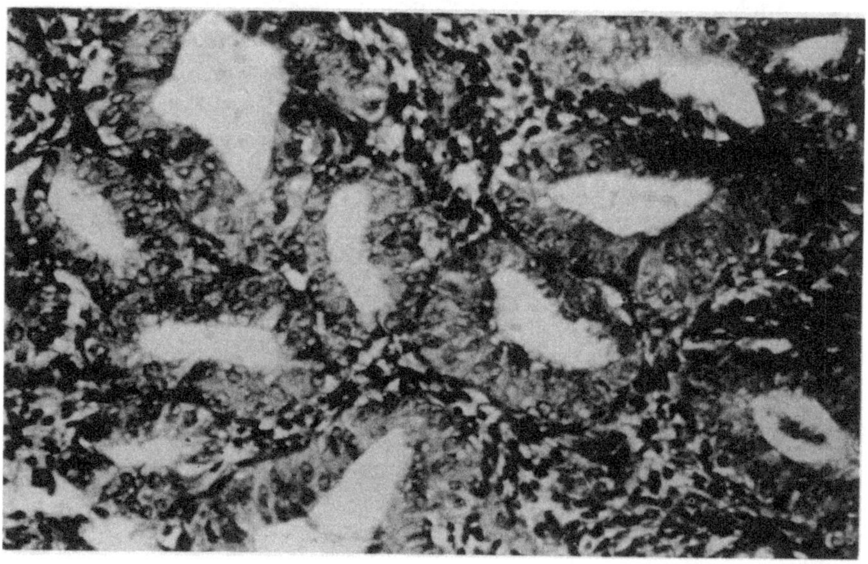

Fig. 7. Adenomatous hyperplasia.

ATYPICAL ADENOMATOUS HYPERPLASIA

When glands are so crowded as to appear back to back with little stroma separating them, the lesion is atypical adenomatous hyperplasia sometimes labelled adenoma malignum. The epithelial cells may stain normally or display an affinity for eosinophil (Fig. 8).

ATYPICAL HYPERPLASIA OR CARCINOMA-IN-SITU

When the morphology of the glands is atypical because of glandular convolutions and staining characteristics and shape and size of nuclei vary markedly, the diagnosis is atypical hyperplasia. This lesion is often referred to as carcinoma-in-situ. The stroma is frequently hyperplastic and possibly includes epithelioid cells and foci of squamous metaplasia (Fig. 9).

ADENOACANTHOMA

When clusters of normal or nearly normal squamous cells intermingle with glandular carcinoma, a diagnosis of adenoacanthoma may be considered. If the squamous cells are atypical and invade the endometrial stroma, the diagnosis becomes adenosquamous carcinoma. At times, the differential diagnosis of severe metaplasia, adenoacanthoma, and adenosquamous carcinoma is difficult (Fig. 10).

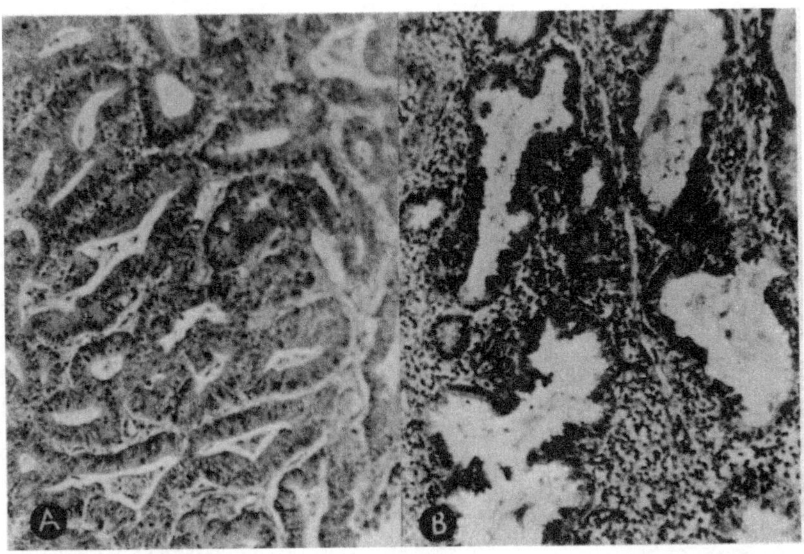

Fig. 8. A, Atypical adenomatous endometrial hyperplasia diagnosed as well differentiated adenocarcinoma; B, converted to a progestational endometrium after a 10-day course of a progestogen.

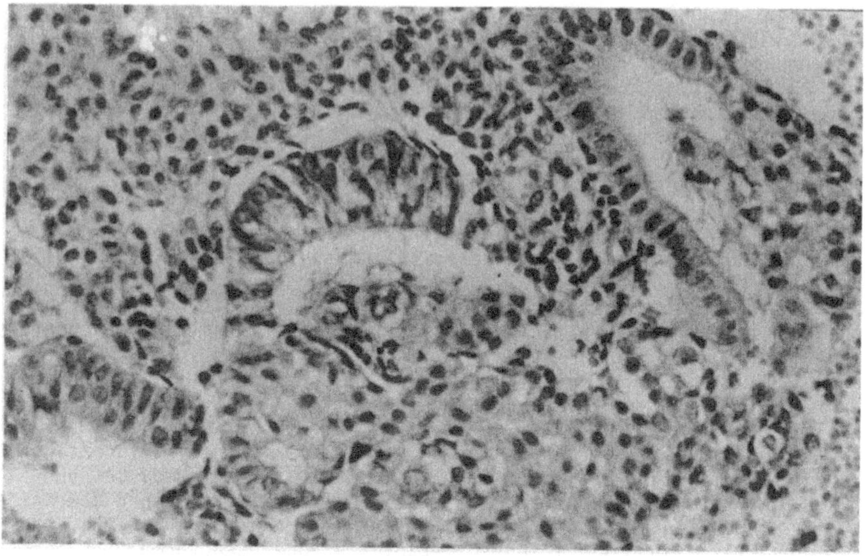

Fig. 9. Atypical hyperplasia diagnosed as adenocarcinoma by one pathologist and carcinoma-in-situ by another.

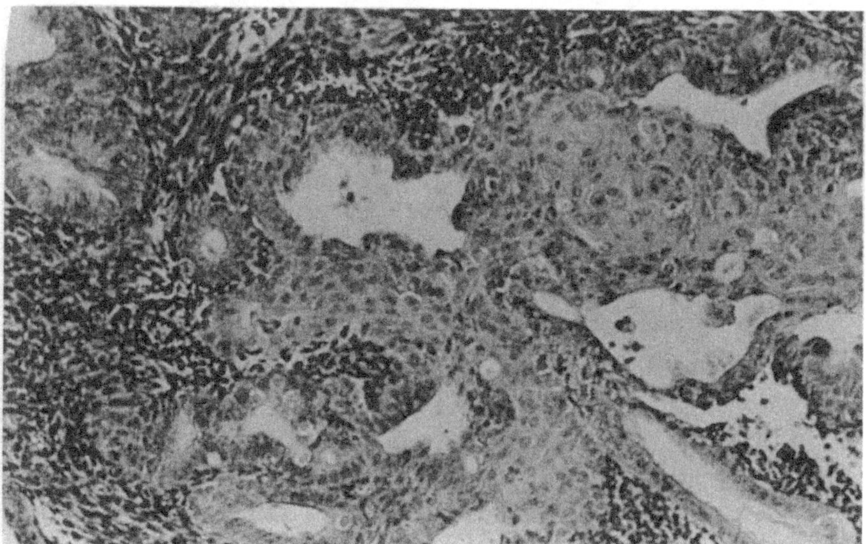

Fig. 10. Severe squamous metaplasia.

ADENOCARCINOMA

Persistent endometrial stimulation may induce changes that may progress from hyperplasia, especially the atypical variety, to malignancy; or the neoplasia may start de novo in a hyperplastic or nonhyperplastic area. Adenocarcinomas of the endometrium vary considerably in degree of differentiation. The microscopic picture is characterized by disorderliness of the glands, the hyperchromatic nuclei, and the abnormal mitotic figures. Papillary projections into the lumen of glands are frequently seen. Having broken through the basement membrane, epithelial cells invade the stroma. The number of dedifferentiated cells increases from 25% in stage I carcinoma to 100% in stage IV. During the reproductive years, such neoplasms occur in some women with the polycystic ovary syndrome of Stein-Leventhal (Fig. 11).

The diagnostic features of adenomatous hyperplasia, atypical adenomatous hyperplasia, carcinoma-in-situ, or atypical hyperplasia may not be distinctive enough for definitive diagnosis. Their atypical features may encourage hysterectomy, thus forever preventing a solution to the infertility.

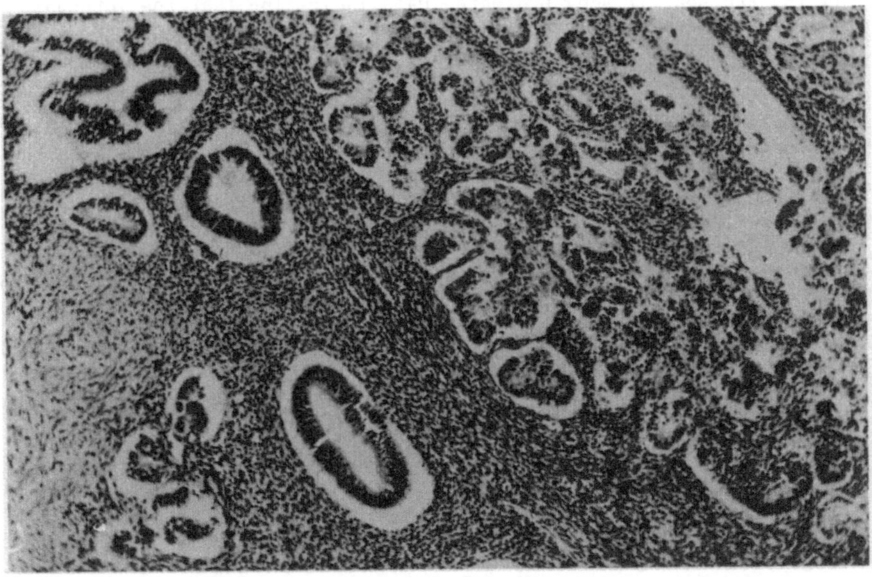

Fig. 11. Adenocarcinoma in a 15-year-old hirsute girl with menorrhagia.

THE FATE OF UNTREATED ENDOMETRIAL HYPERPLASIA

In their reproductive years, women subjected to long, uninterrupted estrogen stimulation are at greater risk of developing endometrial carcinoma. Certain investigators believe the process is ongoing and may take many years (Gusberg, 1976; Wentz, 1966). Shanklin found that focal hyperplasia, hyperplasia, adenomatous hyperplasia, atypical hyperplasia, carcinoma-in-situ, and carcinoma were a steadily rising age function, suggesting that cancer tendencies are set as early as age 30 (Shanklin, 1976).

An association between endometrial hyperplasia and corpus cancer has been suspected ever since Cullen (1900) described a change in atypical hyperplasia as a sign of cancer nearby and Robert Meyer (1923) reported conversion of hyperplasia to carcinoma in some patients (Meyer, 1976). Novak and Woodruff (1962) felt that hyperplasia and endometrial cancer were merely different degrees of similar endocrine or metabolic processes. Many other investigators have discussed precursor cancer lesions. In a prospective study of 562 women with adenomatous hyperplasia, Gusberg (1976) found that 18.5% developed cancer after a few years, but by the tenth year, the incidence rose to 30%. Gambrell believes that any degree of hyperplasia may be significant; 17.4% of 774 patients with varying degrees of hyperplasia progressed to cancer within 1 to 8 years; of these, 1.4% had simple cystic glandular hyperplasia (Gambrell et al, in press). Ng and Richart (1979) and Wentz (1966) presented data indicating that the interval from the diagnosis of hyperplasia to the development of cancer was inversely related to the severity of the hyperplasia.

Persistent estrogen stimulation of the endometrium sooner or later induces abnormal uterine bleeding, varying from irregular spotting to prolonged bleeding episodes. Although dysfunctional uterine bleeding is mostly anovulatory, Gambrell found that in 24% of the patients bleeding was from a secretory endometrium (Table 1) (Gambrell, 1974). He believed that a secretory endometrium in such cases probably indicated inadequate corpus luteum function. Dysfunctional uterine bleeding sometimes follows soon after menarche and unless the bleeding is rapidly arrested with progestational agents, endometrial biopsy is mandatory. The youngest patient one of us (RBG) has studied was a 15-year old hirsute girl who had amenorrhea-menorrhagia and who failed to respond to progestogen therapy. A dilatation and currettage revealed adenocarcinoma. Total hysterectomy was performed; the ovaries were polycystic (Fig. 12).

PROTECTIVE ACTION OF PROGESTERONE IN REVERSING ENDOMETRIAL HYPERPLASIA AND LESSENING THE RISK OF CANCER

Once hyperplasia is identified, the patient should be treated with progestogens or hysterectomy. Most gynecologists prefer hysterectomy, especially for women over 35. Such drastic measures are rarely necessary for the infertile woman wishing to preserve reproductive potential. Ovulation induction is now possible in over 90% of women with responsive ovaries through the use of Clomid®, Parlodel®, or Pergonal®

Table 1

Histopathology of the Endometrium in Women with Dysfunctional Uterine Bleeding*

Findings	<20	21-25	26-30	31-35	36-40	41-45	46-50	>50	Total Number	Total %
Proliferative	10	21	25	34	42	60	45	11	248	44.8
Secretory	5	5	11	20	31	42	17	2	133	24.0
Atrophic	3	2	7	6	8	15	13	10	64	11.6
Endometritis	3	3	2	1	2	2	-	-	13	2.3
Decidua with villi	2	1	-	1	-	-	-	-	4	0.7
Benign hyperplasia (or cystic)	4	-	5	5	10	28	22	2	76	13.7
Adenomatous hyperplasia	-	-	-	-	-	2	1	-	3	0.5
Atypical adenomatous hyperplasia	-	-	1	2	5	2	1	1	12	2.2
Adenocarcinoma	-	-	-	-	-	1	-	-	1	0.2
TOTAL	27	32	51	69	98	152	99	26	554	100.0

*After Gambrell (1974)

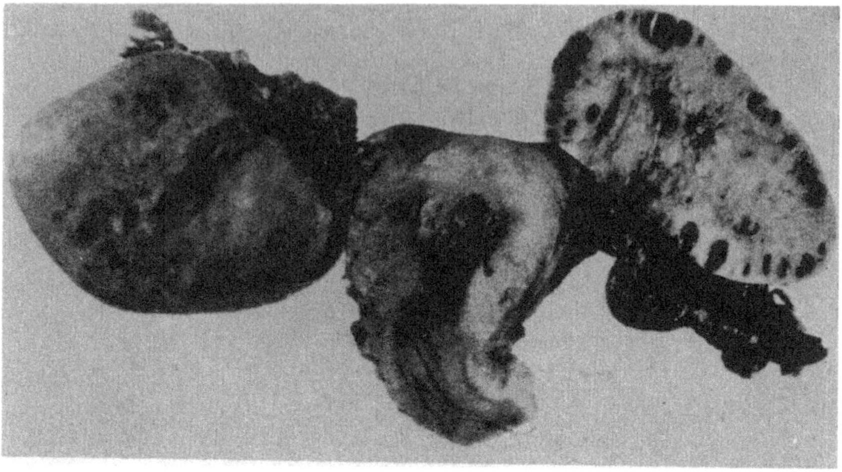

Fig. 12. Typical polycystic ovaries in a young hirsute girl with menorrhagia. Adenocarcinoma of the endometrium (See Fig. 11).

(Greenblatt, 1979). Moreover, cyclic courses of progestogens in adequate doses can reverse the hyperplasia and prevent its recurrence in most instances. Studd et al (1977) have confirmed the advantage of adding a progestogen in the last half of the cycle to avoid "the possibility of endometrial over-stimulation".

From 1972 to 1978, Gambrell and his colleagues at Wilford Hall USAF Medical Center administered progestogens to 258 patients with varying degrees of hyperplasia (Gambrell and Greenblatt, 1979). The histopathology before and after therapy revealed reversal of the hyperplastic endometrium to a normal or atrophic endometrium in 242 (93.5%) of the patients (Table 2). Twelve failed to respond to 7-day and four to 10-day courses administered over a period of 3 to 6 months. Some patients seem to require more than 10 day's therapy even though 5 to 7 day courses of progestogen prevent endometrial hyperplasia in most cases. When hyperplasia persists, 21-day courses may be instituted for another 3 months and curettage repeated. If the hyperplasia does not reverse completely, then hysterectomy is mandatory.

To emphasize the protective action of progesterone, we present our experience in the management of 490 women who were of reproductive age and who received continuous estrogens from pellet implantation of 17β-estradiol for conception control for 1539 woman-years. The progestogen was administered for 5 days at monthly intervals to induce withdrawal periods. If breakthrough bleeding intervened, the dosage was considered inadequate and was increased to 7 to 10 days. Endometrial biopsies were done whenever unusual bleeding occurred. Biopsies were also done at the completion of a course of progestogen or just before its ingestion. We encountered two cases of atypical adenomatous hyperplasia but no endometrial cancers. By increasing the duration of progestogen therapy, we reversed the abnormal hyperplasia (Table 3) (Nezhat and Greenblatt, unpublished). For many years we have maintained that women with adenomatous and atypical hyperplasia may be treated effectively with progestogens (Greenblatt, 1965; Greenblatt et al, 1966; Greenblatt and Stoddard, 1978).

TABLE 2

Effect of Progestogens on Endometrium*

	Before	After
Simple and cystic hyperplasia	186	10
Adenomatous hyperplasia	22	4
Atypical adenomatous hyperplasia	50	2
Total patients	258	16**

* Gambrell and Greenblatt (1979)
** Remaining 242 patients were normal or atrophic

TABLE 3

Endometrial Status After 17β-Estradiol Implantation for Conception Control

	Endometrial Biopsy				
Findings	First	Second	Third	Fourth	Total
Number of biopsies	165	37	11	3	216
Proliferative	64	16	3	1	84
Secretory	44	11	5	2	62
Simple or Cystic Hyperplasia	48	6	2		56
Moderate Hyperplasia	7	4	1		12
Adenomatous Hyperplasia	2*				2

* One of these patients was over 35 years of age, and a course of progestogen was administered prior to hysterectomy. Histologic sections of the uterus revealed that the adenomatous hyperplasia had converted to a progestational endometrium.

The assumption that progesterone does not protect against malignancy is based on several publications (Kelly et al, 1976; Cohen and Deppe, 1977) but particularly that of Silverberg and Makowski (1975). In the Cancer Registry they found 21 cases of endometrial cancer recorded in women taking oral contraceptives when 13 million women in the United States were taking those agents. The number is surprisingly small; seven were taking the classic pill, 13 were taking the sequential pill; and the kind of pill one was taking was not reported. All but one taking the sequential pill received Oracon®, which provides five days' therapy with a weak progestogen, dimethisterone. However, only one woman who used sequential pills, such as C Quens®, containing a more potent progestogen developed endometrial carcinoma, even though the sales of the latter were three-fold greater than those of Oracon. Silverberg and Makowski tried to show that a 5-day course of a progestogen was not completely protective, and they were right. They unwittingly proved that progestogens do partially protect women against development of endometrial cancer, provided the drug is potent enough or is administered for a sufficient length of time.

Several investigators have confirmed in estrogen-treated women the effectiveness of progestogens in reducing the risk of endometrial cancer. Hammond et al (1979), Paterson (1979), and Sturdee et al (1978) found no endometrial cancer in 72, 133, or 325 patients given progestogen for 10 days or more during each cycle. In the double-blind, 10-year prospective study of Nachtigall et al (1979) 84 menopausal women were given a placebo and 84 were given a sequential estrogen-progestogen regimen (7 days of 10 mg of Provera®). Two endometrial and five mammary cancers occurred in the placebo group, none in the other. Gambrell et al (1979) found the incidence of endometrial cancer lower in estrogen-progestogen treated menopausal women than in an untreated group (Table 4).

TABLE 4

Incidence of Endometrial Cancer: 1975-1978*

Patients Treated With:	Patient-Years of Observation	Endometrial Cancers	Incidence (per 100,000)
I Estrogen-progestogen	5,323	3	56.4**
II Estrogen	2,228	8	359.1***
III Estrogen vaginal cream	910	1	109.1
IV Progestogen or androgen	397	0	-
V Untreated	2,014	5	248.3
Totals	10,872	17	156.4

* Gambrell (1979)
** $p < 0.05$ (Difference between Group I and Group V)
*** $p < 0.05$ (Difference between Group I and Group II)

Thom and her co-workers evaluated 74 patients with endometrial disease among 850 climacteric women receiving estrogens (Thom et al, 1979). They concluded that cyclical courses of 7 to 13 days of a progestogen each month should give maximal benefits and minimal risks through prevention or correction of endometrial hyperplasia or both in women receiving oral estrogen or 17β-estradiol implants (Table 5). We agree with Campbell and Whitehead that "epidemiological evidence suggests a true link between unopposed estrogens and early less invasive endometrial cancer," and that "progestogens appear capable of protecting against development of cancer and hyperplasia, although complete protection is yet to be achieved" (Campbell and Whitehead, 1977)

TABLE 5

Prospective Study on Menopausal Women:

Protective Action of Progesterone*

Estrogen Dosage	Progestogen Duration	Hyperplasia %
Low dosage	-	7
High dosage	-	15
High or low dosage	5-10 days	2
Estradiol-17β implants or High or low dosage } **	13 days	0

* Thom et al (1979)
** 200 cases over four years of observation

CASE REPORTS

Four problem cases are presented to highlight the variegated endometrial changes that may be found in the anovulatory infertile woman.

Case 1. O.R., 27 years of age, had oligomenorrhea, hirsutism, and infertility. She was suspected to have had Stein-Leventhal syndrome. An endometrial biopsy in 1958 showed advanced endometrial cancer (Fig. 13). One of us (RBG) challenged the diagnosis and the histologic sections were submitted to a noted professor of pathology in Boston for review. His diagnosis was cancer-in-situ. In the meantime, a wedge resection was done, and several cyclic courses of a progestogen were prescribed. Repeated biopsies over the next few months failed to reveal any atypical endometrium. The patient conceived three times between 1958 and 1966; the first pregnancy ended in abortion and the next two were normal. Fifteen years later, a panhysterectomy was performed because of fibromyomata. The pathologist found no evidence of neoplasia. The patient and her children are alive and well.

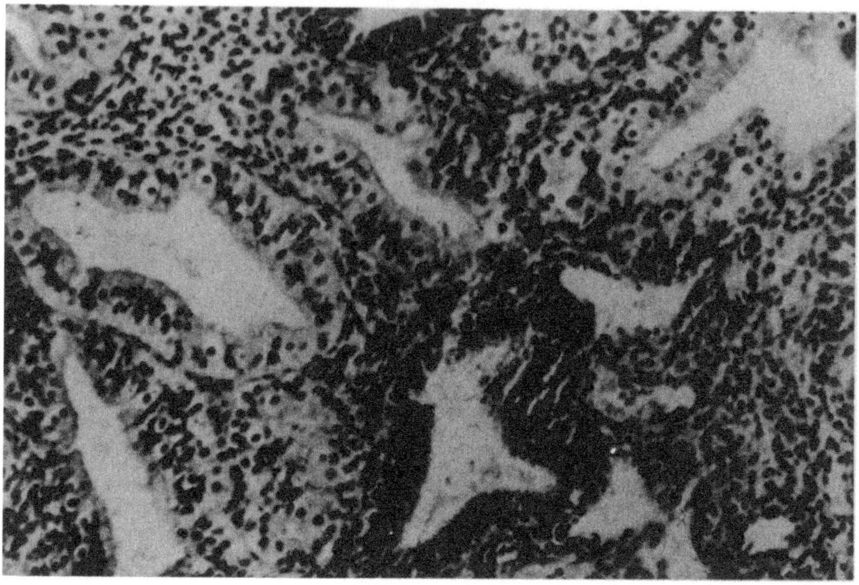

Fig. 13. (Case 1) Atypical hyperplasia.

Case 2. N.H., 28 years of age, had infertility, moderate hirsutism, and menorrhagia. Progestogen therapy began immediately after an endometrial biopsy in 1952. A few days later, the pathologist reported of adenoacanthoma. The patient did not come back as requested because she felt so well; she had no more uterine bleeding. Finally, 4 months later she returned for a total hysterectomy, and the pathology report showed adenoacanthoma. She was followed for many years and remained in good health. On further reflection, we believe that this was a case of severe adenomatous hyperplasia with focal areas of squamous metaplasia (Figs. 14 A and B).

Case 3. B.P., 25 years of age, was evaluated because of infertility and oligomenorrhea in July 1977. An endometrial biopsy revealed moderately severe adenomatous hyperplasia and squamous metaplasia (Fig. 15A). She received cyclic courses of norethindrone acetate in doses ranging from 20 mg for 5 days to 5 mg for 15 days over the next 6 months, and four more endometrial biopsies were done. Progestational endometrial changes were induced, while altered focal adenomatous hyperplasia persisted. In January 1978, she started to take Clomid, 50 mg, one b.i.d. (days 5 to 9), followed by Provera, 10 mg for 10 days (days 16 to 25). A subsequent endometrial biopsy showed only progestational changes. This regimen was repeated, and another biopsy was taken 1 month later (4/13/78). It revealed progestational endometrium without any adenomatous foci (Fig. 15B). She continued to take Clomid therapy and conceived the following month and was subsequently delivered of twins. Eight months after delivery, a follow-up endometrial biopsy showed no evidence of atypia. Both mother and children remain well.

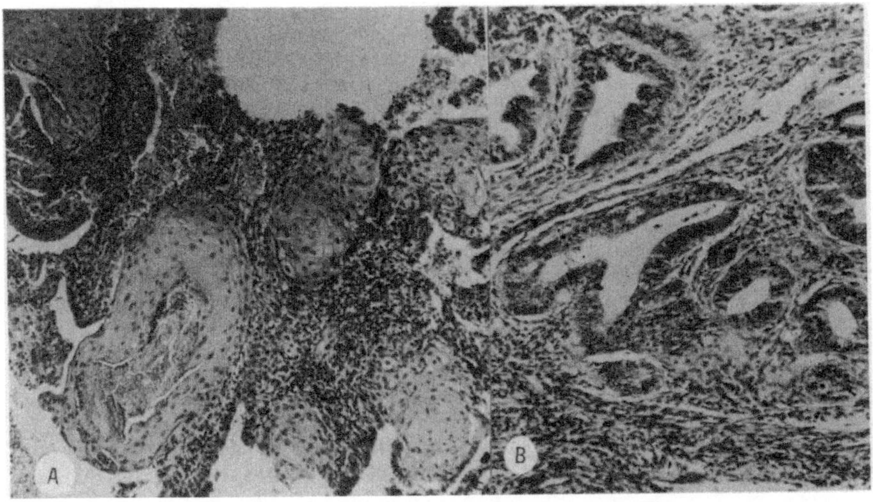

Fig. 14. Hysterectomy specimen diagnosed as adenocanthoma. A, Note focal areas of squamous metaplasia; B, Note atypical hyperplasia.

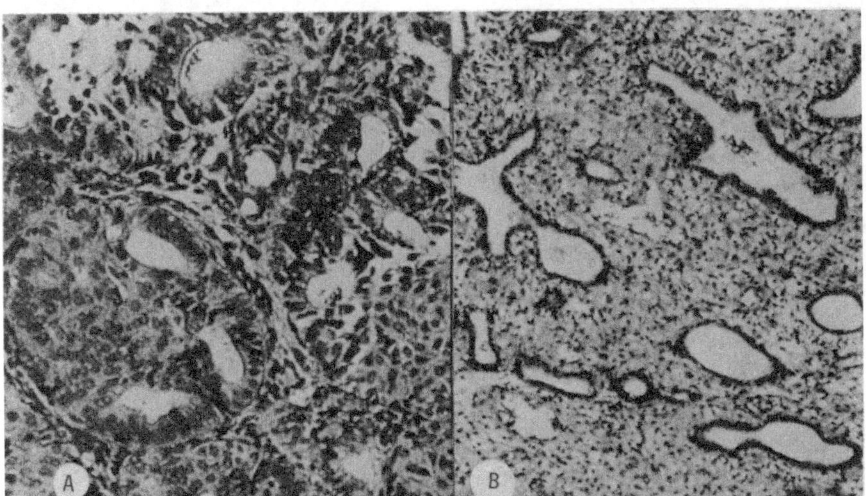

Fig. 15. A, Atypical hyperplasia with squamous metaplasis; B, converted to a progestational endometrium after several months of Clomid® and cyclic progestogen therapy. Patient conceived and bore twins.

Case 4. H.M., 31 years of age, was referred to us because of irregular menses and secondary infertility. Because of anovulation, her gynecologist prescribed 5-day courses of Clomid for 3 months. He performed a dilatation and curettage on 11/22/77 because of vaginal spotting which had lasted for 20 days. Adenocarcinoma with focal stromal invasion was diagnosed (Fig. 16A), and hysterectomy was suggested. We prescribed Clomid, hCG, and Provera, which stimulated ovulation. After several months of this regimen, repeated endometrial biopsies revealed reversal to normal, except for an occasional small focus of atypical endometrium (Fig. 16B). Because of this, we prescribed 100 mg of Depo-Provera® injections at monthly intervals for 3 months and 800 mg of Danocrine® for 1 month, 400 mg for the second month and 200 mg for the third month. A curettage performed on 9/25/79 showed that the endometrium was wholly progestational and no foci of atypia were present. The patient now receives 5-day courses of Clomid, followed by an injection of hCG; if the basal body temperature chart should be uniphasic, then a 10 day course of Provera, 10 mg, is to be added. The patient will be closely watched. Our experience suggests that regular ovulatory menstruation or progesterone-induced withdrawal periods will, in all probability, prevent the recurrence of the atypical adenomatous hyperplasia.

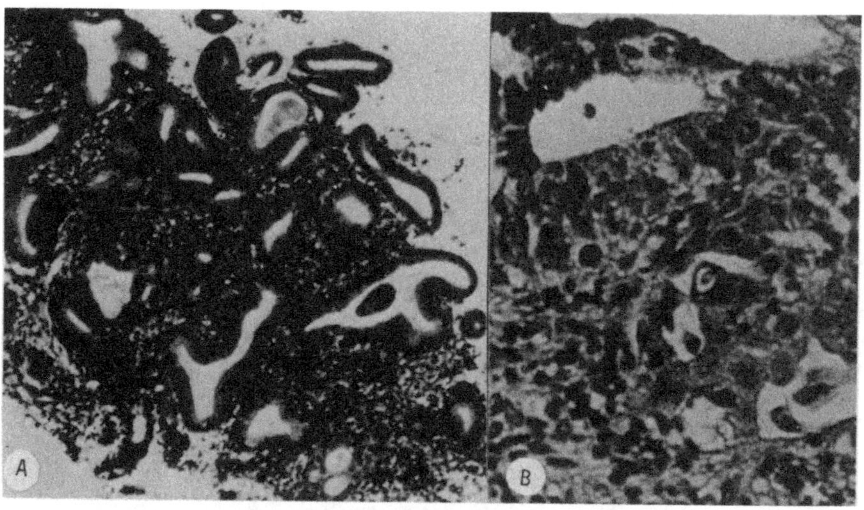

Fig. 16. (Case 4) A, Atypical hyperplasia diagnosed as early adenocarcinoma. B, After three months of cyclic Clomid®, hCG and Provera®, focal areas of atypical cells remained. Large monthly doses of Depo-Provera® and Danocrine® wholly converted the endometrium to a progestational endometrium.

CONCLUSION

The anovulatory infertile woman whose ovaries produce adequate estrogens may develop hyperplasia, adenomatous hyperplasia, atypical hyperplasia, and adenocarcinoma. Adenomatous hyperplasia and atypical hyperplasia need not be precursors of adenocarcinoma. Progression to carcinoma can be minimized if regular ovulation can be induced with ovulatory inducing agents or if the endometrium is shed monthly in response to administration of 7 to 14 day courses of a progestogen.

The histopathologic features of atypical hyperplasia and early adenocarcinoma may at times be so confusing that they cannot be differentiated. In such cases, one or more courses of a progestogen for 10 to 21 days may help distiguish between the two. In our experience, such progestogen dosage has failed to alter the histopathologic appearance of true neoplasia but has helped us to identify the pseudocancers.

REFERENCES

Campbell, S and Whitehead, M: Oestrogen therapy and the menopausal syndrome. Clin Obstet Gynceol 4:31, 1977.

Cohen, CJ and Deppe, G: Endometrial carcinoma and oral contraceptive agents. Obstet Gynecol 49:390, 1977.

Cullen, TS: Cancer of the uterus. (New York; Saunders, 1900).

Gambrell, RD, Jr: Perimenopausal and postmenopausal bleeding: Mechanism, pathology, management with progestational agents. In Greenblatt, RB et al (eds): The Menopausal Syndrome (New York; Medcom Press, 1974) p. 147.

Gambrell, RD, Jr: Workshop report: The endometrium in the menopause. In van Keep, PA, Serr, DM and Greenblatt, RD (eds): Female and Male Climacteric (Lancaster, England; MTP Press Ltd, 1979), p 116.

Gambrell, RD, Jr and Greenblatt RB: The Menopause: Indications for Estrogen Therapy. In Kistner, RW (ed): Current Problems in Obstetrics and Gynecology (Chicago; Year Book Medical Publishers, 1979).

Gambrell, RD, Jr, Massey, FM, Castaneda, TA, et al: Use of the progestogen challenge test to reduce the risk of endometrial cancer. Obstet Gynecol (In Press).

Greenblatt, RB: Current concepts-estrogen therapy for postmenopausal females. N Engl J Med 272:305, 1965.

Greenblatt, RB: Induction of Ovulation (Philadelphia; Lea & Febiger, 1979).

Greenblatt, RB and Roy, S: Virilizing adrenal tumors. In Greenblatt, RB (ed): The Hirsute Female (Springfield, Ill; Charles C Thomas, 1963), p 109.

Greenblatt, RB and Stoddard, LD: The estrogen cancer controversy. J Am Geriatr Soc 26:1, 1978.

Greenblatt, RB, Stoddard, LD, and King PR: Estrogen in endometrial carcinogenesis. In Lewis, CG, Wentz, WB and Jaffe, RB (eds): New Concepts in Gynecological Oncology (Philadelphia; FA Davis Co, 1966), p. 211.

Gusberg, SB: The individual at high risk for endometrial carcinoma. Am J Obstet Gynecol 126:535, 1976.

Halban, J: Quoted by Emil Novak in Gynecologic and Obstetric Pathology, 3rd Ed. (Philadelphia; WB Saunders Co, 1952), p 166.

Hammond, CB, Jelovsek, FR, Lee, KL, et al: Effects of long-term estrogen replacement therapy. II. Neoplasia. Am J Obstet Gynecol 133:537, 1979.

Hertig, AT, Sommers, SC, and Bergloff, H: Genesis of endometrial carcinoma. III. Carcinoma-in-situ. Cancer 2:964, 1949.

Jones, GS: Disordered function of the corpus luteum. In Givens, JR (ed): Endocrine Causes of Menstrual Disorders (Chicago, London; Year Book Medical Publishers, 1979), p 237.

Kelly, WH, Miles, PA, Buster, JE, et al: Adenocarcinoma of the endometrium in women taking sequential oral contraceptives. Obstet Gynecol 47:200, 1976.

Kistner, RW: Histological effects of progestins on hyperplasia and carcinoma in situ of the endometrium. Cancer 12:1106, 1959.

Meyer, R: Quoted by Gusberg SB in The individual at high risk for endometrial carcinoma. Am J Obstet Gynecol 126:535, 1976.

Nachtigall, LE, Nachtigall, RH, Nachtigall, RD, et al: Estrogen replacement therapy. II. A prospective study in the relationship to carcinoma and cardiovascular and metabolic problems. Obstet Gynecol 54:74, 1979.

Ng, APB, Reagan, JW, and Storaagli, JP: Mixed adenosquamous carcinoma of the endometrium. Am J Clin Pathol 59:765, 1973.

Ng, APB and Richart, RM: Recognizing the precursors of endometrial cancer. Contemp Obstet Gynecol 13:183, 1979.

Novak, ER: Gynecologic and Obstetric Pathology, 3rd Ed (Philadelphia; WB Saunders Co, 1952).

Novak, ER and Woodruff, JD: Gynecologic and Obstetric Pathology (Philadelphia; WB Saunders Co, 1962), p 161.

Noyes, RW, Hertig, AT, and Rock, J: Dating the endometrial biopsy. Fertil Steril 1:3, 1950.

Paterson, MEL: Workshop Report: The endometrium in the menopause. In van Keep, PA, Serr, DM and Greenblatt, RB (eds): Female and Male Climacteric (Lancaster, England; MTP Press Ltd, 1979), p 116.

Rabinovitz, D, Spitz, IM, and Beneveniste R: Isolated gonadotropin deficiency. In Givens, JR (ed): Endocrine Causes of Menstrual Disorders (Chicago, London; Year Book Medical Publishers, 1979), p 181.

Shanklin, DR: Correspondence to the Editor. N Engl J Med 294:847, 1976.

Silverberg, SG and Makowski, ED: Endometrial carcinoma in young women taking oral contraceptives. Obstet Gynecol 46:503, 1975.

Studd, JWW, Chakravarti, S, and Oram, D: The climacteric. In Greenblatt, RB and Studd, JWW (eds): Clinics in Obstetrics and Gynaecology (London; WB Saunders Co, 1977), p 3.

Sturdee, DW, Wade-Evans, T, Paterson, MEL, et al: Relationships between bleeding pattern, endometrial histology and oestrogen treatment in menopausal women. Br Med J 1:1575, 1978.

Thom, MH, White, PJ, Sturdee, DW, et al: Prevention and treatment of endometrial disease in climacteric women receiving oestrogen therapy. Lancet. Sept 1, 1979, p 455.

Wentz, WB: Treatment of persistent endometrial hyperplasia with progestins. Am J Obstet Gynecol 6:999, 1966.

DISCUSSION

SHAPIRO: I have two questions. A series of patients who had Turner's syndrome were treated with so-called normal estrogens and nonsteroidal estrogens with different incidence of hyperplasia. Could you comment on that possibility?

GREENBLATT: Yes. The first report in the United States came from Boston (Cutler et al, 1972). Of the three cases reported as adenocarcinoma, at least one appeared to me to be adenomatous hyperplasia. The patients had received stilbesterol and no progestogens. Furthermore, one other case of adenocarcinoma has been reported in an untreated patient with Turner's syndrome. I believe there are now 18 cases in the world literature, but a progestogen was administered only to three. Whether the progestogen dosage was inadequate or regularly administered, I do not know. I've managed about 100 patients with Turner's syndrome during the past 30 years, and none has developed an endometrial carcinoma during cyclic estrogen-progestogen therapy although fibromyomata developed in a few. Maybe women with Turner's syndrome are more prone to neoplasia because of the genetic nature of Turner's syndrome.

SHAPIRO: Clark, a few years ago, reported the administration of clomiphene citrate to rodents and the subsequent development of mullerian problems. I wonder if you'd comment on that in relationship to its use in humans.

GREENBLATT: I do not know anything about the development of mullerian duct anomalies in the offspring following use of clomiphene. We've had a large and long experience with clomiphene; other than multiple births, I'm not aware of any serious anomalies.

GERSCHENSON: The problem with differentiating adenomatous hyperplasia from adenocarcinoma is that surgical pathologists get sections, and they have to make decisions in a short time about a specimen they assume to be representative. Another problem is the fact that we do not know if the so-called preneoplastic lesions really are. Recent experimental information suggests that hyperplastic alveolar nodules in liver and mammary glands might not ultimately be the sites of neoplastic transformation. However, the organs having these lesions are at a higher risk of developing cancer which originated somewhere else.

I would also like to refer to the hypothesis that neoplasms might arise from cells at different stages of differentiation. Many years ago, G.B. Pierce showed experimental evidence for this hypothesis and suggested the possibility that tumors originating from undifferentiated cells could be redirected towards terminal differentiation, which would result in the cure (temporary or final?) of the patient. Maybe when Dr. Greenblatt treats his patients with progestins, this is what he is doing.

Another problem I would like to mention is the possibility, however remote, that similar looking hyperplasias or carcinomas might originate from different cell types. An adenocarcinoma of the endometrium could originate from glandular, luminal, clear, or ciliated, etc. cells. Adenocarcinomas from different cells might look the same, but they will have a completely different biological behavior or hormonal response.

GREENBLATT: Dr. Gerschenson, I agree completely. My plea is this: if the pathologist is uncertain, then try the progestogen test. Today we have a simple test which may help differentiate true cancer from pseudocancers. If a 10 to 21 day course of an oral progestogen induces reversal to secretory change, then, in all probability, the patient does not have a true adenocarcinoma. Even if after one course of therapy only 90% of the glands show progestational changes, repeat the therapy for several more months to learn whether it will completely reverse hyperplasia; if not, then hysterectomy is indicated. We have not reversed true adenocarcinoma after a few courses of an oral progestogen.

GERSCHENSON: I wonder if Dr. Shapiro would elaborate on this since this is what I understood that gynecologists do.

SHAPIRO: I really think it varies around the country and from center to center. Not everyone gives a challenge test. I wonder if the challenge test labels or removes the label of carcinoma. It is possible that these hyperplasias are still carcinoma but treatable because they have receptors, cytoplasmic and nuclear components that will allow response to the progestin. I would be happy to hear your comments on that.

GREENBLATT: Well, yesterday someone mentioned that 30% of metastatic adenocarcinomas respond to Depo-Provera®. The patients who respond evidently have receptors for progesterone. Lesions confined to the uterus may or may not be true neoplasias; perhaps some true neoplasias respond to progestogen. The dosages used in the treatment of metastatic cancer are astronomic in comparison to the more or less physiologic dosages used in the progestogen test. Progestogen therapy reduces the risk of cancer in patients who are anovulatory but produce endogenous estrogens, as well as in patients receiving estrogens. Progestogen therapy reduces the incidence of endometrial cancer to less than that which occurs in untreated women. Progestogens are not completely protective; some women will develop endometrial cancer despite endogenous or exogenously administered progestogens.

FINN: As I'm not a clinician or a pathologist, this may be a simple minded question. What risk are you taking? I've always understood that you remove cancer as soon as possible lest it spread to other parts of the body.

GREENBLATT: Endometrial cancers spread slowly. A good muscular wall confines the endometrial lesion for a long time. As a matter of fact, many menopausal women may have unheralded endometrial cancer which only manifests itself with breakthrough bleeding after the first few months of estrogen therapy. Since several years of estrogen therapy are required to induce adenocarcinoma, a slow growing, silent cancer was probably present in these women for several years before the start of estrogen therapy. Last April we described our series of 1,058 women, 45 and older, who received continuous estrogens from implants of 17β-estradiol pellets for one to 21 years for a total of 9,175 women-years (5,402 had intact uteruses) (Greenblatt et al, 1979). Patients were advised to take a 5 to 7 day course of an oral progestogen monthly to induce orderly withdrawal periods. Endometrial cancers were found in nine of these women. The malignancies were uncovered because of abnormal bleeding in four within the first few months of estrogen therapy. We must conclude that estrogen therapy unmasked an occult cancer in those four. The incidence of five cases of endometrial cancer among women receiving continuous estrogen therapy is less than the expected incidence of eleven.

Giving a course of progestogen to women with suspected adenocarcinoma will not increase the risk of spread by the delay. Smith et al, (1975) alleged a relationship between estrogens and endometrial cancer. They were asked to stage the patients' cancer. There were eight Stage II and III cancers in the estrogen-treated group, and 42 Stage II, III, and IV cancers in the non-estrogen treated control group. The estrogen treated women appear to have been far better off since they had fewer and less aggressive cancers, the diagnoses were probably made earlier, and the prognoses were far better than for the control group. I believe that in patients with Stage III and IV cancers, the cancers have already been present for some time before the diagnoses were finally made.

GLASSER: Dr. Gerschenson has stated and you have agreed that different types of cells might be involved here. I would like to know if either of you has thought about whether we are dealing with a type of cell whose sensitivity may be altered by its stage of the mitotic cycle. I would distinguish here between the stage of the mitotic cycle as opposed to the length of post-mitotic life. A third possible consideration would deal with different subpopulations of really different species of cells. Each of three types of cells could be at risk here, and the risk would be different in each case.

GERSCHENSON: We have published a paper showing two cell populations at least in rabbit endometrium cultures, one that is resting and one that is cycling all the time (Gerschenson et al, 1979). In monolayer cultures the targets of estrogens for proliferation are only the resting cells (G-zero cells). In vivo studies in the rabbit also demonstrate the existence of a resting cell population that is also the target for estrogens (Conti et al, 1979). A target may be the resting cells or the cycling cells.

In terms of differentiation in the uterus different cell types might serve as targets. In humans are a few ciliated cells which have precursor cells and clear cells which are induced by estrogen as well as glandular and luminal cells. An old paper by an Indian author showed at least eight different cell types in the rabbit uterine epithelium, which means that any of these cells could be a target. Each of them can produce a different tumor.

GREENBLATT: During the proliferative phase, numerous mitoses are present in both the stroma and epithelium. During the luteal phase, mitosis is arrested, and mitotic figures are rare. Some pathologists feel that a true carcinoma does not develop from the secretory endometrium. Some carcinomas are called secretory-type carcinomas, but I think it was the nature of the cell that developed in that direction and not due to the influence of endogenous progesterone.

BAULIEU: I agree with many points that you have made, and also I agree with one of the earlier comments that what appears to be cancer can be treated and will regress in response to hormone action. Practically speaking, would you ask someone with endometrial abnormality which may or may not be cancer to undergo progesterone therapy? Would you advise the progestogen test in every case? What would you recommend if you are really sure that it is histologically and cytologically cancer?

GREENBLATT: If the diagnosis is unmistakably cancer, the progestogen test is not undertaken but aggressive therapy is started at once, i.e. radium followed by surgery. Women harboring so-called well-differentiated adenocarcinoma, carcinoma-in-situ, and severe atypical hyperplasia so frequently indistinguishable from endometrial cancer deserve a progestogen test before submitting them to the hazards of radium. If secretory transformation follows progestogen administration, then cyclic courses may be administered for 10 to 14 days every month to prevent progression of the lesion to neoplasia. I've observed several such women for many years, with endometrial biopsies done at yearly intervals. I am satisfied that adenomatous and atypical hyperplasia are not necessarily forerunners or inevitable precursors of cancer. When the pathologist feels as Halban once expressed it - "nicht Karzinom aber besser heraus (not carcinoma but better out)", I wish to use the progestogen test, expecially in women who wish to retain their reproductive potential. Perhaps women over 35 should be encouraged to undergo hysterectomy unless there are cogent reasons against it - not the least of which is psychologic.

References:

Conti, CJ, Gimenez-Conti, IB, Conner, EA and Gerschenson, LE (1979). Hormonal regulation of rabbit uterine epithelium. J Cell Biol 83:253a

Cutler, BS, Forbes, AP, Ingersoll, FM and Scully, RE (1972). Endometrial carcinoma after stilbesterol therapy in gonadal dysgenesis. N Engl J Med 287:628-631.

Gerschenson, LE, Conner, EA, Yang, J and Andersson, M (1979). Hormonal regulation of proliferation in two populations of rabbit endometrial cells in culture. Life Sciences 24:1337-1344.

Greenblatt, RB, Nezhat, C, Roesel, RA and Natrajan, PK (1979). Update on the male and female climacteric. J Am Geriatr Soc 27:481-490.

Smith, DC, Prentice, R, Thompson, DJ and Herrmann, WL (1975). Association of exogenous estrogen and endometrial carcinoma. N Engl J Med 293:1164-1167.

PART II
STEROIDS AND THE ENDOMETRIUM

The Endometrium

5

Estrogen and Progesterone Receptors in Normal and Pathological Human Endometrium

Etienne-Emile Baulieu
Rodrigue Mortel
Paul Robel

ABSTRACT

Cytoplasmic (R_c) and nuclear (R_n) estrogen and progesterone receptors can be measured in endometrial biopsy samples. Total ($R_c + R_n$) receptor concentration (R_t) and receptor subcellular distribution (R_c/R_n) vary during the menstrual cycle, according to the regulatory principles established in laboratory animals. The main methodological principles are reported in this paper, as well as results in normal and anovulatory cycles, cases of luteal insufficiency, early pregnancy and endometrial carcinoma. In the latter disease, tamoxifen (an anti-estrogen) often increases or even induces progesterone receptors. The prognostic and therapeutic implications of this test are discussed.

Measuring steroid receptors reveals an important component of the hormonal responsiveness of the human endometrium which may serve for better patho-physiological understanding and improved treatments.

In the past two decades, the development of saturation analysis methods (Diczfaluzy, 1970 ; Yalow, 1978) has led to specific and accurate measurements of circulating hormone levels and consequently to a better understanding of endocrine regulated phenomena. However, in the last 10 years, study of hormone action at the target cell level has also been considered in practical terms. A large body of evidence has been accumulated, leading to the present concept that hormones interact with receptor systems in order to trigger the responses of the target cells.

In a schematic fashion, a receptor can be represented as a structure having a site _r_ which binds the specific hormone and another site _e_ (effector) which interacts with undefined component(s) of the target cell and originates the hormonal response(s) (Fig. 1). Following these binding and triggering steps, the response will essentially proceed independently of the hormone (Baulieu, 1978).

Hormone receptors were first identified and physiochemically studied for steroids, particularly estradiol in the rat uterus (Jensen & Jacobson, 1962 ; Baulieu et al., 1967 ; Toft et al., 1967). Steroid hormone receptors are intracellular proteins activated by the binding of the proper hormone. The resulting hormone-receptor complexes promote characteristic changes of gene expression, probably by the interaction with the chromosomal machinery. The relevant molecular biology is still in its infancy and continues to be the subject of extensive research (reviews : Jensen & De Sombre, 1972 ; Baulieu et al., 1975 ; Gorski & Gannon, 1976).

Figure 1 : Phenomenological portrait of steroid hormone (H) receptor (R)

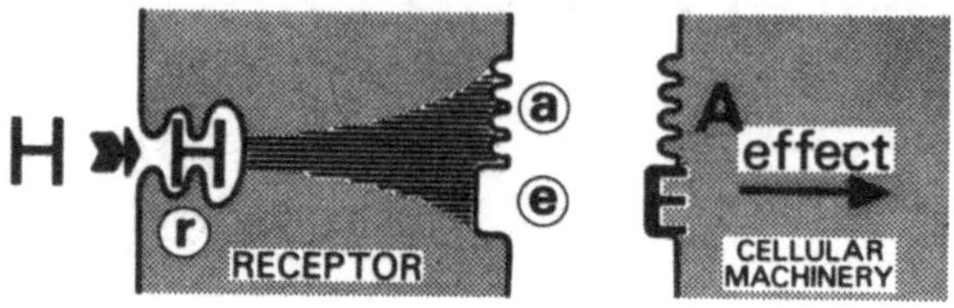

r is the binding site of H, and can stand for receptor , receiving , regulatory . r is hormone specific, binds reversibly and is the last interaction of hormone with the cellular machinery before action is triggered.(This would not be the case if r were the binding site of a transport protein).

The receptor includes a coupling mechanism (transduction) between r and site(s) a and/or e.

The coupling takes place at the level of the effector structure E of the cell machinery. The receptor has a site e (for effect , effector , executive) interacting with E. A is a (another) part of the cellular machinery called Acceptor to which the a site of the receptor can bind. A corresponds operationally to the nuclear positioning of the hormone-receptor complexes. A and E may be either physically distinct or a single entity.

The effect of an antihormone binding to the r site may result in changes in the conformation of the r site, consequently modifying transduction to the a and/or e sites, and thus abolishing hormone effect.

STEROID HORMONE RECEPTORS

Steroid hormone receptors share common properties. They are acidic proteins, containing no sugar or lipid. They are easily denaturated by heat, and in addition, the binding of hormone to the receptor can be prevented or disrupted by SH-blocking agents. Information remains ambiguous about their molecular weight. The only well known calf uterine estradiol receptor has a binding unit of ∿ 70,000 daltons and appears to be a single polypeptide chain (Soulignac et al., 1977 ; Sica & Bresciani, 1979, Secco et al., 1979). The affinity measured at equilibrium for the specific hormone corresponds to a K_d ∿ 0.1-1 nM, and this very high affinity is responsible for the selective recognition of the hormone. Interestingly, steroids of lower biological activity than the natural hormone have lower affinity. Essentially the high affinity of steroid-receptor interaction is dependent upon the dissociation rate of the ligand. The slower the dissociation rate, the higher the affinity. At low temperatures, the dissociation rate of a high affinity steroid from the receptor may be so slow (half-life greater than 1 day) that it is possible to label receptor with radioactive (tritiated) hormone and measure easily the resulting hormone-receptor complexes (Baulieu et al., 1970).

The quantitation of receptor molecules through the number of bound steroid molecules has indicated a limited number of binding sites per target cell, in the order of 10,000+ This level is relatively low. It represents approximately a concentration in the range of 10 nM in the cell and is responsible for difficulties encountered in biochemical studies of receptor proteins.

All target cells of a given steroid do not contain the same number of receptor binding sites. The relationship between receptor concentration and the response to the hormone has not been definitively established, but a variety of physiological, pathological, pharmacological and genetic observations are compatible with the schematic equation :

$$\text{response} = f(H)(R)$$

indicating the dependence of response size to both hormone (H) and receptor (R) concentrations. This equation does not say that besides receptor concentration, there are no other parameters of the hormone response, but it indicates that in most circumstances, more receptor will make the target cell more responsive to hormone. Incidently, no modification of the receptor affinity has yet been involved in receptor regulatory mechanisms.

Subcellular distribution of steroid receptors

The subcellular distribution of steroid receptors has been the subject of many interesting observations. The initially described case of the uterus of immature or castrated rats, indicated that, in absence of steroid, the estradiol receptor is found entirely in the cytosoluble fraction (cytosol) of the tissue. However, following exposure to estradiol, the cytoplasmic receptor concentration decreases while hormone-receptor complexes appear in the nucleus. This is taken as evidence for intracellular translocation of the receptor (Jensen et al., 1968 ; Gorski et al., 1968). In human endometrium, the distribution of the receptor apparently does not follow this clear-cut pattern. Indeed, in no circumstance human endometrium can be obtained in complete absence of circulating estrogen. Consequently, the presence of some nuclear estradiol receptor is always expected. It should also be noted that unoccupied hormone receptor sites have been discovered in the nucleus of various tissues, including normal human endometrium (Levy et al., 1979a). It is not clear at this point whether or not these non occupied sites may have been translocated by a ligand secondarily released, or if they were present in the nucleus in absence of a translocation process*. Indeed, it has been also demonstrated that in absence of hormone, a fraction and eventually the quasi-totality of the estradiol receptor in the young male chicken liver cells is initially located in the nucleus (Mester & Baulieu, 1972). Moreover, experiments with a non steroidal antiestrogen in the chick oviduct (tamoxifen), have demonstrated translocation of cytoplasmic receptor by tamoxifen and subsequent

---

+In published reports, numbers of receptor binding sites differ for at least three sorts of reasons : 1. technical problems ; 2. pathophysiological variations, as described later ; 3. mode of expression, referring to weight (mg) of DNA or of protein from a given fraction. The latter is particularly dependent of the pathophysiological state and of cellular heterogeneity of the tissue sample.

*It should also be realized that in most instances steroid concentrations in human are such that not all sites of both cytoplasmic and nuclear receptors are saturated.

formation of tamoxifen-receptor complexes in the nucleus although there was no estrogenic response (Sutherland et al., 1977). These findings suggest that the presence of nuclear receptor does not necessarily mean triggering of action. Experiments again in the chick oviduct system have indicated that estradiol effect can be immediately stopped by tamoxifen and that conversely the inhibition of estrogen effect by tamoxifen can be rescued by adequate amounts of estradiol (Mester et al., 1977 ; Palmiter et al., 1978). These results suggest that nuclear estradiol receptor sites, free or occupied by a ligand, can be reached by another compound if its affinity for the sites and its concentration are appropriate for an exchange Previous depletion of the cytoplasmic receptor does not seem to preclude access of hormonal ligand to the nucleus and formation of nuclear receptor complexes.

Progesterone receptor is much less studied in this respect. It was discovered in the uterus of castrated guinea pig treated with estradiol (Milgrom et al., 1970), and most of it was found in the cytoplasm. A systematic search for unoccupied nuclear progesterone receptors has not been undertaken in human endometrium. Results reported in Table 1 indicate that nuclear progesterone receptor is found even at the beginning of the normal menstrual cycle, but the technique utilized does not differentiate between free sites or those occupied by hormone.

In conclusion, while the importance of measuring both cytoplasmic and nuclear receptors is being stressed in order to obtain the total concentration of intracellular receptors, the significance of subcellular distribution of the receptor should be interpreted with caution. Although it may be stated that no steroid action occurs in absence of nuclear receptor, it should be also understood that the presence of nuclear receptor does not prove that the receptor is engaged in hormone activity. Consequently, it is misleading to use the word activation as synonymous for translocation, if by activation one implies the idea of action. Along the same line, the word acceptor means only a structure accepting and then binding in the nucleus the translocated cytoplasmic receptor. It should not be used as synonymous of effector site (Baulieu, 1978), because as previously indicated, translocation of the receptor may occur in absence of the triggering of hormone action. Having all these reservations in mind, it remains that physiologically in human endometrium the cytoplasmic to nuclear ratios of receptors vary during the menstrual cycle according to the rather simple principle that active hormone promotes receptor translocation to the nucleus (see Table 1).

ESTRADIOL AND PROGESTERONE RECEPTORS

Estradiol receptor

Estradiol receptor is specific for estrogens. It binds estradiol, the natural hormone, with high affinity ($K_d \sim 0.1$ nM) whereas metabolites of estradiol, namely estrone and estriol, display approximately 2 and 10 times lower affinity, respectively (Baulieu et al., 1967). Synthetic steroidal estrogens like 17α-ethynyl estradiol, 11β-methoxy-17α-ethynyl-estradiol (moxestrol) and a non-steroidal estrogen, diethylstilbestrol, bind to the receptor with an affinity nearly similar to that of estradiol itself. However, the affinity of triphenyl-ethylene antiestrogens is 10-100 times less. Some C19-steroids of the androgen series, mainly 3β,17β-dihydroxy-5α-androstane and 3β,17β-dihydroxy-Δ^5-

Table 1 : Estradiol and progesterone receptors : concentration and subcellular distribution in the endometrium during normal menstrual cycle.

	Estradiol receptor				*Progesterone receptor*			
	Total	*Cytosol*	*Nuclei*	R_c/R_n	*Total*	*Cytosol*	*Nuclei*	R_c/R_n
I	*1.5*	*1.1*	*0.4*	*2.7*	*1.5*	*1.2*	*0.2*	*6.0*
II	*1.9*	*1.0*	*0.9*	*1.1*	*3.0*	*3.0*	*0.5*	*4.8*
III	*1.2*	*0.4*	*0.8*	*0.5*	*1.9*	*0.9*	*1.0*	*0.9*
IV	*0.7*	*0.3*	*0.4*	*0.7*	*0.9*	*0.7*	*0.2*	*3.5*

The results are expressed in pmol per mg DNA. Figures have been obtained from 54 biopsies reported in Bayard et al., 1978. Number of cases : I : 10 ; II : 12 ; III : 10 ; IV : 22.

androstene, have low affinity for the receptor, corresponding to $K_d \sim 0.1\ \mu M$; testosterone and dihydrotestosterone bind even less. Incidently, the question has been raised whether estrogenic or antiestrogenic effects resulted from androgen binding to estradiol receptors. The subject is still being investigated, but present results indicate that at least in the rat uterine system (Rochefort & Garcia, 1976), an estrogenic effect results from the binding of androgens to the estradiol receptor. Corticosteroids and progesterone have no affinity, but several progestagens of the 19-nor series (and their metabolites) used in contraception interact to some extent with the estrogen receptor, contrary to what is observed with C21 compounds.

An interesting question has been raised concerning the biological activity of estrogens in relation to their affinities for the receptor. For instance, estriol is a weaker estrogen than estradiol when tested by a single injection to the laboratory animal. A large dose also impeded to reach the level of response to estradiol (Huggins & Jensen, 1955). This has been explained on the ground of the faster dissociation of estriol from the receptor. It is also accepted that the persistence of the agonist-receptor complexes in the nucleus is a factor determining the importance of the hormonal response (Anderson et al., 1974). In fact, when fractioned doses of estriol were injected, the estrogenic activity obtained was comparable to that of estradiol given in a single injection. Conversely, it should be stressed that a compound can have a high affinity for the receptor (due to slow dissociation rate) without displaying any hormonal activity and consequently be used as a competitive antagonist. This is illustrated by the activities of hydroxytamoxifen recently described in the chick oviduct system (Binart et al., 1979). However, as tamoxifen itself, hydroxytamoxifen in the rat uterus is also a mixed agonist-antagonist. Thus, it can be concluded that the affinity and the dissociation rate of a ligand from the receptor do not indicate directly whether or not the activity will be agonistic or antagonistic.

In addition to the affinity, the general metabolism of a compound is must also be considered. For example, although its affinity for the receptor is relatively low, tamoxifen is a very powerful antiestrogen. This is mainly due to its very prolonged half life because of its slow metabolism (review in Jordan et al., 1978). Therefore it remains at a cellular concentration high enough to compete sucessfully with estrogens.

Progesterone receptor

Progesterone has high affinity for the progesterone receptor with a K_d on the order of 1 nM. However, the complex it forms with the receptor dissociates relatively rapidly and such situation creates a serious difficulty for labeling hormone binding sites in the human endometrium. The rate of dissociation is slower when glycerol is added to the incubation medium, and this is of practical use. Alternatively, synthetic steroids of the 19-norprogesterone series, such as R 5020 (Raynaud, 1977) and ORG 2058 (Isomaa et al., 1979), may be prefered because they have slower dissociation rates from the receptor than progesterone itself. It is rather interesting that the C19-progestagens used in contraception, in which 17β-hydroxy-17α-alkyl chains are substituted for the 17β-(CH_3-CO) chain of progesterone, bind to the receptor equally well. All metabolites of progesterone have less affinity than progesterone; and other hormones, namely estradiol, cortisol and testosterone, have negligible affinity for the progesterone receptor.

STEROID BINDING PLASMA PROTEINS IN HUMAN ENDOMETRIUM

Human endometrial biopsies are necessarily contaminated to some extent by blood. Such a contamination brings into the homogenate and particularly the cytosol fraction, a number of plasma proteins, some of which of high specificity for steroid hormones. Two plasma proteins have been described in this respect.

Cbg or transcortin binds cortisol and progesterone with an affinity (K_d of the order of 1 nM) similar to that of the progesterone receptor. In contrast to Cbg contained in the rat uterus (Milgrom & Baulieu, 1970), the wide variations reported for concentrations of Cbg in human endometrium were found to be unrelated to the phase of menstrual cycle (Kreitmann et al., 1978). The concentration of Cbg binding sites in human endometrium is usually greater than that of progesterone receptor. Consequently, in order to insure specificity of the progesterone receptor binding site measurements, one may use a synthetic ligand such as R 5020 which has high specificity for progesterone receptor and minimal binding to Cbg. However, it has been demonstrated that R 5020 has also some affinity for the glucocorticosteroid receptor also present in human endometrium. Therefore, to obliterate non-specific binding, the addition of an excess of cortisol is always recommanded in assays using radioactive R 5020 or progesterone to determine progesterone receptor concentrations in human endometrium. Another method which distinguishes between progesterone receptor and Cbg binding is the use of SH-group blocker which inhibits only the binding to the receptor.

The other protein is sex steroid binding plasma protein (Sbp) (Mercier-Bodard et al., 1970) (also called testosterone-estradiol binding globulin, Tebg, or sex hormone binding globulin, Shbg). It binds testosterone, dihydrotestosterone and 5α-androstanediols with a K_d of the order 0.1 nM and estradiol with a lower affinity but still K_d in the range of 1 nM. The concentration of Sbp in the plasma is 1/10 that of Cbg and the binding of estradiol to Sbp in cytosol preparations can be generally considered as negligible. However, when particular precautions are to be taken, it is suggested either to use moxestrol which does not bind to Sbp or to load the system with a concentration of 0.1 µM dihydrotestosterone which will block Sbp but not receptor binding of estradiol. The use of diethylstilbestrol is not advisable because although it does not bind Sbp, radioactive diethylstilbestrol is unstable; and in addition it binds heavily to numerous non-specific proteins.

Actually in working with endometrial extracts, the binding to other non-specific proteins of plasmatic and tissular origin also poses a problem for all steroids (see practical implications later).

METHODOLOGY FOR MEASURING STEROID RECEPTORS

It should be realized that the labelling of receptors with radioactive ligand represents the only way receptors can be measured at the present time. Therefore, the specificity of this labelling should be strictly insured. Undoubtedly, progress will be made when antibodies to the receptor will become available enabling the assay of receptor protein itself. The problem related to the elimination of binding due to plasma proteins has already been discussed and in addition all non-specific low affinity and abundant sites should be taken into account. Practically, in most instances, the isotopic dilution method has to be used. A double measurement is performed at each point-one with the radioactive tracer (total binding) and the other with the same radioactive hormone at the same concentration plus an additional excess (usually 100 times) of the same radioinert compound (non-specific binding). Specific binding is then obtained by subtracting the non-specific from the total binding. For current endometrial studies, due to the limited amount of material, a single point determination at saturating concentration of radioactive ligand is performed with the appropriate isotopic dilution. When systematic studies are to be conducted, Scatchard plots are preferably constructed following measurements of specific binding at various concentrations of isotopic ligands (Soutter et al., 1979). From the curve obtained, the concentration of specific sites may be obtained and an apparent value for K_d determined.

Several problems are encountered in the use of radioactive hormones. 1. One of them addresses the metabolism of the radioactive ligand and/or its non radioactive counterpart. This represents an important consideration because if, under the experimental conditions, the radioactive ligand is metabolized into products of different affinities, the results will be usually underestimated. 2. The possible presence of endogenous ligands in the endometrial extract is to be considered in terms of labelling technique. Particularly in the case of progesterone during the secretory phase of the menstrual cycle or during pregnancy, the radioactive tracer may be diluted several times leading to an underestimation of the number of the binding sites in the case of single point saturation or to an apparent decrease of the affinity when Scatchard plot is performed. 3. Endogenous hormones present in endometrial extracts may occupy partly the receptor binding sites. Particularly in the case of estradiol where the dissociation rate from the receptor is slow, the radioactive ligand cannot readily occupy the binding sites. To get all the binding sites occupied by radioactive hormone, the so-called exchange technique must be performed. It consists of an exchange of the non-radioactive ligand initially bound to the receptor with the radioactive hormone introduced experimentally. This is usually accomplished by incubating the biological extract with the radioactive hormone at appropriate temperature and for a short time (0°C 3 h for progesterone, and 30°C 3 h for estradiol in our method (Bayard et al., 1978)). In this fashion, there will be dissociation of the non radioactive ligand from the sites mixing with the incubated radioactive steroid which is in large excess, providing an opportunity for the radioactive ligand to bind secondarily and to label the sites. Such a maneuver is critical because partial degradation or inactivation of the receptor is a possibility. Therefore, quantitative controls have to be established very carefully: 4. Finally, the method for measuring the bound radioactive steroid to the receptor after incubation has to be also controlled. The procedure mostly used is the so-called charcoal-dextran technique which adsorbs the unbound ligand. However, as indicated previously (Milgrom & Baulieu, 1969), the time of exposure to the adsorbant is very critical and should be carefully chosen in order to keep at minimum the dissociation of the ligand-receptor complexes and to eliminate the maximum of non-specifically bound ligand. From the precedent discussion on subcellular distribution of receptor, it is not surprizing that we suggest to measure systematically total receptors in both the cytosol and the nuclear fractions of the homogenates. To obtain the cytosol fractions, homogenate is first recentrifuged at 105,000 x g for 60 min. This high speed supernatant is called cytosol (also cytoplasmic : for a discussion see Baulieu et al., 1975). The crude nuclear fraction obtained from the low speed centrifugation is properly washed, incubated with the appropriate hormone(s) and secondarily treated with Triton containing buffer in order to eliminate most non-specific binding. As previously discussed, if theoretically all nuclear receptors should be in the form of hormone-receptor complexes, there are in fact and very often free receptor sites present in the nuclei. For estradiol, studies have indicated that free sites can be distinguished from occupied sites by labelling at low temperatures (0-4°C). The free sites will be readily occupied by the radioactive tracer, whereas the occupied sites should be exchanged. In the assay methods leading to the results presented in the next sections (Bayard et al., 1978), we have only considered total binding sites (free + occupied), using a technique including an exchange step.

HORMONAL REGULATION

For pathophysiological, endocrine-regulated phenomena, a fundamental question is raised as to whether or not, the number of receptor units per target cell can vary. In fact, receptor concentration in target cells changes with hormonal levels. The basic features of such an important regulatory mechanism has been first observed in studying precisely estradiol and progesterone receptors in the uteri of the laboratory animals. Such findings add a new dimension to Endocrinology, which up to now essentially was considering the changes in hormone levels.

Briefly, the classically described priming of progesterone action by estradiol in the uterus correlates with the increase of progesterone receptor by estradiol (Milgrom et al., 1970), the first well established regulatory mechanism concerning the hormonal control of receptor concentration. Actually, the situation is rather complex because other experiments have also indicated that estradiol increases the synthesis of its own receptor (Jensen & De Sombre, 1972) and that progesterone seems to inactivate its own receptor (Milgrom et al., 1973). This latter finding provides a remarkable example of negative regulation of binding site availability by its own hormone. In addition, progesterone antagonizes the estrogen induced increase of the estradiol receptor (Mester et al., 1974 ; Hsueh et al., 1975 ; Tseng & Gurpide, 1975), and there is a positive effect of progesterone on estradiol receptor concentration f.i. in the castrated rat endometrium (Mester et al., 1974). Besides these complex changes in receptor concentrations, the homologous hormone causes, as previously indicated, a change of receptor cellular distribution between cytosol and the nucleus. Essentially in presence of the hormone, the ratio of cytoplasmic to nuclear receptors (R_c/R_n) decreases.

Results presented in the next paragraph concerning the changes of receptor observed during the normal menstrual cycle in human endometrium are essentially in agreement with these laboratory animal observations, and correlate well with hormonal steroid levels.

NORMAL MENSTRUAL CYCLES

The cycle can be divided into 4 periods defined in relation to the day of ovulation, indicated as day 0. They are :
I. Early proliferative phase, days - 7 and - 6 (8 patients) ;
II. Late proliferative phase, days - 4 to 0 (21 patients) ;
III. Early secretory phase, days + 1 to + 6 (16 patients) ;
IV. Late secretory phase, days + 7 to + 12 (56 patients). No biopsies were available for day - 5.

The sum of receptors sites measured in the cytosol and nuclear fractions represents total cellular receptor sites (free and occupied by endogenous hormones). Since the precision of dating was $\pm$ 1 day, the values for total estradiol or progesterone receptors for each day of the cycle were pooled with those of the adjacent days (Fig. 2). The mean values of plasma estradiol and progesterone are given for comparison.

Estradiol receptor

During the early proliferative phase, the concentration of total estradiol receptor sites is about 1.5 pmol/mg DNA, with a tendency to increase in the late proliferative phase to $\sim$ 2.0 pmol/mg DNA. Analysis of this preovulatory increase by examining the cytoplasmic and nuclear receptors separately shows that the concentration of cytoplasmic receptor sites does not change, whereas the nuclear receptor sites more than doubles (0.4 to 0.9 pmol/mg DNA) (Table 1). Thus the ratio R_c/R_n decreases. Both increase of total estradiol receptor and decrease of R_c/R_n are expected when estradiol increases in the blood.

After ovulation, a rapid and large decrease in total estradiol receptor to 1.2 pmol/mg DNA occurs early in the secretory phase, followed by a greater diminution in the late secretory phase, resulting in a concentration (0.7 pmol/mg DNA) well below that at the beginning of the cycle. Analysis of these decreases shows that the cytoplasmic receptor sites decrease very early in the secretory phase while nuclear receptor sites decrease later. In summary, the most striking change during the proliferative phase involves the nuclear receptor, while the most significant modification in the post-ovulatory period is that of the cytoplasmic receptor.

Figure 2 : Estradiol and progesterone receptors in endometrial cells during the normal menstrual cycle.

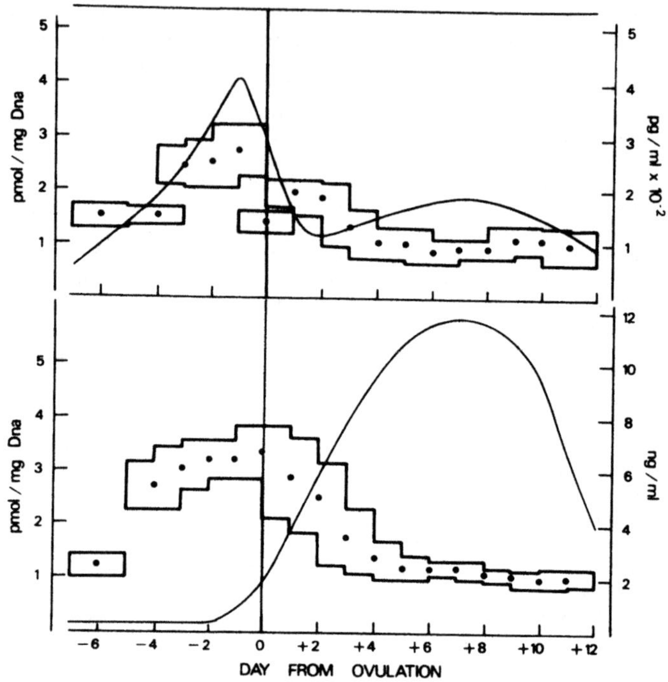

The concentrations of estradiol receptor (upper panel), and of total progesterone receptor (lower panel) for each day of the cycle were pooled with those of the adjacent days. Each point represents the mean of pooled values obtained from 101 biopsies (see Levy et al., 1979b). It is surrounded by a rectangle with its abscissa extending from the preceding to the following day to account for the imprecision of dating and with its ordinate equal to twice the standard error of the mean. When rectangles overlap, only the external contour is drawn. No biopsies were available for day -5. The curves represent the mean values of plasma estradiol and progesterone taken from Frolich et al. (1976).

Progesterone receptor

In the early proliferative phase, the cellular concentration of progesterone receptor (1.5 pmol/mg DNA) is slightly lower than that of estradiol receptor. However the preovulatory rise is very large and reaches about 3.0 pmol/mg DNA. This increase is mainly due to the large rise in cytoplasmic receptor with some elevation in nuclear receptor concentration (0.2 to 0.4 pmol/mg DNA), but no change occurs in the cytoplasmic/nuclear ratio. These results are expected from endometrium under estrogen stimulation and virtual lack of exposure to progesterone.

During the secretory phase until day + 4, total progesterone receptor concentration decreases gradually reaching a concentration similar to or even lower than that of early proliferative phase. After ovulation, there is an immediate and large decrease in cytoplasmic sites (2.4 to 0.9 pmol/mg DNA), whereas the concentration of nuclear receptor is at its highest (∿ 1 pmol/mg DNA). These results correlate well with the luteal progesterone output and designate the nuclear progesterone receptor as a important component of the physiological changes undergone by the endometrium during the luteal phase in preparation for implantation. In the late secretory phase, nuclear receptor concentration decreases to values similar to those found in proliferative phase.

Correlation of estradiol and progesterone receptors with circulating hormones and with endometrial 17β-hydroxysteroid oxidoreductase activity

The high concentrations of estradiol and progesterone receptors in the late proliferative phase correlate with the plasma estradiol surge. Indeed in 13 cases where the endometrium was in proliferative phase and plasma estradiol was measured, a significant positive correlation was observed between total progesterone receptor and circulating estradiol ($p < .01$) Fig. 3), and between total estradiol receptor and circulating estradiol ($p \sim .05$). No correlation between receptor and either circulating estradiol and progesterone was found in secretory endometrium, in part probably because of the opposing effects of the 2 hormones. Although statistical analysis cannot validly be performed on the R_c/R_n ratios, it can be observed that their changes follow rather closely the hormonal plasma levels. An additional significant finding was a negative correlation ($p = .05$) between cytoplasmic progesterone receptor and 17β-hydroxysteroid oxidoreductase activity in the microsomal pellets.

Figure 3 : Correlation of total progesterone receptor and estradiol during the proliferative phase of normal menstrual cycle.

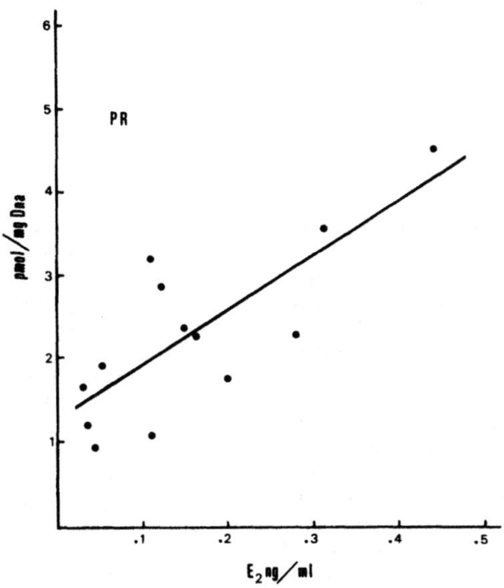

PR ($y = 6.61x + 1.283$; $r = .775$; $p < .01$).

This enzyme catalyzes the conversion of estradiol into estrone, and its increase under progesterone and progestagen stimulation may account partly for the antiestrogenic activity of these hormones (Tseng et al., 1977).

ANOVULATORY CYCLES

All cases were considered as a single group, independently of age, etiology, duration, frequency or regularity of menses. The concentration of estradiol in plasma (103 ± 68 pg/ml, mean ± sd, n = 10), was slightly lower than that recorded in late proliferative phase of normal menstrual cycle (145 ± 117 pg/ml, n = 10). Nevertheless, high concentrations of estradiol and progesterone receptors were generally found, similar to those of late proliferative phase. The cytoplasmic/nuclear ratio of the estradiol receptor was smaller than in normal pre-ovulatory phase. On the contrary, the concentration of nuclear progesterone receptor was significantly lower than in preovulatory endometrium. One should recall that these patients have undetectable plasma progesterone, in contrast to the small but significant increase in plasma progesterone which occurs just before ovulation.

LUTEAL INSUFFICIENCY

This is a rather heterogeneous group of patients, diagnosed on the basis of histological abnormalities (sparse glandular tubes, low glycogenic charge, lack of intraluminal secretion, small number of convoluted arteries), decreased mean concentrations of plasma progesterone and estradiol, and in some cases short luteal phases. A detailed clinical description is reported elsewhere (Levy et al., 1979b).

The receptor concentrations are quite different from those found for anovulatory cycles. The concentration of estradiol receptor, in particular of nuclear receptor, is even lower than in late secretory phase. The level of progesterone receptor is also relatively low and similar to that found in late secretory phase.

EARLY PREGNANCY

Abortion was performed by aspiration at 8 to 10 weeks of gestation. Endometrium was then removed by curettage, and careful histological examination was performed. Only samples which contained more than 90 % intact gestational endometrium were used for receptor measurements. Most of the biopsies weighed only 25 to 60 mg (fresh weight), and therefore only the progesterone receptor was systematically measured in both cytoplasm and nuclei. Cytoplasmic progesterone receptor was barely detectable (0.10 ± 0.15 pmol/mg DNA, mean ± sem), whereas nuclei contained a high concentration of progesterone receptor (3.9 ± 0.6 pmol/mg DNA, mean ± sem), which is significantly above the concentration of not only nuclear, but also total progesterone receptor in preovulatory endometrium. Correlation with the very low ornithine decarboxylase activity (see next paragraph and table 3) remains to be established.

In the four cases where estradiol receptor could be measured, it was also barely detectable in cytoplasm and present in nuclei at concentrations similar to those found in early secretory phase.

Table 2 : Estradiol and progesterone receptors : concentration in normal and malignant endometrium.

Normal cycle periods	Number of cases	Estradiol receptor	Progesterone receptor
II	21	2.2	3.1
IV	56	0.9	1.1
Carcinoma grades			
G 1	21	2.3	2.2
G 2	13	0.8	0.7
G 3	3	2.5	0.9

The results are expressed in pmol/mg DNA. Details will be found in Mortel et al. (in preparation).

ENDOMETRIAL CARCINOMA

Receptors were measured in post menopausal women with endometrial carcinoma. Nearly all tumors contained variable but often large amounts of total estradiol receptor (mean ∿ 1.8 pmol/mg DNA), comparable to those observed in late proliferative phase of the cycle. Total progesterone receptor concentration (mean ∿ 1.5 pmol/mg DNA) was in the range of late secretory phase and considered undetectable or insignificant (< 0.3 pmol/mg DNA) in 10 cases of a series of 43 patients. Although higher levels of receptors were found in well differentiated cancers, no significant correlation was found between receptor concentrations and histologic grading (Table 2). Both receptors concentrated mostly in the cytoplasm, but in 11 cases for estradiol and 5 for progesterone, the totality or majority of receptors was located in the nuclei. From this generally high estradiol receptor concentration and low progesterone receptor concentration, it appears that endometrial carcinoma are particularly susceptible to the influence of estrogens. However, prediction of hormone responsiveness by receptor measurement alone is unlikely. In 15 patients, estradiol and progesterone receptor concentrations were measured before and after an antiestrogen (tamoxifen) to evaluate hormone responsiveness of the tumors. Forty mg daily x 5-7 days of tamoxifen were given. The progesterone receptor increased significantly ($p < 0.05$). This "estrogenic" response of the antiestrogen contrasted with the lack of change in ornithine decarboxylase activity (table 3). This latter enzymatic activity is associated with growth, and an increase would have been expected in case of full estrogenic stimulation (Robel et al., 1978, Mortel et al., in preparation). On the other hand, progestagens (used in the treatment of advanced or metastatic endometrial carcinoma) decrease the progesterone receptor (Tseng et al., 1977). Therefore with this in vivo challenge test, it is possible to delineate cases in which tamoxifen may rescue the progesterone receptor and constitute an important component of the treatment to restore possible sensitivity to progestins. These results indicate the potentiality of in vivo pharmacology based on the measurement of receptors.

Table 3 : Ornithine decarboxylase activity in normal and malignant endometrium.

	Early pregnancy	Normal Endometrium II	Normal Endometrium IV	Hyperplasia	Cancer	Cancer + tamoxifen Controls	Cancer + tamoxifen After
Number of cases	6	4	2	1	22	4	
Arbitrary units	1	10	8	23	62	30	24

The results are reported here in arbitrary units of activity. Details will be found in Mortel et al. The tamoxifen test is described in the text.

CONCLUSIONS AND AREAS OF FUTURE RESEARCH

The results reported here indicate that a cycle of estradiol and progesterone receptors is indeed involved in the normal menstrual cycle and probably in the determination of the implantation time of the fertilized ovum. They also confirm the findings obtained with laboratory animals dealing with the hormonal control of the subcellular distribution and of the concentration of both receptors by circulating hormones. It is important to note that, besides obvious differences of reproductive physiology in mammals, the regulatory controls of steroid receptors follow essentially the same basic rules at the cellular level. Indeed, several medical aspects of sex hormone regulatory mechanisms may even be studied profitably in avian species (i.e. chick). The problem of model systems to study in a meaningful fashion hormones, drugs and other contraceptive means should take these considerations into account. This is not to deny the search for animal systems directly useful for the human needs. However, we propose that well-planned and detailed studies in the rat, the chick or even in tissue culture, may be more helpful than experiments in a limited number of higher apes for designing actual therapeutic agent. Conversely it remains that one should have in mind specific species differences : for instance implantation in baboons and humans differs histologically, and it is not easy to study the closest to human chimpanzee. Therefore, the strategy proposed considers the establishment of basic principles in the usual laboratory systems, and when they are well understood, their transfer under appropriate precautions to the human. This is obviously necessary in order to work out the pharmacological problems (doses, timing, etc...).

In vitro binding studies with steroid receptors can be and are used efficiently to design new molecules having hormonal/antihormonal properties. This is of great help for chemists, and the availability of purified receptors will make these studies even more profitable. Paradoxically, the most important information may turned out to be a negative one. The lack of binding indicates that a compound will not display agonistic or antagonistic activity related to the studied receptor (even it could naturally interfere more or less specifically with other part of the cellular machinery). Two points of caution : 1. One cannot predict from binding parameters whether the steroid will have agonistic or antagonistic activities. 2. Whereas all estradiol receptors look very similar in mammals and even in avians as far as binding properties and even antigeneicity (Greene et al., 1977 ; Radanyi et al., 1979), it is not the case for progesterone receptor since significant differences have been observed between different mammals (Kontula et al., 1975) and human vs chick (Smith et al., 1974).

Can we consider the development of new methods of fertility control based on interference with physiological properties and cyclic variations of the receptor, particularly the progesterone receptor ?

It is conceivable that the administration of progesterone at mid cycle, when endogenous progesterone level is increasing but still low, would lead to set a premature negative effect on progesterone receptor concentration and render abnormal the secretory transformation phase of the endometrium (Baulieu, 1975). It is known that implantation occur even in guinea pigs castrated 3 days after ovulation (implantation takes normally place on the 7th day) (Deanesly, 1960). It is also possible that the use of an antiestrogen would prevent the synthesis of cytoplasmic progesterone receptor during the late proliferative phase of the cycle and therefore inhibit the development of an endometrium favorable to implantation. Moreover, it appears that the use of a specific antiprogestin at any time between the end of the proliferative phase and early weeks of pregnancy would be of some contraceptive interest by occupying the progesterone receptor site without progestational effect and side effects.

Knowledge is lacking about the relationship among female hormone receptor concentration, subcellular distribution and bleeding from the endometrium occurring during the normal cycle in absence of treatment or under the various contraceptive methods presently used. Measuring receptor gives an information which may help to predict what could occur in the following days. Therefore, it would be of great importance to systematically undertake measurements of steroid receptors in order to explore the implications of contraceptive preparations and mechanical devices on their hormonally regulated equilibrium in the endometrium.

As far as endometrial pathology is concerned, the receptor pattern found in carcinomas favours a systematic search for elevated estradiol receptor concentration and/or estradiol receptor/progesterone receptor ratio in perimenopausal and menopausal women at risk of cancer. Further work may help to detect women who may benefit from progestin or antiestrogen administration, and those who should not be exposed to estrogen alone. The high risk of endometrial hyperplasia and adenocarcinoma in anovulatory cycles (Gusberg, 1976) may prove to be related to unopposed prolonged estradiol secretion, which in turn creates sustained high concentrations of nuclear receptor-estradiol complexes and thus a state of estrogen hyper-receptivity. The observation of low receptor concentrations in luteal insufficiency was unexpected, since low plasma progesterone might have allowed higher concentrations of receptors. Therefore it is likely that estradiol insufficiency, starting at the preovulatory period, is a constitutive feature of most of these cases. The relatively low level of progesterone receptors may also be related to the low level of estradiol (Gautray et al., 1978) and of estradiol-receptor complexes. Finally, measurements of receptors, if necessary before and after administration of a drug challenging their concentration (for instance progestin or antiestrogen), may, in correlation to the blood hormonal levels, be helpful for a better understanding of cases of amenorrhea, bleeding, infertility, etc...

Receptor determinations may, in the eighties, become an important tool for better medical care, as the histological examination of endometrial biopsies and the radioimmunoassays of hormones in the blood are recognized as useful indicators by the gynaecologists in the precedent decades.

REFERENCES

Anderson, J.N., Peck, Jr. E.J. and Clark, J.H. (1974) Nuclear receptor estradiol complex : a requirement for uterotrophic responses. Endocrinology 95, 174-178.

Baulieu, E.E., Alberga, A. and Jung, I. (1967) Récepteurs hormonaux. Liaison spécifique de l'oestradiol à des protéines utérines. C.R. Acad. Sci. Paris 265, 354-357.
Récepteurs hormonaux. Liaison de divers oestrogènes à des protéines utérines. Une méthode de dosage de l'oestradiol. C.R. Acad. Sci. Paris 265, 501-504.

Baulieu, E.E., Raynaud, J.P. and Milgrom, E. (1970) Measurement of steroid binding proteins. Acta Endocrinol. 64, suppl. 147, 104-121.

Baulieu, E.E. (1975) Antiprogesterone effect and midcycle (periovulatory) contraception. Eur. J. Obst. Gynecol. Reprod. Biol. 4, 161-166.

Baulieu, E.E., Atger, M., Best-Belpomme, M., Corvol, P., Courvalin, J.C., Mester, J., Milgrom, E., Robel, P., Rochefort, H. and De Catalogne, D. (1975) Steroid hormone receptors. Vitamins and Hormones 33, 649-731.

Baulieu, E.E. (1978) Current approaches to steroid hormone-cell interactions. In "Central Regulation of the Endocrine System" (K. Juxe, T. Hökfelt and R. Luft, eds.), pp. 239-260, Plenum Publishing Corporation, New York.

Bayard, F., Damilano, S., Robel, P. and Baulieu, E.E. (1978) Cytoplasmic and nuclear estradiol and progesterone receptors in human endometrium. J. Clin. Endocrinol. Metab. 46, 635-648.

Binart, N., Catelli, M.G., Geynet, C., Puri, V., Hähnel, R., Mester, J. and Baulieu, E.E. (1979) Monohydroxytamoxifen : an antioestrogen with high affinity for the chick oviduct oestrogen receptor. Biochem. Biophys. Res. Commun. (in press).

Deanesly, R. (1960) Implantation and early pregnancy in ovariectomized guinea-pig. J. Reprod. Fertil. 1, 242-248.

Diczfalusy, E., ed. (1970) Steroid assay by protein binding. Acta Endocrinol. suppl. 147.

Frölich, M., Brand, E.C. and van Hall, E.V. (1976) Serum levels of unconjugated aetiocholanolone, androstenedione, testosterone, dehydroepiandrosterone, aldosterone, progesterone and oestrogens during the normal menstrual cycle. Acat Endocrinol. 81, 548-562.

Gautray, J.P., De Brux, J., Azadian-Boulanger, G., Jolivet, A., Colin, M.C. and Margenet-Baudry, M. (1978) Hormonal and endometrial aspects of the human menstrual cycle at the time of implantation. In "L'implantation de l'oeuf" (F. Mesnil du Buisson, A. Psychoyos and K. Thomas, eds.) Masson, Paris, p. 35.

Gorski, J., Toft, D.O., Shyamala, G., Smith, D. and Notides, A. (1968) Hormone receptors : studies on the interaction of estrogen with the uterus. Rec. Progr. Hormone Res. 24, 45-72.

Gorski, J. and Gannon, F. (1976) Current models of steroid hormone action : a critique. Ann. Rev. Physiol. 38, 425-450.

Greene, G.L., Closs, L.E., Fleming, H., De Sombre, E.R. and Jensen, E.V. (1977) Antibodies to estrogen receptor : immunochemical similarity of estrophilin various mammalian species. Proc. Natl. Acad. Sci. USA 74, 3681-3685.

Gusberg, S.B. (1976) The individual at high risk for endometrial carcinoma. Am. J. Obstet. Gynecol. 126, 535-542.

Hsueh, A.J.W., Peck, E.J. and Clark, J.H. (1975) Progesterone antagonism of the oestrogen receptor and oestrogen-induced uterine growth. Nature 254, 337-339.

Huggins, C. and Jensen, E.V. (1955) The depression of estrone-induced uterine growth by phenolic estrogens with oxygenated functions at positions 6 or 16. The impeded estrogens. J. Expr. Med. 102, 335-346.

Isomaa, V., Tostalo, H. and Jänne, O. (1979) Regulation of cytosol and nuclear progesterone receptors in rabbit uterus by estrogen, antiestrogen and progesterone administration. Biochim. Biophys. Acta 585, 24-33.

Jensen, E.V. and Jacobson, H.I. (1962) Basic guides to the mechanism of estrogen action. Rec. Progr. Hormone Res. 18, 387-314.

Jensen, E.V., Suzuki, T., Kawashima, T., Stumpf, W.E., Jungblut, P.W. and De Sombre, E.R. (1968) A two-step mechanism for the interaction of oestradiol with the rat uterus. Proc. Natl. Acad. Sci. USA 59, 632-638.

Jensen, E.V. and De Sombre, E.R. (1972) Mechanism of action of the female sex hormones. Ann. Rev. Biochem. 41, 203-230.

Jordan, V.C., Dix, C.J., Naylor, K.E., Prestwich, G. and Rowsby, L. (1978) Non steroidal antiestrogens : their biological effects and potential mechanisms of action. J. Toxicol. Environ. Health 4, 363-390.

Kontula, K., Jänne, O., Vihko, R., De Jaer, E., De visser, J. and Zeelen, F. (1975) Progesterone-binding proteins : in vitro binding and biological activity of different steroidal ligands. Acta Endocrinol. 78, 574-592.

Kreitmann, B., Derache, B. and Bayard, F. (1978) Measurement of the corticosteroid binding globulin, progesterone and progesterone "receptor" content in human endometrium. J. Clin. Endocrinol. Metab. 47, 350-353.

Levy, C., Mortel, R., Eychenne, B., Robel, P. and Baulieu, E.E. (1979a) Unoccupied nuclear oestradiol-receptor sites in normal human endometrium. Biochem. J. in press.

Levy, C., Robel, P., Gautray, J.P., de Brux, J., Verma, U., Descomps, B. and Baulieu, E.E. (1979b) Estradiol and progesterone receptors in human endometrium. Normal and abnormal menstrual cycles and early pregnancy. Am. J. Obstet. Gynecol. in press.

Mercier-Bodard, C., Alfsen, A. and Baulieu, E.E. (1970) Sex steroid binding plasma protein (SBP) Acta Endocrinol. 64, suppl. 147, 204-224.

Mester, J. and Baulieu, E.E. (1972) Nuclear estrogen receptor of chick liver. Biochim. Biophys. Acta 261, 236-244.

Mester, J., Martel, D., Psychoyos, A. and Baulieu, E.E. (1974) Hormonal control of oestrogen receptor in uterus and receptivity for ovoimplantation in the rat. Nature 250, 776-778.

Mester, J., Geynet, C., Binart, N. and Baulieu, E.E. (1977) Retarded administration of an antagonist stops steroid hormone action. Biochem. Biophys. Res. Commun. 79, 112-118.

Milgrom, E. and Baulieu, E.E. (1969) A method for studying binding proteins, based upon differential dissociation and small ligand. Biochim. Biophys. Acta 194, 602-605.

Milgrom, E., and Baulieu, E.E. (1970) Progesterone in uterus and plasma. I. Binding in rat uterus 105,000 g supernatant. Endocrinology 87, 276-287.

Milgrom, E., Atger, M. and Baulieu, E.E. (1970) Progesterone in uterus and plasma. IV. Progesterone receptor(s) in guinea pig uterus cytosol. Steroids 16, 741-754.
Milgrom, E., Luu Thi, M., Atger, M. and Baulieu, E.E. (1973) Mechanisms regulating the concentration and the conformation of progesterone receptor(s) in the uterus. J. Biol. Chem. 248, 6366-6474.
Mortel, R., Lévy, C., Wolff, J.P., Nicolas, J.C., Robel, P. and Baulieu, E.E. Female sex steroids and post-menopausal endometrial carcinoma. II. Assessment of hormone responsiveness by the use of an antiestrogen, in preparation.
Palmiter, R.D., Mulvihill, E.R., Mac Knight, G.S. and Senear, A.W. (1978) Regulation of gene expression in the chick oviduct by steroid hormones. Cold Spring Harbor Symposia on Quantitative Biology : Symposium on Chromatin 1977, vol. 42, pp. 639-647.
Radanyi, C., Redeuilh, G., Eigenmann, E., Lebeau, M.C., Massol, N. Secco, C., Baulieu, E.E. and Richard-Foy, H. (1979) Production et détection d'anticorps antirécepteur de l'oestradiol d'utérus de veau. Interaction avec le récepteur d'oviducte de poule. C.R. Acad. Sci. Paris 288, 255-258.
Raynaud, J.P. (1977) R 5020 a tag for the progestin receptor. In "Progesterone receptors in normal and neoplastic tissues" (W.L. Mac Guire, J.P. Raynaud and E.E. Baulieu, Eds.) Progress in Cancer Research and Therapy, vol. 4, pp. 9-21, Raven Press, New York.
Robel, P., Levy, C., Wolff, J.P., Nicolas, J.C. and Baulieu, E.E. (1978) Réponse à un anti-oestrogène comme critère d'hormonosensibilité du cancer de l'endomètre. C.R. Acad. Sci. Paris 287 1353-1356.
Rochefort, H. and Garcia, M. (1976) Androgens on the estrogen receptor. I. Binding and in vivo nuclear translocation. Steroids 28, 549-560.
Secco, C., Redeuilh, G., Radanyi, C., Baulieu, E.E. and Richard-Foy, H. (1979) Purification en deux étapes du récepteur cytosoluble de l'oestradiol d'utérus de veau. C.R. Acad. Sci. Paris, in press.
Sica, F. and Bresciani, F. (1979) Estrogen-binding proteins of calf uterus. Purification to homogeneity of receptor from cytosol by affinity chromatography. Biochemistry 18, 2369-2378.
Smith, H.E., Smith, R.G., Toft, D.O., Neergaard, J.R., Burrows, E.P. and O'Malley, B.W. (1974) Binding of steroids to progesterone receptor in chick oviduct and human uterus. J. Biol. Chem. 249, 5924-5932.
Soulignac, O., Secco-Millet, C., Rocher, P., Baulieu, E.E. and Richard-Foy, H. (1977) Filtration of calf uterine cytosol on Ultrogel AcA 34 prevents aggregation of the estradiol receptor. Febs Letters 74, 129-134.
Soutter, W.P., Hamilton, K. and Leake, R.E. (1979) High affinity binding of oestradiol-17β in the nuclei of human endometrial cells. J. Ster. Biochem. 10, 529-534.
Sutherland, R., Mester, J. and Baulieu, E.E. (1977) Tamoxifen is a potent "pure" anti-oestrogen in chick oviduct. Nature 267, 434-435.
Tseng, L. and Gurpide, E. (1975) Effect of progestins on estradiol receptor in levels in human endometrium. J. Clin. Endocrinol. Metab. 41, 402-404.
Tseng, L., Gusberg, S.B. and Gurpide, E. (1977) Estradiol receptor and 17β-dehydrogenase in normal and abnormal human endometrium. Ann. N.Y. Acad. Sci. 286, 190-198.
Toft, D., Shyamala, G. and Gorski, J. (1967) A receptor molecule for estrogens : studies using a cell free system. Proc. Natl. Acad. Sci. USA 57, 1740-1743.
Yalow, R.S. (1978) Radioimmunoassay : a probe for the fine structure of biologic systems. Science 200, 1236-1245.

DISCUSSION

LOBL: I was interested in the fact you found there were 4,000 nuclear sites for the estrogen receptor. Do you think that there are 4,000 different genes activated, proteins initiated or other events? What are all those sites doing in the nucleus? Is it correct to think that one nuclear receptor initiates one activity?

BAULIEU: No one can properly answer that question today. The molecular biology of steroid hormone action in the nucleus is not yet understood. I can give you a few personal views. For instance, I do not think that the control of transcription in mammalian tissue occurs as it does in bacteria, i.e. by interaction of the regulatory protein (receptor) with a well-defined site situated at the 5'-end extremity of the gene coding for the regulated protein. Coordination of the expression of a domain influenced by a given hormone-receptor complex may be due to an effect upon a sector of the chromatin made available by interaction with this hormone-receptor complex. It does not follow that the interaction of the hormone-receptor complex has to take place with a unique specific DNA sequence. That the receptor binds to a protein component of the chromatin or even that the receptor is an enzyme has not been disproven. The number of 10^3-10^4 sites does not necessarily mean there are 10^3 or 10^4 interactions, but I believe that more receptor molecules will provoke a more intense response whatever the detailed mechanism of action for reasons related to the law of mass action.

GERSCHENSON: I remember three or four years ago I talked with Dr. Robel in your institute when you were starting your clinical studies using specimens from patients with endometrial cancer. We discussed whether or not the pieces of endometrium that one gets from human specimens are representative. We who spend a small part of our time looking at histological sections know that sometimes we get 90% stroma and 10% tumor, and sometimes we get 90% tumor and 10% stroma. In many cases of endometrial cancer there is a lot of histiocytic infiltration. When you mentioned quantitative studies of receptors, how do you know the cell population of specimens that you analyze are homogeneous without doing a careful histological sampling. This is, in a way, a classical question for this kind of study.

BAULIEU: Naturally I know the remarkable heterogeneity of the tumors and biopsies we are dealing with. It is extraordinarily remarkable, in my opinion, that in samples from normal and diseased endometrium we can see some definitive trend and even some highly significant statistical correlations. We cannot explain such a remarkable result. In spite of the problem you cite, I feel that many different cell types in a given tissue or tumor could share a similar receptor content. Naturally this is only one possibility; we may have data soon to prove or disprove this hypothesis. We plan to do quantitative histo-immunological studies with antibodies against the receptor.

GERESCHENSON: Do you have histological controls for the specimens in which you measure the receptor?

BAULIEU: Certainly we have histological controls. Again I do not want to underestimate the problem, but I have also been impressed recently by receptor measurements in separate nodules of cutaneous metastases of breast cancer; results in two different nodules are very similar in most cases.

BARKER: I'd like to ask you one question that relates to some experiments we've done. In an in vitro organ culture system using rat uterus, we can induce glucose-6-phosphate dehydrogenase by estradiol. During a study of steroid specificity, we added some tamoxifen at concentrations of 2×10^{-6}M and 2×10^{-8}M. At the highest dose of tamoxifen, we saw no response, but the lower dose of tamoxifen was a good inducer of this enzyme. I wonder if you have tried a number of tamoxifen doses in your chick oviduct system in which tamoxifen could induce ovalbumin synthesis.

BAULIEU: Your observations are very interesting. In mammalian systems the onset of the antiestrogenic effect of tamoxifen is slow as if the estrogenic component was secondarily antagonized by the antiestrogenic properties of the compound. We do not understand the molecular biology of this double aspect of tamoxifen in mammalian systems, and indeed we do completely understand the chick system in which, up to now, we have always seen an antiestrogenic effect of tamoxifen and no estrogen activity. However, recently, my colleagues M.G. Catelli and N. Binart have observed a sort of potentiation of progesterone effects by tamoxifen, an unexpected and as yet unexplained result.

KATZENELLENBOGEN: If I could just respond to your question. There are very marked species differences in estrogenic and antiestrogenic potencies of the so-called antiestrogens. What you report for glucose-6-phosphate dehydrogenase and tamoxifen appears very similar to tamoxifen induction of progesterone receptors in MCF-7 cells. In this case, some progesterone receptors are induced at certain concentrations of tamoxifen and then inhibited at higher concentrations. In the chick, compounds like tamoxifen seem to be nearly pure antagonists, but in the rat, they have some estrogenic activity.

BAULIEU: I may add that in the chick, not only tamoxifen, but other antiestrogens such as those of the nafoxidine series behave similarly; they are not estrogenic. This is true not only in the chick oviduct but also in the chick liver.

MILGROM: We have been very much interested in the transfer of the receptor from the cytosol to the nuclei. This phenomenon is called activation. You have shown transfer of the receptor to the nucleus in conditions linked to some biological activity and also in conditions where no response was observed. This is an important issue because if such a transfer using active or inactive ligands is possible, then, of course, two different conformations of activated receptor must bind to the nuclei: one which will lead to the hormonal response and the other one which will not lead to such a response. On the other hand, you probably will have two different kinds of acceptors in the nuclei: one for the active form of the receptor and one for the inactive form. Therefore, this question is very important from a theoretical point of view.

Unfortunately, I am not sure that experimentally the situation is clear. All these antiestrogens are always both antagonists and agonists. If you look carefully enough one or several specific agonistic effects may be observed, even though others are not present. So you are never sure that what receptor interaction you observe with nuclei is due to the antagonistic effects of the compound and not its agonistic activity.

BAULIEU: I agree completely with this argument because in mammalian systems, studying an antiestrogen devoid of estrogenic effects has been impossible. However, I don't eliminate the possibility that in the chick tamoxifen could have some estrogenic effect via the receptor, and that effect would be negated, let us say, by a toxic effect of tamoxifen. The toxicity is highly improbable but, until we disprove that sort of possibility, to definitely say that tamoxifen provokes an inactive conformation of the receptor in contrast to estrogen is difficult. We probably will have the answer to these questions in the near future.

Characterization of Estrogen Receptors and Biological Responses to Estrogen in Human Endometrium

Benita S. Katzenellenbogen Nancy C. Lan
Edward J. Pavlik Richard L. Eckert

Many of the studies in this laboratory are aimed at trying to understand how estrogens modulate the growth of uterine and mammary tissue. While much is known about the details of estrogen interaction with uterine cells, almost all of this information comes from studies in experimental animals such as the rat. In these studies, the general model of initial steroid hormone interaction with a cytoplasmic receptor, followed by activation of the hormone receptor complex and its translocation to the nucleus where its interaction alters the pattern of gene expression, appears to provide a suitable outline for receptor interactions at the target cell level (Gorski and Gannon, 1978; Katzenellenbogen, 1980). One of our interests has been to apply this information to analyze and compare these receptor interactions in human endometrium, and to study the regulation of biological responses by steroid hormones in human endometrium. We, therefore, have utilized tissue culture and cell culture of human endometrium towards this end.

This chapter will report our studies on the characterization of estrogen receptors in human endometrium with particular emphasis on the nuclear estrogen receptor, and will describe some cell culture studies employing human endometrium.

It is generally agreed that steroid hormone action depends, at least in part, upon interaction of a steroid hormone-receptor complex with chromatin sites in target cells. Although an understanding of this ternary chromatin-nuclear receptor-hormone complex is crucial to an understanding of the mechanism of steroid hormone action, difficulties in extractability of the nuclear receptor have made analysis and characterization of this receptor difficult. In studies of hormone action in the uterus, salt extraction of nuclear receptor and analysis on sucrose gradients has been the most common method of analysis. This technique is not ideal, as in rat tissue only a portion of nuclear receptor is readily salt extractable, and some of this receptor-estradiol complex undergoes dissociation during the high salt extraction (Clark and Peck, 1976; Zava et al., 1976; Barrack et al., 1977; Muller et al., 1977; Katzenellenbogen et al., 1978). These problems are magnified in human uterine tissue, in which salt extraction of nuclear receptor is even less efficient (Evans and Hahnel, 1973; and this report). Hence, the report of Rat et al. (1974) that mild trypsinization produces a stable form of the cytoplasmic receptor in calf uterus was of interest in that it suggested that mild proteolysis might be effective in releasing nuclear receptor from chromatin "acceptor" sites without impairment of estradiol binding activity. Such an approach has been employed by others (Lebeau et al., 1974) in attempts to characterize the estrogen receptor from chick liver.

In this chapter, we report an adaptation of the trypsinization procedure for solubilization of nuclear estrogen receptor from human endometrium and rat uterus which gives a greatly improved efficiency of extraction and minimizes dissociation of the steroid-receptor complex. The physicochemical characteristics and binding parameters of these trypsin released nuclear receptors are analyzed by sucrose density gradient ultracentrifugation, isoelectric focusing, and polyacrylamide gel electrophoresis, and are compared to those of the salt extractable nuclear estrogen receptor and to a trypsinized form of the cytoplasmic estrogen receptor from human and rat uterine tissue. Our studies document that these trypsin-solubilized nuclear receptor complexes are of high affinity and are stable, and provide a method that may be useful in analyzing the molecular properties of estrogen receptors in a variety of estrogen target tissues.

EXPERIMENTAL

Materials

Studies employed uteri from immature female rats, 20-24 days old (Holtzman; Madison, Wisconsin), and noncancerous human endometrium from patients (35-54 years of age) undergoing hysterectomy for therapeutic reasons totally unrelated to this research that included uterine prolapse, fibroids, endometriosis, and adenomyosis.

Cytosol Preparation and Trypsinization Conditions

Cytosols from rat and human uterine tissue were prepared at 0-4°C in 0.01 M Tris, 0.0015 M EDTA, 0.02% sodium azide (TEA) buffer, pH 7.4. Uteri from immature rats were homogenized at 8 uteri per 2.4 ml TEA buffer; human endometrium was minced and then homogenized at 200 mg tissue per 1 ml TEA buffer using a Polytron PT-10 homogenizer. The homogenate was centrifuged at 226,000 x g for 1 h to yield the resulting supernatant (cytosol) which routinely was ca. 3 mg protein/ml. Cytosols were generally treated with charcoal-dextran slurry (1 part slurry to 10 parts of cytosol) to adsorb unbound steroids, and then were incubated with 10^{-8} M ^{3}H-estradiol with and without 10^{-6} M diethylstilbestrol for 2 h at 0°C to deterine total and low affinity, nonspecific binding, respectively. Parallel incubations were also done with 10^{-8} M ^{3}H-estradiol plus 10^{-6} M dihydrotestosterone to ensure that the binding observed was not due to any contaminating sex steroid binding protein in the cytosol preparation.

A trypsin solution was prepared immediately before use at 8 mg/ml in 0.001 M HCl. For rat receptor preparations, 40 µg of trypsin was then added for each mg of protein, and the proteolysis maintained at 0°C for 1 h. Human endometrial cytosol preparations required 20 µg trypsin per mg of protein for 1 h. Trypsinization was stopped by the addition of 2 µg soybean trypsin inhibitor for each µg of trypsin. Samples were then treated with charcoal dextran (10% vol/vol, 15 min, 0°C) and analyzed further as described below (sucrose density gradients, polyacrylamide gels, and isoelectric focusing). Although trypsin undergoes rapid autolysis in the absence of Ca^{2+} (TEA buffer), the conditions described above appear optimal for effecting receptor disaggregation while minimizing loss of binding activity (Rat et al., 1974; Carlson et al., 1977).

Incubation of Uterine Tissue In Vitro and Preparation of Nuclear Extracts

Rat uteri (ca. 30 mg wet weight each) or human endometrial tissue slices (ca. 25 mg each) were incubated in Eagle's HeLa medium (3 uteri/3 ml or 150 mg endometrial tissue/3 ml) with 3×10^{-8} M ^{3}H-estradiol (E_2) to determine total binding, or with 3×10^{-8} M ^{3}H-estradiol plus 3×10^{-5} M unlabeled diethylstilbestrol to determine nonspecific binding (Ruh et al., 1973). Incubations were conducted for 1 h at 37°C (rat) or 30°C (human) in stoppered 10-ml-capacity Erlenmeyer flasks, under an atmosphere of 95% O_2-5% CO_2. Uterine tissue was then thoroughly rinsed with iced 0.01 M Tris-HCl-0.0015 M EDTA, pH 7.4 (TE buffer) and homogenized with Kontes glass tissue grinders. The 800 x g x 20 min pellet was obtained and washed three times with 3 ml of TE buffer, each wash followed by centrifugation at 800 x g for 10 min. This washed nuclear pellet was then extracted with various solutions for 1 h at 0°C, unless otherwise indicated, followed by a 180,000 x g (46,000 rpm, Beckman Ti 50 rotor), 15 min centrifugation, and the counts in the supernatant were then measured to determine extraction efficiency. In the case of trypsin-KCl extraction, the nuclear pellet was treated with trypsin, 20 or 40 μg/rat uterine nuclear equivalent (containing ca. 250 μg DNA) or 50 μg per nuclear pellet from 150 mg endometrial tissue (containing ca. 400 μg DNA) in 0.5 ml TE buffer for 1 h at 0°C, and then 0.5 ml of 0.8 M KCl in TE buffer per nuclear equivalent was added for another hour at 0°C. To the final solution, a quantity of soybean trypsin inhibitor equal to twice the trypsin concentration was added before centrifugation. For DNase extractions, nuclear pellets were prepared in 0.01 M Tris buffer, pH 7.4 and extractions with DNase were performed in this buffer at 0°C. Further details for particular experiments are given in the Table and Figure Legends.

Preparation of Purified Uterine Nuclei

Buffers used for nuclei isolation were 0.25 M S-TKM (0.01 M Tris-HCl, 0.025 M KCl, 0.005 M $MgCl_2$, 0.25 M sucrose, pH 7.5 at 20°C), 0.5 M S- TKM (0.01 M Tris- HCl, 0.025 M KCl, 0.005 M $MgCl_2$, 0.5 M sucrose, pH 7.5 at 20°C), and 2.1 M S-TKM (0.01 M Tris, 0.25 M KCl, 0.005 M $MgCl_2$, 2.1 M sucrose, pH 7.5 at 20°C) (Blobel and Potter, 1966). After exposure to radiolabeled estradiol in vitro as described above, uterine tissue was washed and minced finely in 0.5 M S-TKM and homogenized (4/1 v/v, buffer:tissue) slowly with a Polytron PT- 10 homogenizer for 3 min with intermittent cooling. The homogenate was homogenized further in a Potter-Elvehjem teflon-glass homogenizer and then filtered through 5 layers of prewetted cheesecloth, then through one layer of 100 mesh organza cloth. The resulting filtrate was then spun at 800 x g for 15 min and then resuspended in 8 vol of 2.1 M S-TKM. The suspension was then centrifuged for 30 min at 22,000 x g using an L5-50 Beckman ultracentrifuge with SW-56 rotor. The supernatant was then removed and the inside of all centrifuge tubes wiped clean. The resulting purified nuclei were then washed twice and finally suspended in 0.25 M S-TKM for further use. Nuclei were judged to be free of cytoplasmic contamination by phase-contrast microscopy. Yields of nuclei ranged from 23-44%.

Determination of Receptor-bound ^{3}H-estradiol

Two methods were used to measure the receptor-estrogen complexes after extraction. The nuclear extract (180,000 x g x 15 min supernatant) was treated with charcoal dextran (10% vol/vol, 15 min at 0°C) to remove dissociated or free estradiol, or an equal volume of hydroxylapatite slurry was added to the supernatant to adsorb the estrogen-receptor complexes. The hydroxylapatite was then washed 3 times with iced 0.05 M Tris-HCl buffer, pH 7.2 and then ethanol extracted for 20 min at room temperature.

Sucrose Density Gradients

Linear 5-20% sucrose density gradients (3.6 ml) were prepared in polyallomer tubes in TE buffer (low salt) or TKE buffer (TE buffer containing 0.4 M KCl, high salt) and were kept at 0-4°C for 3-6 h before use. ^{14}C-labeled marker proteins (ovalbumin, twice recrystallized from Worthington, and bovine γ-globulin, crystallized and lyophilized, fraction II, from Nutritional Biochemicals) were prepared according to the procedure of Rice and Means (1971). Samples (300 μl) containing 10 μl of marker proteins were layered onto gradients and centrifuged at 308,000 x g for 16 h at 4°C (56,000 rpm, SW Ti 56 rotor in a Beckman L2-65B centrifuge; high salt gradients) or at 246,000 x g for 13 h (50,000 rpm, SW Ti 56 rotor; low salt gradients). Three drop fractions were collected from the top of the gradient. The recovery of counts on the gradient was always near 100%. Sedimentation coefficients were determined according to Martin and Ames (1961), relative to the internal γ-globulin marker (7.0S) and ovalbumin marker (3.6S low salt, 4.1S high salt).

Electrophoresis

Gels were cast in 12 cm long x 6 mm I.D. glass tubes. The tubes had been cleaned in a 6% KOH-methanol bath for ~30 min, rinsed, coated with a 0.5% aqueous solution of Kodak Photo-Flo 200, and oven dried. The catalyst solution (0.28% ammonium persulfate) was prepared fresh daily.

A neutral pH system described by Rodbard and Chrambach (1971; System d) was modified by substituting N,N'-diallyltartardiamide (DATD) for methylene-bisacrylamide to cross-link the separation gel (Anker, 1970). The gel composition is designated as %T [total acrylamide; (gm acrylamide + gm DATD)/100 ml solution] and %C [cross-linker: gm DATD per (gm acrylamide + gm DATD) x 100]. The separation gel was prepared at 4,6,8,10, or 12%T and 7.35%C and had a running pH of 7.8.

A Searle Analytic-Buchler electrophoresis apparatus (Polyanalyst) was used. The lower buffer reservoir is jacketed, and the lower buffer is magnetically stirred and cooled to 0-2°C by circulation of chilled methanol from a Lauda Kryomat. The gel tubes are immersed in the lower buffer so that the entire gel is surrounded by the cooled solution. The electrophoresis was conducted at 2 ma/gel. Following electrophoresis, gels for radioactivity determinations were frozen on dry ice and sliced into 2.15 mm slices. Each slice was dissolved in 0.5 ml of 2% periodic acid at room temperature and counted in 5 ml of a xylene-Triton X-114 based scintillation fluid as described (Katzenellenbogen et al., 1978). Gels containing proteins used as standards to estimate molecular radii ($\bar{R}$) were fixed overnight in 12.5% trichloroacetic acid and the positions of the white precipitated marker proteins relative to the bromophenol blue tracking dye were noted. To visualize higher oligomers of bovine serum albumin, gels were stained for 1 h at room temperature in 0.05% Coomassie blue in 12.5% trichloroacetic acid and destained in 7% acetic acid.

Isoelectric Focusing

Isoelectric focusing was done in polyacrylamide gels containing 5%T, 15%C (Baumann and Chrambach, 1976) and 2% w/v pH 5-8 range ampholytes (Ampholine, LKB). The experiments were performed in the same jacketed bath assembly used for electrophoresis. The focusing was initiated at 0.5 ma/gel until a voltage of 200 V was reached; the voltage was then maintained at 200 V for 8-10 h. Focusing of the receptor proteins was complete within 8 h and the pI values were stable up to 20 h. After focusing, the gels were frozen on dry ice and sliced into 2.15 mm sections. The pH profile was determined by suspending each slice from a gel in 1.0 ml of 0.02 M KCl for 2 h at 4°C. The gel slice, together with the KCl eluant, was counted in 10 ml of scintillation fluid. Profiles of radioactivity and pH were determined on the same gels.

Establishment of Human Endometrial Cell Cultures and Cell Culture Conditions

Studies utilized relatively normal premenopausal uterine specimens obtained immediately after hysterectomy. Part of the fresh tissue was fixed for histological examination; the rest was returned to the laboratory in sterile Dulbecco's modified Eagle's medium (MEM) containing 10% fetal calf serum (FCS), 200 U/ml penicillin, and 200 μg/ml streptomycin. All procedures were conducted under a sterile biological containment hood. Endometrium was dissected free, cut into small pieces, and incubated in Dulbecco's MEM containing 200 U/ml penicillin and 200 μg/ml streptomycin for 30 min at room temperature to reduce the possibility of contamination. Free cells were then obtained by trypsinization (0.25% trypsin in Ca^{++}- and Mg^{++}-free Hank's balanced salt solution) for _ca_. 1 h at room temperature. The cell solution was poured through two layers of sterile gauze to remove tissue fragments; FCS (15%) was added to inactivate the trypsin, and free cells were pelleted at 300 x g (10 min) and plated in Dulbecco's MEM containing 10% FCS, 100 U/ml penicillin, and 100 μg/ml streptomycin. A sealed flask system, buffered with Hepes and bicarbonate (0.01 M HEPES, 1.8 g/liter $NaHCO_3$ found to be optimal), was used for standard growth conditions.

Cells (_ca_. 5-10 x 10^5) were plated in 75 or 150-cm^2 sealed plastic flasks (Costar) and were incubated at 37°C. Attachment was complete in about 10 h, and the attachment efficiency was usually about 60%. At confluence, cells were harvested by treatment for 5-10 min at room temperature with sterile 0.05% trypsin-0.02% EDTA. Trypsinization was halted by making the suspension 15% in FCS and cooling to 0-2°C. Cells were recultured at a 1:4 or 1:5 dilution.

Cell Growth Curves

The effects of hormones on cell proliferation were monitored with cells grown at 37°C in 25-cm^2 plastic flasks with Dulbecco's MEM as the nutrient medium. For 3-5 days before the start of growth experiments, the growth medium of the cells was changed from Dulbecco's MEM containing 10% FCS to medium containing serum (10%) from castrate-adrenalectomized calves (steroid-free serum; SFS), kindly supplied by Dr. W. C. Wagner, College of Veterinary Medicine. This serum, as opposed to FCS, is low in estrogen, androgen, and progesterone, as determined by RIA, and it was used in preference to charcoal dextran-stripped FCS because the charcoal dextran adsorbs some 5-10% of proteins in addition to the steroids. RIAs indicated this serum to contain barely detectable (ca. 6×10^{-11} M) concentrations of estrogen, progesterone, or androgen, as opposed to batches of FCS which contained significant, (ca. 6×10^{-10} M) concentrations of estrogen (estradiol plus estrone), and androgen (3×10^{-9} M; T plus DHT), but lower ($2\text{-}3 \times 10^{-10}$ M) progesterone.

After growth in Dulbecco's MEM-10% SFS for 3-5 days, cells were harvested by trypsinization, seeded into 25-cm^2 plastic flasks at $2\text{-}4 \times 10^3$ cells/cm^2, and allowed to attach for 24 h. The hormones to be tested, dissolved in ethanol, were then added to the cell cultures in 1 µl ethanol/ml culture medium.

Cell proliferation was scored as the percentage of initial cell number, monitored either by electronic Coulter counting of trypsinized cells at fixed times over the 7 to 15 -day culture period, or by *in situ* cell counting (when cells were limiting) using an inverted phase contrast microscope, graduated counting reticle, and adhesive template which allowed for relocation of specific counting fields on successive days of growth determination.

RESULTS AND DISCUSSION

Extraction of Nuclear Estrogen Binding Protein

Table 1 summarizes data on the efficiency of extraction of the nuclear estrogen receptor from rat uterus and human endometrium by different agents. Procedures for the extraction of nuclear estrogen receptors have been characterized by a "radioactive ligand extraction efficiency" which is the fraction of the specific nuclear receptor associated radioactivity that is found in the extract (Table 1, column labeled Radioactivity) and a "receptor solubilization efficiency" which is the fraction of estradiol-receptor complexes found in the extract (Table 1, column labeled Receptor-Bound Radioactivity). Since assay of the extracts for receptor binding (by hydroxylapatite) generally indicates that not all the extracted ligand is still bound to receptor, the receptor solubilization efficiency is less than the ligand extraction efficiency.

As seen in Table 1, a single extraction of the rat uterine nuclear fraction with high salt (line 2a) a commonly used method for solubilization of the nuclear estrogen receptor, results in a ligand extraction efficiency of 65% and a receptor solubilization efficiency of only 48%. In human endometrium (line 1a), this procedure results in even lower yields, with ligand extraction efficiency being 40% and receptor solubilization only 15%.

A striking increase in extraction efficiency is seen, however, with mild trypsin treatment of both rat and human uterine nuclei

Table 1. Extraction of the Estrogen Receptor from Human Endometrial or Rat Uterine Nuclei

Treatment.	Extraction Efficiency Radioactivity(%)*	Receptor-Bound Radioactivity(%)*
Human Endometrium		
(1a) 0.4 M KCl, 1 or 2 h	40.2 ± 7.0(6)	14.6 ± 3.8(6)
(1b) Trypsin alone, 1 or 2 h	71.8 ± 6.1(4)	45.0 ± 2.8(4)
(1c) Trypsin 1 h → + KCl 1 h**	84.0 ± 7.2(6)	52.1 ± 4.0(6)
Rat Uterus		
(2a) 0.4 M KCl, 1 or 2 h	65.2 ± 5.5(11)††	47.8 ± 3.2(11)
(2b) Trypsin alone, 1 or 2 h**	73.5 ± 3.3(4)	51.0 ± 2.8(4)
(2c) Trypsin, 1 h → + KCl 1 h**	93.7 ± 4.6(8)	75.2 ± 4.0(8)
(2d) DNase alone, 0.5 h§	78.9 ± 5.4(3)	52.4 ± 2.3(3)
(2e) DNase alone, 1.5 h	56.3 ± 3.6(3)	34.0 ± 1.2(3)
(2f) DNase + 10 mM Mg++, 0.5 or 1.5 h	22.1 ± 0.9(4)	0.5 ± 0.1(4)
(2g) DNase, 0.5 h → + KCl, 1 h	79.5 ± 4.5(3)	53.5 ± 1.7(3)
(2h) 0.025 M to 2 M NaSCN, 1 h	19 to 84%	5 to 16%
(2i) 1 M or 2 M $NaClO_4$, 1 h	71 to 76%	5 to 13%

† Endometrial tissue slices or immature rat uteri were incubated in Eagle's HeLa medium with 3×10^{-8} M ^{3}H-estradiol or 3×10^{-8} M ^{3}H-estradiol plus 3×10^{-5} M unlabeled diethylstilbestrol for 1 h at 30°C (human) or 37°C (rat). Uterine nuclear fractions were then prepared. A portion was ethanol extracted to determine total binding and the remainder extracted with the indicated extractant for the indicated time at 0°C as described in Methods prior to centrifugation at 180,000 x g for 15 min. The supernatant was counted directly to obtain the efficiency of extraction of radioactivity, and the hydroxylapatite (HAP) adsorption assay was used to measure the ^{3}H-labeled nuclear receptor complexes after extraction. In all cases, values are based on the difference between ^{3}H-estradiol and ^{3}H-estradiol plus unlabeled DES incubations.

* Data have been corrected for nonspecific binding (less than 10% of total binding) and all are expressed as % of ethanol extractable counts (set at 100%). Receptor-bound radioactivity was assayed by hydroxylapatite binding. Recharging of soluble nuclear extracts from rat uterus with ^{3}H-estradiol prior to HAP assay indicated that none of the extracts contained receptor that had lost ligand during solubilization and was still in a form capable of binding ^{3}H-estradiol.

** Optimal trypsin found to be 40 μg/250 μg DNA = 1 rat uterine nuclear fraction/ml, and 50 μg/400 μg DNA = nuclear pellet from 150 mg human endometrium/ml. At the end of the extraction with trypsin, a concentration of soybean trypsin inhibitor twice that of the trypsin was added prior to centrifugation at 180,000 x g for 15 min.

§ Optimal DNase found to be 50 μg/rat uterine nuclear fraction/0.5 ml 0.01 M Tris buffer, pH 7.4.

†† Mean ± SEM (number of experiments).

(lines b and c). Treatment for 1-2 h (line 2b) with concentrations of trypsin found to be optimal (see Table 1 footnote) resulted in extraction of ca. 75% of the radioactive ligand and solubilization of 50% of the receptor from rat uterine nuclei. Treatment with trypsin for 1 h at 0°C, followed by 0.4 M KCl for 1 h (line 2c), was even more effective; nearly complete (94%) extraction of radioactivity from the rat nuclear fraction was obtained, with 75% estrogen receptor solubilization. This value is 150% of that seen after either KCl extraction alone or trypsin treatment alone. Studies have indicated that under our extraction conditions, as little as 2 μg of trypsin per uterine nuclear pellet (ca. 250 μg DNA) gives maximal solubilization of receptor. At high concentrations of trypsin (>80 μg per uterine nuclear pellet), however, the receptor-estradiol complex is destroyed.

Quantitation of total proteins extracted by KCl or trypsin → KCl (lines 2a and 2c) indicates that KCl alone extracts 283 ± 26 μg protein/rat uterine nuclear pellet whereas 40 μg trypsin → KCl extracts twice as much protein, 573 ± 44 μg per uterine nuclear pellet.

It should be noted that all of the values for estrogen receptor complexes reported in Table 1 are from assays employing hydroxylapatite (HAP) adsorption. Although trypsin-KCl extracted receptor sites were assayed equally well by the HAP or charcoal dextran (CD) assay, we have found that nuclear receptor sites extracted with KCl are underestimated by the CD assay, as documented by Peck and Clark (1977). Under our conditions of assay with CD (1 uterine equivalent/ml, 0.5% charcoal - 0.05% dextran, 10 min, 0°C), 25-30% of ligand was "stripped" from the KCl-extracted nuclear receptor sites. However, KCl-extracted estrogen receptor complexes could be assayed accurately by HAP adsorption. It is interesting that trypsinized nuclear receptor or trypsin-KCl extracted receptor was protected from this stripping effect of CD even in very dilute extracts (low protein concentrations), so that similar values were determined by either the CD or HAP assay.

Solubilization of the human endometrial estrogen receptor is also greatly improved by mild trypsin treatment (line 1b) or by a combined trypsin treatment followed by salt extraction (line 1c). In the latter case, 84% of the specific nuclear radioactivity is extracted and 52% of estrogen-receptor complexes are solubilized. This receptor solubilization (52%) is therefore three times as efficient as is extraction with salt alone (15%).

DNase was also effective in solubilizing a substantial portion of the nuclear estrogen-receptor complexes. Studies in the rat uterus indicated that DNase, in the absence of Mg^{2+} (line 2d), extracts ca. 80% of radioactivity, (as reported also for the mouse uterus (Harris, 1971), and solubilizes 50% of the receptor. Treatment with 0.4 M KCl after prior treatment with DNase (line 2g) does not increase further the solubilization of receptor; and both treatments (lines 2d, 2g) extract nuclear estrogen receptor complexes only as well as KCl alone (line 2a).

Since chaotropic salts have been used for the resolution of membrane proteins and multicomponent enzymes and especially for increasing the water solubility of proteins (Hatefi and Hanstein, 1969), the two most powerful chaotropic reagents - NaSCN and $NaClO_4$ - were tested in this study. Although the extraction of nuclear radioactivity is increased from 19% to 84% as the concentration of NaSCN is increased from 0.025 M to 1 M (line 2h) and is ca. 70-75% after 1 M or 2 M $NaClO_4$-extraction (line 2i), most of the extracted counts are not receptor associated. Addition of glycerol (25%) or urea (2 M or 4 M) to the chaotropic agent extraction solution did not improve the efficiency of solubilization of estrogen receptor complexes (data not shown).

Limited studies with intact, purified nuclei from rat uterus yielded results similar to those reported in Table 1. Treatment with trypsin (20 μg trypsin/200 μg nuclear DNA) followed by KCl solubilized nearly all (up to 96%) of the radioactivity and 75-80% of this radioactivity was present in a receptor bound form as determined by the hydroxylapatite method, whereas salt extraction resulted in solubilization of only 53-57% of the total receptor complexes.

Analyses of Extracted Nuclear Estrogen Receptor-Complexes by Sucrose Density Gradient Centrifugation

Fig. 1 compares by sucrose density gradient centrifugation the sedimentation behavior of 0.4 M KCl extracted nuclear receptor and of trypsin-KCl extracted nuclear receptor from rat and human uterine tissue. On high salt gradients, salt extracted rat nuclear receptor sediments at 5.6S as previously reported (Schmidt et al., 1976; Katzenellenbogen et al., 1978), while trypsin-KCl extracted nuclear receptor sediments at 4.0S, as does nuclear receptor extracted with trypsin alone (data not presented). The sedimentation behavior of the salt extracted [3.8S; a value reported also for human myometrial receptor (Notides et al., 1976)] and trypsin-salt extracted (3.5S) nuclear receptors from human endometrium are more similar, although the trypsin treated form sediments slightly more slowly, as seen also for rat uterine receptor (right panel). The salt extracted nuclear receptor forms of both rat and human uterus aggregate when subjected to low salt gradient conditions (Fig. 2); all counts are found at the bottom of the gradient when centrifugation was run for 13 h at 246,000 x g. Interestingly, under the same conditions, trypsin-KCl extracted receptor does not aggregate but instead sediments at 3-4S (Fig. 2) as it did under high salt conditions (Fig. 1). Furthermore, a similar (3-4S) form of the rat uterine receptor is generated when nuclear receptor extracted by high salt is subsequently exposed to mild trypsin treatment (KCl → trypsin, Fig. 2).

Rates of Dissociation of Trypsin-KCl and KCl Extracted Nuclear Estrogen Receptor

The rates of dissociation of the trypsin-KCl and KCl extracted nuclear estrogen receptors were determined at 0-4°C in the presence of a large excess of unlabeled estrogen (Fig. 3). Although there is a small fraction of rapidly dissociating sites in trypsin-KCl solubilized receptors, dissociation of the major portion of the extracted nuclear receptor complexes appears monophasic, and the half-times for dissociation for the three solubilized rat and human nuclear receptors are 55-60 h. The rate constant of dissociation k_{-1} is 3.5×10^{-6}/sec for KCl extracted receptor, 3.3×10^{-6}/sec for trypsinized rat receptor, and 3.2×10^{-6}/sec for trypsin-KCl extracted nuclear receptor from human endometrium. At this temperature (0-4°C), all the receptor preparations were very stable over the long time course of the assay showing less than 5% loss of activity.

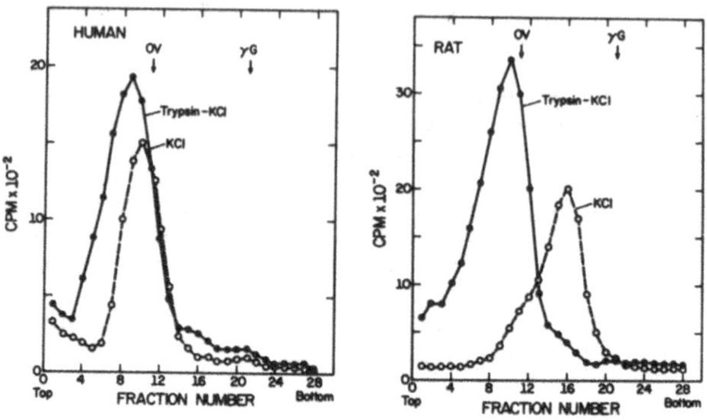

Fig. 1. High salt sucrose density gradient analyses of human endometrial (left panel) and rat uterine (right panel) nuclear estrogen receptors. Human endometrial tissue slices or immature rat uteri were incubated in vitro with 3×10^{-8} M ^{3}H-estradiol or 3×10^{-8} M ^{3}H-estradiol plus 3×10^{-5} M unlabeled diethylstilbestrol for 1 h at 30°C (human) or 37°C (rat) and the 3-times washed nuclear pellet was prepared. Salt (0.4 M KCl) extracted and trypsin- KCl extracted nuclear receptors were prepared as described in Methods and were subjected to centrifugation on 5-20% sucrose density gradients containing 0.4 M KCl. ^{14}C-labeled marker proteins ovalbumin (OV) and γ-globulin (γG) were added to all samples as internal standards and their positions are designated by arrows. The graphs represent high affinity binding, namely the difference between hot gradients (total binding) and hot plus cold gradients (low affinity, "nonspecific" binding).

Analysis of Estrogen Binding to Trypsin Extracted Nuclear Receptor; K_d Determinations

It has been shown previously (Rochefort et al., 1972; Ruh et al., 1975; Schmidt et al., 1976) that high concentrations of androgens in vitro translocate the estrogen receptor from the cytoplasmic to the nuclear fraction of the immature rat uterus. These androgen-moved estrogen receptor sites are either unfilled with hormone at the estrogen binding site or contain very weakly associated androgen as these sites moved to the nucleus by androgen are able to directly bind or exchange with ^{3}H-estradiol at 0°C (Schmidt et al., 1976). Taking advantage of this, we have used the androgen movement of estrogen receptor sites as a means of directly determining the K_d of the solubilized nuclear receptor-estradiol complex. For this analysis of binding of estradiol to trypsinized nuclear receptor, rat uteri or human endometrial tissue slices were incubated in vitro with 3×10^{-6} M DHT for 1 h at 37°C (rat) or 30°C (human) and washed nuclear pellets were prepared and extracted with trypsin and KCl. Trypsin-KCl extracted nuclear receptor was then incubated with $0.44\text{-}9.2 \times 10^{-9}$ M ^{3}H-estradiol and ^{3}H-estradiol plus 100-fold unlabeled estradiol for 17 h at 0°C and estradiol bound nuclear receptor was then measured. As seen in Fig. 4, where data are plotted

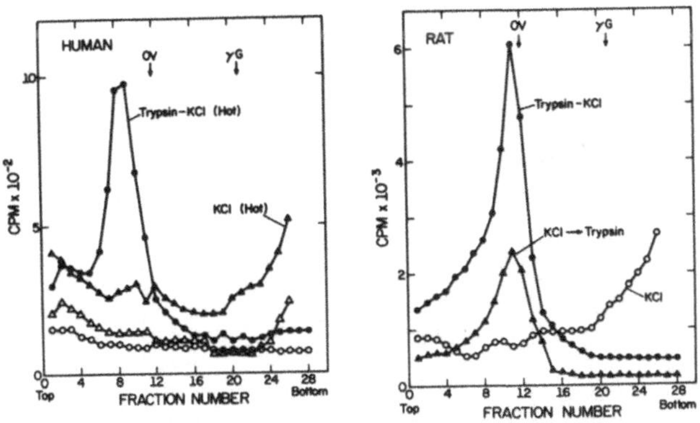

Fig. 2. Low salt sucrose density gradient analyses of human endometrial (left panel) and rat uterine (right panel) nuclear receptors. Human endometrial tissue slices were incubated with 3 x 10^{-8} M ^{3}H-estradiol or 3 x 10^{-8} M ^{3}H-estradiol plus 3 x 10^{-5} M diethylstilbestrol for 1 h at 30°C. The 3-times washed nuclear pellets were prepared and extracted with 0.4 M KCl in TE buffer (KCl) for 1 h at 0°C or with trypsin followed by 0.4 M KCl (trypsin- KCl) and addition of soybean trypsin inhibitor as described in Methods. Samples were treated with charcoal dextran (10% vol/vol) prior to layering on to gradients. In the left panel, filled symbols show gradients of extracts derived from hot, ^{3}H-estradiol alone endometrial tissue incubations. Unfilled symbols show gradients representing low affinity binding derived from ^{3}H-estradiol plus 1000-fold unlabeled diethylstilbestrol tissue incubations. The right panel shows sucrose density gradient centrifugation profiles of rat nuclear receptor extracted for 1 h with trypsin followed by 1 h with 0.4 M KCl in TE buffer (trypsin-KCl); or extracted for 1 h with 0.4 M KCl in TE buffer (KCl); or extracted for 1 h with 0.4 M KCl in TE buffer followed by exposure of the KCl soluble extract to trypsin (50 μg trypsin/1 mg protein) for 1 h at 0°C (KCl → trypsin). Profiles shown represent specific binding, the difference between hot (total binding) and hot plus cold (low affinity binding) gradients.

according to the method of Scatchard, the K_d for the rat receptor was determined to be 2.6 x 10^{-10} M and for the human receptor, 9.0 x 10^{-10} M. Hence, the nuclear receptors in both species have a very high affinity for estradiol.

Isoelectric Focusing and Electrophoretic Properties of Nuclear and Cytoplasmic Receptor Complexes

In further studies, we compared the physical properties of the trypsin extracted nuclear estrogen receptors of rat and human uterus with those of trypsin-treated forms of the cytoplasmic estrogen receptors in these species. When trypsinized nuclear and cytoplasmic human estrogen receptors are subjected to isoelectric focusing in polyacrylamide gels in pH gradients of 5-8 (Fig. 5), the ^{3}H-labeled receptor

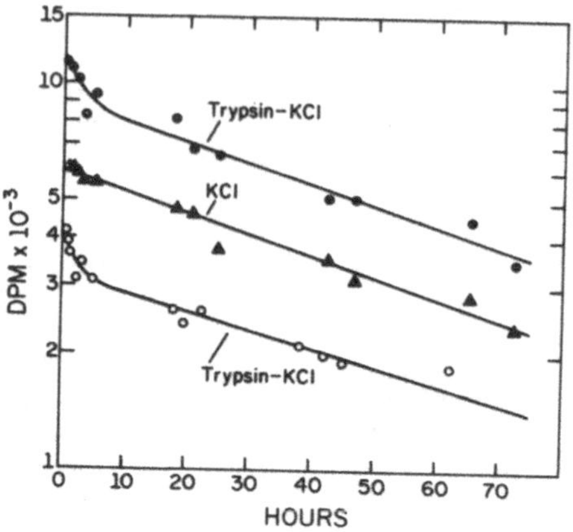

Fig. 3. Rates of dissociation of solubilized nuclear estrogen receptors. Human endometrial tissue slices or immature rat uteri were incubated _in vitro_ with 3 x 10^{-8} M ^{3}H-estradiol or 3 x 10^{-8} M ^{3}H-estradiol _plus_ 3 x 10^{-5} M diethylstilbestrol as described in Methods. Nuclear fractions were prepared and extracted with 0.4 M KCl or with trypsin followed by KCl and addition of soybean trypsin inhibitor. The 180,000 x g x 15 min supernatants were then treated with charcoal-dextran (10% vol/vol, 10 min, 0°C) prior to the addition of 3 x 10^{-6} M unlabeled estradiol (or buffer alone for stability determinations). At time intervals thereafter, triplicate samples were subjected to hydroxylapatite assay for receptor measurement. Filled symbols represent rat uterine nuclear estrogen receptor preparations, and open symbols, human endometrial nuclear receptor.

forms migrate sharply and to very similar positions coincident with isoelectric points of 6.3-6.4 (and this peak is competable with 100-fold excess unlabeled estradiol or diethylstilbestrol but not dihydrotestosterone, not shown). The rat cytoplasmic estrogen receptor shows a similar isoelectric point near 6.4, but the rat nuclear receptor consistently focused at a slightly higher pH (6.6) indicative of a slightly less acidic isoelectric point. (The radioactivity peak at gel slice 36 represents free ^{3}H-estradiol.)

The molecular sizes of these receptor proteins were estimated by determining the extent to which their electrophoretic mobility is retarded by increasing acrylamide gel concentrations (Ferguson, 1964). On a plot of log relative mobility, R_f vs % gel concentration, T at constant %C (a Ferguson plot) proteins appear as lines. Minus the slope of a line (called the retardation coefficient, K_R) is related to the molecular size of the protein, and the ordinate intercept depends on its charge to surface area ratio and is a measure of its free electrophoretic mobility. A Ferguson plot of the human and rat receptor forms on 4-10% acrylamide gels is shown in Fig. 6 (left panel). A linear plot relating the square root of the retardation coefficient of standard proteins to their anhydrous molecular radii ($\bar{R}$) shown in Fig. 6 (right panel), was used to estimate the molecular weights of the different receptor forms as described by Rodbard and Chrambach (1971). By this method, the four receptor forms appear nearly

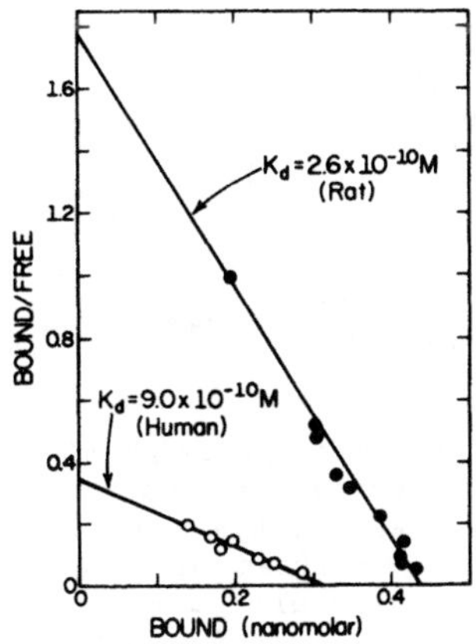

Fig. 4. Scatchard analysis of the binding of estradiol to trypsin-KCl solubilized nuclear receptor from human endometrium or rat uterus. Rat uteri or human endometrial tissue slices were incubated in vitro with 3 x 10^{-6} M DHT at 30°C (human) or 37°C (rat) for 1 h. Washed nuclear pellets were then prepared and extracted with trypsin and then KCl as described in Methods. Trypsin inhibitor was added before centrifugation to obtain the 180,000 x g x 15 min supernatant. The extracted estrogen receptor sites were then incubated with various concentrations of ^{3}H-estradiol (0.44-9.2 x 10^{-9} M) and ^{3}H-estradiol plus 100-fold excess unlabeled estradiol for 17 h at 0°C and receptor binding was assayed by charcoal-dextran. All points are corrected for nonspecific binding and slopes calculated by linear regression analysis.

identical in size. Molecular weights have been calculated using the relationship $MW = (4\pi N\bar{R}^3)/3\bar{v} = 3456\ \bar{R}^3$ where N is Avogadro's number, $\bar{v}$ (partial specific volume) is assumed to be 0.73 cm^3g^{-1}, and $\bar{R}$ is in nanometers. The calculated molecular weights of these four trypsinized receptor forms vary between 45,000 and 50,000.

From the very similar slopes of the Ferguson plot (Fig. 6, left panel), it is evident that the molecular weights of the four trypsinized receptor forms are quite close. However, the slight differences in the ordinate intercepts suggest slight differences in relative free charge mobilities which are consistent with the pI's of the receptor forms determined by isoelectric focusing. Hence, the human nuclear receptor had the lowest pI (6.3), and the rat nuclear receptor the highest pI (6.6), with the cytoplasmic receptors of both species having intermediate pI values of 6.4.

These studies document that mild trypsinization treatment of nuclear and cytoplasmic estrogen receptors from both human and rat uterine tissue produces very similar, stable forms of the receptors. These trypsinized receptor forms can be readily characterized because they do not aggregate under low ionic strength conditions, as opposed to the salt-extracted nuclear (Fig. 2) and untreated cytoplasmic receptors. Our analyses presented here indicate that the nuclear and

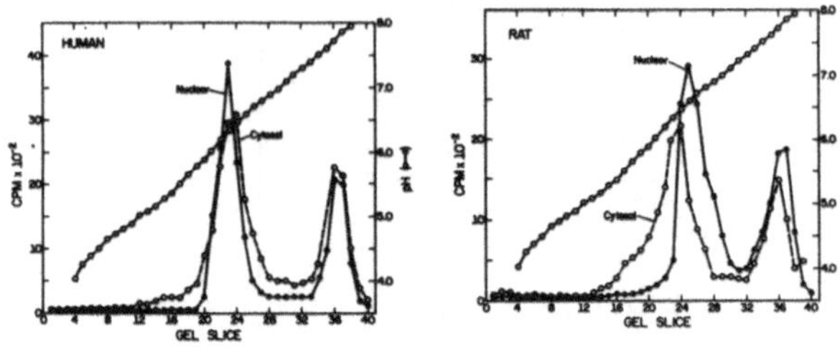

Fig. 5. Gel isoelectric focusing patterns of human (left panel) and rat (right panel) uterine nuclear and cytosol estrogen receptors. Receptor preparations were subjected to mild trypsinization as described in Methods and freed of unbound steroid by charcoal adsorption. Samples (50 µl) were layered onto 6 x 85 mm polyacrylamide gels (5% T, 15% C) containing 2% of the pH 5-8 range ampholines. After focusing for 10 h, gels were processed as described in Materials and Methods. The radioactivity and pH measurements were done on the same gel. Essentially identical pH profiles were obtained from the two gels used to construct each panel.

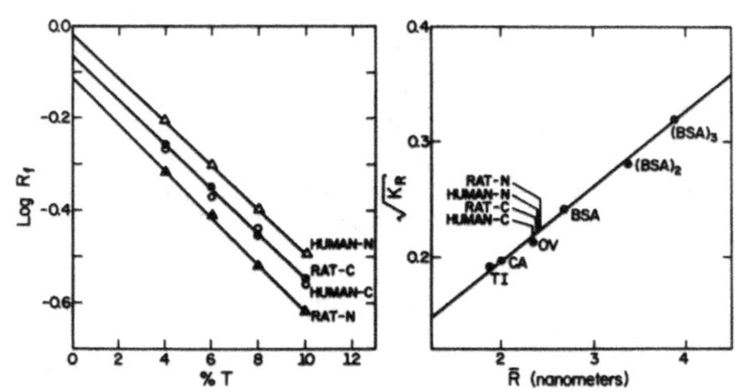

Fig. 6. Estimation of molecular radii (R̄) of human endometrial and rat uterine nuclear and cytoplasmic receptor species by electrophoretic mobility. (Left panel) Ferguson plot (log relative mobility vs. % gel concentration) of the trypsinized forms of the nuclear (N) and cytoplasmic (C) estrogen receptors. Minus the slope of each line is designated as the retardation coefficient K_R. (Right panel) Standard curve relating $(K_R)^{1/2}$ of several standard proteins to their molecular radii. R̄ (as nm) are 1.89, soybean trypsin inhibitor (TI); 2.03, carbonic anhydrase; 2.36, ovalbumin (OV); 2.69, bovine serum albumin monomer (BSA); 3.39 BSA dimer (BSA_2); and 3.88 BSA trimer (BSA_3). The vertical lines indicate the positions of the four receptor species on the standard curve (means of 2 determinations each). The calculated R̄'s for uterine receptors are 2.35 nm, human cytoplasmic receptor; 2.39, rat cytoplasmic receptor; 2.40, human nuclear receptor; and 2.43, rat nuclear receptor.

cytoplasmic receptors from both animal species have similar molecular weights and isoelectric points and retain radiolabeled estradiol with high affinity. In addition, treatment with low concentrations of trypsin is a simple procedure that results in a greatly improved solubilization of nuclear estrogen receptor, particularly in the case of the human endometrial nuclear receptor in which only a portion of the receptor population is readily extracted by salt.

Effects of Estrogens on Human Endometrial Cells in Primary Tissue Culture

We have been using short-term culture of human endometrial cells to characterize the biological potencies of a variety of steroidal and nonsteroidal estrogens in the human as monitored by their effects on cell proliferation and responses *in vitro*. We have found that approximately 60% of the cultures show increased rates of proliferation in response to the addition of estrogen, as shown in a representative experiment depicted in Fig. 8. When this cell strain was exposed to Dulbecco's-10% SFS containing different concentrations of the natural estrogen, E_2 or the synthetic estrogen, DES, increases in proliferation over control levels were observed (Fig. 7, A and B). Addition of 2×10^{-7} M E_2 or DES resulted in a 2- to 5-fold, optimal acceleration in the rate of proliferation, with stimulation first being detected at 2-4 days (Fig. 7). Ten-fold higher or lower concentrations of E_2 or DES resulted in little stimulation, and high (2×10^{-5} M) concentrations of either estrogen stopped cell proliferation in this cell strain. In recent studies we find stimulation of some cell strains by concentrations of estradiol between 1 and 10×10^{-9} M. This stimulation is accompanied by increases in the cellular content of progesterone receptor (R. L. Eckert and B. S. Katzenellenbogen, in preparation).

In a putative nontarget cell line, the human sternum transformed cell line Detroit-98, the addition of estradiol or DES failed to elicit any increase in the rate of proliferation, although high (2×10^{-5} M) concentrations of E_2 and DES also terminated proliferation in this cell line.

Metabolism of Estradiol by Human Endometrial Cell Cultures

Since uterine tissue *in vivo* is able to metabolize estradiol, we investigated the metabolic fate of E_2 after interaction with the uterine cells. For this experiment (Fig. 8), cells were grown to confluency and ^3H-E_2 was then added. At successive intervals of time after the addition of steroid (day 0 measurement is taken after 1 h), media and cells were extracted separately, and the extracts were subjected to thin layer chromatographic analysis. The results of these determinations, shown in Fig. 8, indicate that progressive conversion of E_2 to estrone rapidly occurred within cells (Fig. 8A). By 2 days, more than half of the cellular radioactivity was present as estrone, and even significant conversion of E_2 to estrone had occurred by 1 h (plotted as day 0; Fig. 8A). Likewise, the ^3H-E_2 present in the media in which the cells had been grown was also converted to estrone; 50% conversion was seen by 2 days, and nearly complete conversion occurred by 10 days. As would be expected, culture medium alone (without cells) showed no conversion of E_2 to estrone over the 10-day period (data not shown).

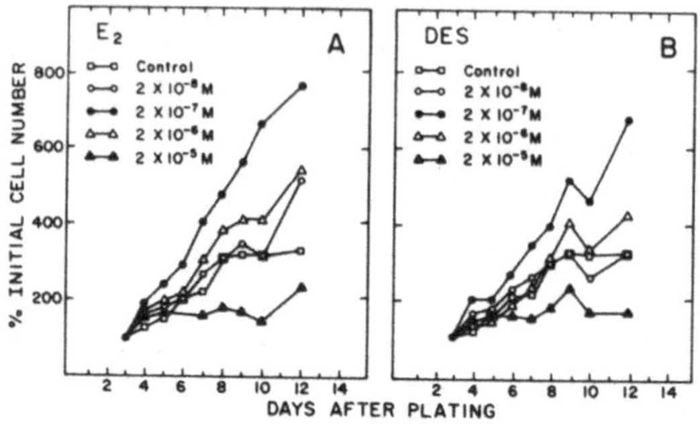

Fig. 7. Growth of human endometrial cells under estrogen-supplemented conditions. A and B, Tissue was from a 48-yr-old patient with multiple fibroids and menorrhagia. Cells were grown in culture for 5 days before being used in these determinations. In all growth curves, cells were allowed to attach for 24 h before hormone was added. The cell count, taken on day 3 after plating, is set at 100% (From Pavlik and Katzenellenbogen, 1978).

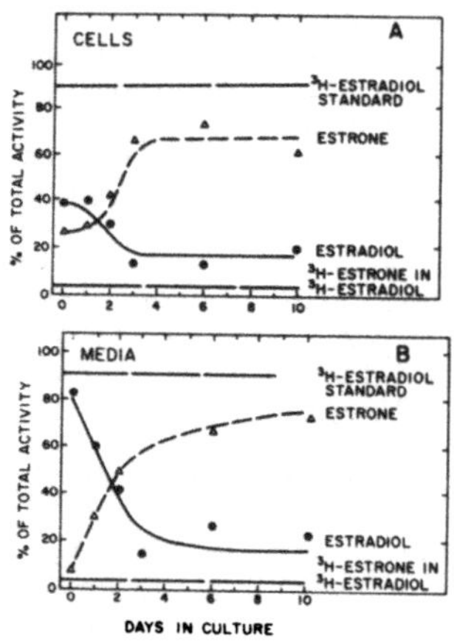

Fig. 8. The conversion of $^3H\text{-}E_2$ to ^3H-estrone by human endometrial cells. Cells were grown to confluence in 25-cm^2 flasks and held in medium containing SFS for 5 days. Medium was then made 2×10^{-8} M in $^3H\text{-}E_2$ and at indicated times thereafter, cells were freed by trypsinization and washed one time. Both the media and the cells were extracted twice with ethyl acetate; the extracts were evaporated to dryness and chromatographed in a silica gel thin layer chromatographic system containing benzene-ethanol (95:5, vol/vol) plus 1% triethylamine. Authenticity of E_2 and estrone was established by the comigration of nonradioactive E_2 and estrone identified under iodine vapor (From Pavlik and Katzenellenbogen, 1978).

These studies provide evidence that estrogens in vitro are able to directly enhance the rate of proliferation of human endometrial cells in tissue culture. Biologically active estrogens, such as DES and E_2, are effective cell stimulants, whereas the very weak estrogen, 17α-estradiol, was inactive at equivalent concentrations. The endometrial cells also retain the ability to convert E_2 to estrone in vitro, probably through activity of the enzyme estradiol dehydrogenase.

We are currently using tissue and cell culture to evaluate the activities of a variety of estrogens, including the zearalenone estrogens (Katzenellenbogen et al., 1979), in human uterine tissue in vitro. In addition, high affinity cytoplasmic estrogen binding has been detected in some human uterine cell strains, and further studies we are pursuing are aimed at characterizing estrogen receptors in these cells and relating estrogen receptors with cell responsiveness. We are also currently attempting to understand why a sizeable number of cell strains (ca. 40%) do not respond to estrogens in vitro.

The methodological advantages offered by cell culture, which enables hormone responsiveness to be studied for rather prolonged periods, should allow assessment of both short and long term estrogen-induced physiological changes and their relationship to nuclear and cytoplasmic hormone receptor levels and period of receptor occupancy. This system should, therefore, eliminate the necessity of extrapolating to human tissue information obtained solely with other experimental animal systems; it also may provide a valuable complement to clinical studies and thus, may obviate some of the difficulties inherent in obtaining information about human reproduction from in vivo studies.

ACKNOWLEDGMENTS

This work was supported by National Institutes of Health Grants USPH HD06726 and CA18119 (to B.S.K.), NIH Postdoctoral Fellowship CA06149 and HD07028 (to E.J.P.), and Ford Foundation Grant 700-0333 (postdoctoral traineeship, N.C.L.). We greatly appreciate the assistance of the Gynecology and Pathology Departments, and thank Dr. Merrill Huffman for his interest in these studies. We also thank Susan Rutledge and Kathryn Carlson for assistance in some of these studies.

REFERENCES

Anker, H. S. (1970). A solubilizable acrylamide gel for electrophoresis. FEBS Lett. 7, 293.

Barrack, E. R., Hawkins, E. F., Allen, S. L., Hicks, L. L., and Coffey, D. S. (1977). Concepts related to salt resistant estradiol receptors in rat uterine nuclei: Nuclear matrix. Biochem. Biophys. Res. Commun. 79, 829-836.

Baumann, G. and Chrambach, A. (1976). A highly cross-linked, transparent polyacrylamide gel with improved mechanical stability for use in isoelectric focusing and isotachophoresis. Anal. Biochem. 70, 32-38.

Blobel, G. and Potter, V. (1966). Nuclei from rat liver: Isolation method that combines purity with high yield. Science 154, 1662-1665.

Carlson, K. E., Sun, L-H. K., and Katzenellenbogen, J. A. (1977). Characterization of trypsin-treated forms of the estrogen receptor from rat and lamb uterus. Biochemistry 16, 4288-4296.

Clark, J. H., and Peck, E. J., Jr. (1976). Nuclear retention of receptor-oestrogen complex and nuclear acceptor sites. Nature 260, 635-637.

Evans, L. H. and Hahnel, R. (1973). Distribution of oestrogen receptors in cell fractions of human uterine tissue. J. Endocrinol. 56, 503-528.

Ferguson, K. A. (1964). Starch-gel electrophoresis: Application to the classification of pituitary proteins and polypeptides. Metabolism 13, 985-1002.

Gorski, J. and Gannon, F. (1976). Current models of steroid hormone action: A critique. Ann. Rev. Physiol. 38, 425-450.

Harris, S. G. (1971). Nature of oestrogen specific binding sites in the nuclei of mouse uteri. Nature New Biol. 231, 246-248.

Hatefi, Y. and Hanstein, W. G. (1969). Solubilization of particulate proteins and nonelectrolytes by chaotropic agents. Proc. Nat. Acad. Sci. U.S.A. 62, 1129-1136.

Katzenellenbogen, B. S. (1980). Dynamics of steroid hormone receptor action. Ann. Rev. Physiol. 42, 17-35.

Katzenellenbogen, B. S. and Gorski, J. (1975). Estrogen actions on syntheses of macromolecules in target cells. Biochem. Actions Hormones 3, 187-243.

Katzenellenbogen, B. S., Katzenellenbogen, J. A., Ferguson, E. R., and Krauthammer, N. (1978). Anti-estrogen interaction with uterine estrogen receptors: Studies with a radiolabeled anti-estrogen (CI-628). J. Biol. Chem. 253, 697-707.

Katzenellenbogen, B. S., Katzenellenbogen, J. A., and Mordecai, D. (1979). Zearalenones: Characterization of the estrogenic potencies and receptor interactions of a series of fungal β-resorcylic acid lactones. Endocrinology 105, 33-40.

Lebeau, M. C., Massol, N., and Baulieu, E. E. (1974). Extraction, partial purification, and characterization of 'the insoluble estrogen receptor' from chick liver nuclei. FEBS Lett. 43, 107-111.

Martin, R. and Ames, B. (1961). A method for determining the sedimentation behavior of enzymes: Application to protein mixtures. J. Biol. Chem. 236, 1372-1379.

Muller, R. E., Traish, A. M., and Wotiz, H. H. (1977). Interaction of receptor-estrogen complex (R-E) with uterine nuclei. J. Biol. Chem. 252, 8206-8211.

Notides, A. C., Hamilton, D. E., and Muechler, E. K. (1976). A molecular analysis of the human estrogen receptor. J. Steroid Biochem. 7, 1025-1030.

Pavlik, E. J. and Katzenellenbogen, B. S. (1978). Human endometrial cells in primary tissue culture: Estrogen interactions and modulation of cell proliferation. J. Clin. Endocrinol. Metab. 47, 333-344.

Peck, E. J., Jr. and Clark, J. H. (1977). The effect of ionic strength on charcoal adsorption assays of receptor-estradiol complexes. Endocrinology 101, 1034-1043.

Rat, R. L., Vallet-Strouve, C., and Erdos, T. (1974). The properties of a uterine oestradiol receptor after limited proteolysis. Biochimie 56, 1387-1391.

Rice, R. and Means, G. E. (1971). Radioactive labeling of proteins in vitro. J. Biol. Chem. 246, 831-833.

Rochefort, H., Vignon, F., and Capony, F. (1972). Formation of estrogen nuclear receptor in uterus: Effect of androgens, estrone, and nafoxidine. Biochem. Biophys. Res. Commun. 47, 662-670.

Rodbard, D. and Chrambach, A. (1971). Estimation of molecular radius, free mobility, and valence using polyacrylamide gel electrophoresis. Anal. Biochem. 40, 95-134.

Ruh, T. S., Katzenellenbogen, B. S., Katzenellenbogen, J. A., and Gorski, J. (1973). Estrone interaction with the rat uterus: In vitro response and nuclear uptake. Endocrinology 92, 125-134.

Ruh, T. S., Wassilak, S. G., and Ruh, M. F. (1975). Androgen-induced nuclear accumulation of the estrogen receptor. Steroids 25, 257-273.

Schmidt, W. M., Sadler, M. A., and Katzenellenbogen, B. S. (1976). Androgen-uterine interaction: Nuclear translocation of the estrogen receptor and induction of the synthesis of the uterine-induced protein (IP) by high concentrations of androgens in vitro but not in vivo. Endocrinology 98, 702-716.

Zava, D. T., Harrington, N. Y., and McGuire, W. L. (1976). Nuclear estradiol receptor in the adult rat uterus: A new exchange assay. Biochemistry 15, 4292-4297.

DISCUSSION

LOBL: The Ferguson analysis showed that the cytoplasmic receptor and the nuclear receptor were about the same size. Does this indicate that the binding of steroid to the cytoplasmic receptor does not significantly change either the size or the shape of the estrogen receptor?

KATZENELLENBOGEN: These Ferguson analyses were all done on trypsin treated preparations, not with the native receptor which is an aggregated form and very difficult to analyze using acrylamide gel electrophoresis, although one can do so to a limited extent. The Ferguson plots indicate that these proteolyzed forms of receptor were very similar in both charge and molecular weight. We can't say anything about the conformation of receptor, etc., based on this type of analysis. The differences in Y intercept in the Ferguson plots indicate there are slight differences in the charge of the proteins which is reflected in the minor differences in isoelectric focusing positions.

LOBL: Are the receptors made up of aggregates of similar or identical subunits?

KATZENELLENBOGEN: Yes. These data suggest that at least a portion of nuclear and cytoplasmic receptor that remains after this limited proteolysis is probably very similar. In addition, they suggest that the native receptors have at least a portion of receptor that is very similar. Studies from Bill Schrader's lab have also indicated that limited proteolysis of progesterone receptor subunits A and B, with an endogeneous protease generates a Form IV receptor. The physical properties of the Form IV progesterone receptor are quite similar to what we see with the estrogen receptor. The important thing is that both of the progesterone receptor subunits as well as the nuclear and cytoplasmic estrogen receptors contain at least a significant portion of receptor that appears to be virtually identical.

GERSCHENSON: How long can you keep your endometrial cells going in culture? Do the cells show the same degree of responsiveness during the time you keep them in culture? If you culture cells in the presence of estradiol, do they develop refractoriness?

KATZENELLENBOGEN: In general we try to work with the human endometrial cell cultures within one to two weeks after culturing. There is a tremendous variation with time in the loss of estrogen receptor in different cell cultures. Some cells lose estrogen receptors very quickly after culture, some seem to retain receptor for as long as two months. We are working with short term cultures. We have not yet examined whether the presence of continual estrogen makes these cells refractory, but it is something we have been interested in doing. These are mixed cell populations, which we are trying to separate into epithelial and stromal components. The method is very effective in separating the components, but we have had very poor luck in maintaining the epithelial cells in culture for any period of time.

The Endometrium

7

Uterine Progesterone Receptors During Pregnancy

Frederique Logeat
Mai T. Vu Hai
Pierre Sartor
Edwin Milgrom

The mechanisms of endocrine control of pregnancy are still poorly understood. Hormone concentrations in blood have been determined in various species throughout pregnancy, but questions still remain. For instance, how are implantation and parturition triggered? One reason for these uncertainties is the fact that circulating steroids represent only a portion of the hormones which reach the uterus. Local secretions from the placenta (Csapo, 1969) and from the blastocyst (Dickman et al, 1976, George and Wilson, 1978) have been implicated in the control of uterine functions.

Moreover, the response of target cells to hormonal stimuli depends not only on the magnitude of the stimuli but also on the cellular receptivity. Receptor concentrations can be assessed. Quantitation of steroid-receptor complexes in nuclei is particularly important since these complexes reflect the magnitude of the biological effect of a given steroid at a defined moment (King and Mainwaring, 1974).

At parturition in the rat nuclear progesterone-receptor complexes disappear, implying that the cellular activity of progesterone has ended. This is clearly related to the drop in plasma progesterone which occurs at this stage since cytosol receptors are still available, in fact, in increased concentration. It is unknown how the progesterone block is removed in other species, such as the human, in whom serum progesterone concentration does not decrease before parturition (Heap et al, 1973). In these species the regulation of progesterone receptor at parturition may differ from that of the rat.

Only one-fifth to one-third of the cellular progesterone receptors move into the nucleus from the cytoplasm during pregnancy. Whether this is due to heterogeneity of receptors or is related to the strikingly low affinity of the hormone for this progesterone receptor (K_A = 1 - 1.7 x $10^8 M^{-1}$ at 0^oC) (Vu Hai and Milgrom, 1978a) when compared to other receptors is unknown. Finally progesterone may be bound by nonreceptor proteins, such as albumin and CBG known to be in uterus. Therefore, the concentration of available, free hormone may not be sufficient to saturate the receptor.

The uterus is of course, a heterogeneous organ, composed of various cell types, and one might expect that in each compartment receptor concentrations were varying independently. Experiments have shown that at least during the estrous cycle this is not the case. In guinea pigs, biochemical (Milgrom et al, 1972) and autoradiographic (Warembourg and Milgrom, 1977) studies performed in parallel showed that receptor concentrations differed from one cell type to another, but that variations during the estrous cycle were parallel in all cells. Apparently, similar control mechanisms operate in various cell types. Such studies must now be performed in pregnant animals to determine whether there is heterogeneity of receptor distribution in different cells.

We shall discuss here the special difficulties in the measurement of steroid hormone receptors during pregnancy and the possible biological significance of some of the results obtained to date.

I - METHODS FOR PROGESTERONE RECEPTOR ASSAY IN THE PREGNANT RAT UTERUS

Extremely high concentrations of progesterone in blood make accurate measurement of the progesterone receptor difficult. Exchange assays, in which nonradioactive endogenous hormone is replaced by radioactive steroid must be used. However for determination of cytosolic receptor such exchange is insufficient since the added radioactive hormone is diluted by an undetermined high concentration of endogenous hormone. It is thus preferable to assay after as much endogenous hormone as possible is removed.

Measurement of cytosol receptor (Vu Hai and Milgrom, 1978a)

This assay (Table 1) is based on the finding that progesterone-receptor complexes in rat uterine cytosol are very unstable even at low temperature. Exposure to dextran-coated charcoal for 60 minutes at $0^{o}C$ removes about 90% of endogenous progesterone without making the receptor unstable. The cytosol is then incubated at $0^{o}C$ with a saturating concentration of $[^{3}H]$R5020 (17,21-dimethyl-19-norpregna-4,9-diene-3,20 dione), a synthetic progestin with high affinity for the receptor. Parallel incubations are performed in the presence of 2 μM unlabeled progesterone to measure nonspecific binding. During incubation, progesterone is replaced by $[^{3}H]$R5020 in the few remaining progesterone-receptor complexes.

Assay of nuclear receptor (Vu Hai and Milgrom, 1978b)

Since the progesterone receptor is thermolabile, the assay must be performed at $0^{o}C$. Nuclear receptor assay is facilitated by the fact that the progesterone-receptor complex dissociates readily even at low temperature. Complete exchange is obtained in about 6 hours at $0^{o}C$ (Figure 1). The main technical problem in assaying progesterone-receptor complexes in nuclei is nonspecific binding. This binding tends to be high and to obscure the saturable, specific binding. Various methods of minimizing this nonspecific binding have been defined (Table 2), and it can be decreased to about 10-30% of total binding.

Table 1

Assay of Total Progesterone Receptor Concentration (hormone-bound and free) in the Rat Uterine Cytosol

1. Each uterus was homogenized in 4 vol of buffer (10 mM-Tris-HCl buffer, pH 7.4, containing 1.5 mM-EDTA, 1 mM-β-mercapto-ethanol, and 10% (v/v) glycerol).
2. The homogenate was centrifuged at 800 g for 10 minutes.
3. The supernatant was centrifuged at 105,000 g for 90 minutes.
4. The cytosol was diluted with buffer to obtain a protein concentration of 4 mg/ml.
5. One volume of 0.05% dextran-0.5% charcoal was added. Agitation for 60 minutes, centrifugation at 3,000 g for 10 minutes.
6. The supernatant was incubated for 2 hours at $0^{o}C$ either with a saturating concentration of [^{3}H]R5020 (10 nmol/l) or with varying concentrations of [^{3}H]R5020. Parallel incubations in the presence of 2 μM-unlabeled progesterone were also carried out.
7. One volume of dextran-coated charcoal was added. The suspension was agitated for 10 minutes and centrifuged at 3,000 g for 3 minutes. Radioactivity was counted in the supernatant.
8. Receptor concentration was obtained either by Scatchard (1949) plot analysis or as the difference between total and nonspecific binding at hormone saturation.

The temperature was kept at $0^{o}C$ throughout the procedure.

Table 2

Assay of Progesterone-Receptor Complexes in Nuclei of Rat Uterus

1. Each uterus was homogenized in 4 vol of 10 mM Tris-HCl buffer containing 1.5 mM-EDTA, 1 mM-β-mercaptoethanol, and 10% (v/v) glycerol.
2. The homogenate was centrifuged at 800 g for 10 minutes.
3. The precipitate of the 800 g centrifugation was washed with 6 ml buffer and then resuspended in 6 ml buffer.
4. Aliquots (1 ml) of the suspension were added to 1 ml buffer containing the steroids with final steroid concentrations of either 10 nM [^{3}H]R5020 or 10 nM [^{3}H]R5020 plus 2 μM unlabeled progesterone. Incubation was 6 hours at $0^{o}C$.
5. The incubates were centrifuged at 3,000 g for 10 minutes. The precipitate was washed three times with 5 ml buffer containing bovine serum albumin (10 mg/ml) and once with 5 ml buffer.
6. The precipitate was suspended in 1.5 ml buffer and transferred into a counting vial.
7. After radioactivity was counted, DNA concentration was measured in the nuclear pellet. DNA concentration was also measured in an aliquot of the initial suspension.
8. Receptor concentration = [total binding]-[nonspecific binding, incubation in presence of unlabeled progesterone].

The temperature was kept at $0^{o}C$ throughout the procedure.

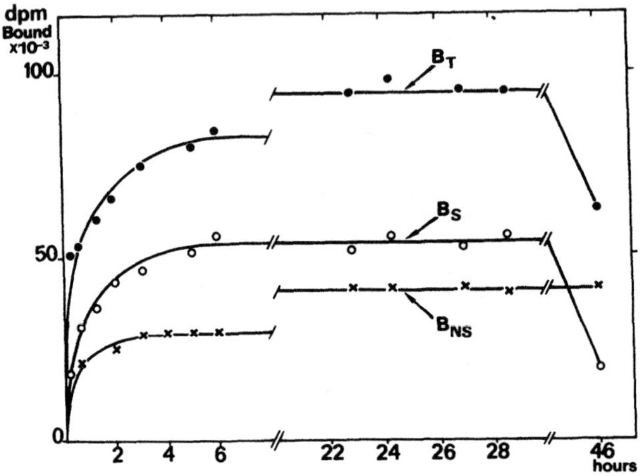

Figure 1. Time-course of the exchange of the synthetic progestin [^{3}H] R5020 with unlabeled progesterone in rat uterine nuclear progesterone-receptor complexes. Nuclei were incubated for varying periods of time at 0^{0}C with either 10 nM [^{3}H]R5020 (total binding, B_T) or 10 nM [^{3}H] R5020 and 2 μM unlabeled progesterone (nonspecific binding, B_{NS}). Specific binding (B_S) = (B_T) - (B_{NS}).

II - PROGESTERONE RECEPTORS IN THE RAT UTERUS DURING PREGNANCY

Results

Initial experiments were performed on total, nonfractionated, uteri (Vu Hai et al, 1978). The animals had been killed at various stages of pregnancy, and progesterone receptors were measured in cytosol and nuclei. Progesterone concentrations in blood were also determined.

The concentration of cytosol receptors was low at the beginning of pregnancy (about 1.5 pmoles/mg DNA on day 3) (Figure 2 and Table 3). This confirms previous observations of receptor levels in the guinea pig (Milgrom et al, 1972). Cytosol receptors decreased sharply on day 5, corresponding to an increase in nuclear progesterone-receptor complexes. The correspondence suggests a transfer of receptor from cytosol to nuclei. The concentration of cytosol receptors remained low until day 12 and then increased progressively from day 15 to 22, reaching about 6.5 pmoles/mg DNA. This increase was probably related to increased estradiol and decreased progesterone concentrations in blood. Either

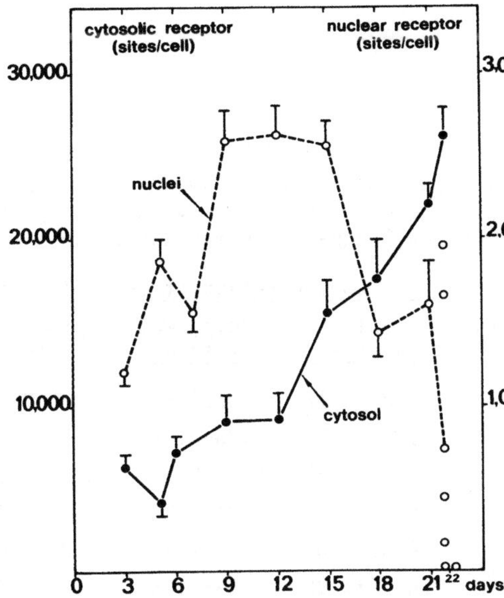

Figure 2. Variations in the concentration of uterine cytosolic (•) and nuclear (o) progesterone receptors during pregnancy in the rat. Day 1 of pregnancy was taken as the day of appearance of spermatozoa in the vagina. Results are means ± S.E.M., and the numbers of measurements are given in Table 3.

situation leads to stimulation of uterine receptor concentration (Milgrom et al, 1973, Vu Hai et al, 1976). On day 22 of pregnancy, cytosol receptor concentration was about 6.7 pmoles/mg DNA. This is comparable to the highest concentration observed during estrous cycle, about 7.6 pmoles/mg DNA, at proestrous.

Nuclear receptors followed a different pattern (Figure 2 and Table 3). Receptor concentration was low on day 3, increased slightly on day 5, peaked between days 9 and 15, and decreased to very low levels on day 22. Some animals probably on the verge of parturition had no detectable receptors in the nuclei on that day.

Discussion

The biological significance of cytosol and nuclear progesterone receptors still remains somewhat problematic. The concentration of nuclear steroid-receptor complexes reflects the magnitude of the biological effect of the hormone at a given moment. The concentration of nuclear complexes is a function of at least two factors: the concentration of hormone arriving at the target cell and the concentration of available cytosol receptor.

Table 3

Variations in the Concentrations of Progesterone in the Plasma and Uterine Progesterone Receptors in the Nuclei and Cytosol During Pregnancy in the Rat (means±S.E.M.)

Day of pregnancy	Number of rats	Concentration of Cytosolic Receptors: pmol/ uterus	pmol/g wet tissue	pmol/mg protein	pmol/mg DNA
3	4	1.81±0.17	6.05±0.52	0.30±0.02	1.57±0.20
5	7	1.19±0.15	3.73±0.54	0.14±0.02	1.01±0.14
6	6	2.02±0.26	5.47±0.51	0.22±0.04	1.78±0.22
9	7	5.04±0.95	6.91±1.28	0.28±0.04	2.27±0.40
12	7	8.67±2.04	6.01±1.16	0.22±0.05	2.28±0.40
15	7	20.76±3.30	9.54±1.35	0.31±0.03	3.97±0.48
18	7	27.22±4.08	6.55±0.85	0.23±0.02	4.47±0.55
21	6	28.60±3.17	8.54±0.59	0.29±0.03	5.59±0.28
22	7	39.42±4.80	9.99±0.56	0.36±0.04	6.67±0.60

Day of pregnancy	Number of rats	Concentration of Nuclear Receptors: pmol/ uterus	pmol/g wet tissue	pmol/mg DNA	ng/ml plasma progesterone
3	4	0.38±0.04	1.29±0.15	0.30±0.03	36.65±3.42
5	7	0.56±0.05	1.82±0.17	0.47±0.03	40.47±8.83
6	6	0.50±0.05	1.41±0.18	0.40±0.02	33.78±5.36
9	7	1.50±0.16	1.88±0.14	0.66±0.05	35.47±5.49
12	7	2.30±0.30	1.78±0.17	0.67±0.05	57.69±6.73
15	7	3.47±0.31	1.66±0.13	0.65±0.03	98.76±6.85
18	7	2.25±0.47	0.58±0.07	0.36±0.04	90.88±8.93
21	6	2.33±0.38	0.65±0.10	0.41±0.06	47.49±4.74
22	7	0.88±0.35	0.24±0.11	0.18±0.08	7.14±0.90

The concentration of the cytosol receptor reflects the cell's ability to respond to hormonal stimuli. When many cytosol receptors are present, a low concentration of hormone will elicit a marked biological response. Such an interpretation suggests that the low concentrations of progesterone prevailing during the last part of pregnancy may still provoke important biological effects since many receptors are present.

Two stages of pregnancy appear interesting in terms of receptor variations. At implantation receptors shift from cytosol to nuclei. The relationship of this translocation to blastocyst physiology will be discussed below.

III - PROGESTERONE AND ESTROGEN RECEPTORS AT IMPLANTATION SITES AND IN DECIDUALIZED ENDOMETRIUM

Hormones control implantation (Psychoyos, 1973), but the precise mechanism of this control is still poorly understood. Very little is known in particular about receptor concentrations during implantation. Previous experiments in which progesterone receptors were measured in whole uteri were clearly only a preliminary approach since differences are expected to arise between implantation sites and nonimplantation regions. Thus we have measured progesterone receptors separately in these two regions. Moreover, the role of estrogens in blastocyst implantation has been emphasized (Psychoyos, 1973) and it was necessary to consider the receptor for these hormones, as well.

Pregnant rats

Six-day pregnant rats were injected with Trypan blue. Thirty minutes after injection, the animals were killed. Implantation sites colored blue were excised in the cold, and endometrium was gently scraped off. Interimplantation regions of endometrium were similarly obtained. Estrogen (Anderson et al, 1972) and progesterone receptors (Tables 1 and 2) were measured in cytosol and nuclei.

For both estrogen and progesterone receptors, the concentration of nuclear receptors (expressed per mg DNA) was two-fold higher at implantation sites (Table 4). Concentration of cytosol receptors was only slightly higher in nonimplantation regions than in implantation sites. Concentration of proteins was considerably higher at implantation sites, probably due to local vascular changes. The qualitative characteristics of cytosol receptors in both implantation and nonimplantation regions were similar. Sedimentation on density gradients yielded similar patterns, and Scatchard analysis of the affinity for the hormone gave similar values for all regions of the endometrium ($K_D = 1.7 \times 10^{-9}$M for estradiol and $K_D = 3.3 \times 10^{-9}$M for R5020).

Thus the only difference observed between implantation zones and the remaining part of the endometrium is that more receptors were found in the nuclei of the nonimplantation endometrium. One explanation of this finding might be that more estrogen and progesterone are delivered to endometrial cells at implantation sites than to other regions. These hormones could be of maternal origin, brought through the vascular changes accompanying decidualization. Alternatively, the steroids could be supplied by the blastocyst, as Dickman et al (1976) suggested.

Table 4

Estradiol and Progesterone Receptors at Ovo-Implantation Sites in the Rat Endometrium*

	Implantation sites	Nonimplantation sites	Statistical significance of difference (pmoles/mg DNA)
Estradiol receptors			
In the cytosol			
pmoles/mg DNA	11.33±1.73	12.11±1.05	N.S.
pmoles/mg protein	0.42±0.03	0.96±0.06	
In the nuclei			
pmoles/mg DNA	8.83±0.34	4.62±0.33	p<0.001
Progesterone receptors			
In the cytosol			
pmoles/mg DNA	1.41±0.04	1.74±0.39	N.S.
pmoles/mg protein	0.17±0.03	0.35±0.10	
In the nuclei			
pmoles/mg DNA	0.86±0.07	0.45±0.02	p<0.001

*Rats were killed on the morning of the 6th day of pregnancy after receiving an intravenous injection of Trypan Blue. Implantation and nonimplantation regions of the endometrium were dissected. Progesterone and estradiol receptors were measured in cytosol and nuclei. The results given are the mean ± S.E.M. of 5 measurements for estradiol receptor and 6 for progesterone receptor. 30 animals were used for each measurement. N.S. = not significant.

Pseudopregnant rats

To answer the question about steroids from the blastocyst, receptors were measured after decidualization occurred but in the absence of a blastocyst. Rats were mated, and oviducts sectioned on day 1 of pregnancy. On the morning of day 5, a cotton thread was introduced into one of the uterine horns to provoke decidualization. Twenty-four hours later the animals were killed, and endometria were analyzed as described above. The concentrations of nuclear and cytosolic receptors per milligram of DNA were equal in the decidualized and the nondecidualized horns Table 5). This experiment showed that decidualization in the absence of the embryo was not accompanied by an increase in nuclear accumulation of estrogen and progesterone receptors. Strikingly the total cellular concentration of estradiol receptors was markedly lower in pseudopregnant than in pregnant rats (Table 4).

Table 5

Estradiol and Progesterone Receptors in Decidualized and Nondecidualized Endometrium of Pseudopregnant Rats*

	Decidualized horn	Nondecidualized horn
Estradiol receptors		
In the cytosol		
pmoles/mg DNA	1.23 ±0.12	1.33±0.17
pmoles/mg protein	0.093±0.001	0.38±0.07
In the nuclei		
pmoles/mg DNA	1.43 ±0.14	1.38±0.16
Progesterone receptors		
In the cytosol		
pmoles/mg DNA	2.25 ±0.21	2.27±0.23
pmoles/mg protein	0.161±0.016	0.44±0.06
In the nuclei		
pmoles/mg DNA	0.94 ±0.09	0.93±0.05

*Oviduct was sectioned on day 1 of pregnancy. On the morning of day 5 a cotton thread was introduced into one of the uterine horns. The animals were killed 24 hours later. Results are given as the mean ± S.E.M. 4 determinations were performed in each case. 20 rats were used for each determination. The differences between receptor concentration (pmoles/mg DNA) were not statistically significant.

Castrated pregnant rats

Another series of experiments was designed to examine whether or not the increased transfer of receptors to the nuclei at implantation zones was due to steroids of maternal origin. Castration on the morning of day 5 of pregnancy does not prevent implantation (P Sartor, manuscript in preparation). (In the absence of treatment by progesterone, however, the pregnancy will not be maintained.)

In the castrated animal most steroids of maternal origin are suppressed; only adrenal steroids are maintained. In spite of this, the 2-fold difference in nuclear receptors for both progesterone and estradiol was still observed in the castrated animals when comparing implantation and nonimplantation regions on the morning of day 6 (Table 6).

Table 6

	Implantation sites	Nonimplantation sites	Statistical significance of difference (pmoles/mg DNA)
Estradiol receptors			
In the cytosol			
pmoles/mg DNA	4.49±0.38	2.99±0.81	N.S.
pmoles/mg pr' ein	0.54±0.07	0.81±0.19	
I the nuclei			
pmoles/mg DNA	5.49±0.45	2.42±0.33	$p<0.001$
Progesterone recept			
In the cytosol			
pmoles/mg DNA	4.17±0.09	2.23±0.26	$p<0.05$
pmoles/mg protein	0.44±0.08	0.40±0.05	
In the nuclei			
pmoles/mg DNA	1.11±0.02	0.67±0.05	$p<0.001$

*Animals were castrated on the morning of day 5 of pregnancy. Endometrium from implantation zones and nonimplantation regions was obtained on the morning of day 6 and analyzed as described in Table 4. Results are given as the mean ± S.E.M. of 4 determinations. Thirty rats were used for each determination.

Another striking phenomenon was the increase in the total cellular concentration of progesterone receptors at implantation sites (from 9,200 to 21,300 sites/diploid genome) provoked by the castration of pregnant animals. The mechanism of this change is not well understood. It may be due to the suppression of most of the progesterone of maternal origin. Progesterone does decrease the concentration of its own rece (Milgrom et al, 1973).

Discussion

The concentration of nuclear receptors for estradiol and progesterone is twice as high at implantation sites as at nonimplantation regions of the endometrium in 6-day pregnant rats. One possible explanation for this finding is that a higher concentration of steroids is supplied to the cells in these endometrial regions. The steroids may originate from the blastocyst since receptor distribution does not differ when decidualization occurs in the absence of the embryo. Moreover, the difference between implantation and nonimplantation regions of the endometrium still persists even when most steroids of maternal origin are eliminated.

Other explanations of these results, for example, the secretion by the blastocyst of a factor favoring nuclear transfer of steroid receptors, seem less likely. In any case, the blastocyst appears to exert a local effect on the subcellular distribution of estradiol and progesterone receptors in the adjacent endometrium.

ACKNOWLEDGMENTS

This work was supported by the INSERM, the DGRST and the Fondation pour la Recherche Médicale Francaise. Y. Douillet has typed the manuscript.

REFERENCES

Anderson J, Clark JH and Peck EJ (1972). Oestrogen and nuclear binding sites. Determination of specific sites by [^{3}H] oestradiol exchange. Biochem J 126, 561-567.

Csapo AI (1969). The four direct regulatory factors of myometrial function. In: Progesterone: its regulatory effect in the myometrium (GEW Wolstenholme and J Knight, eds), Churchill, London, pp. 13-42.

Dickmann Z, Dey SK and Gupta J (1976). A new concept: control of early pregnancy by steroid hormones originating in the preimplantation embryo. Vitam Horm 34, 215-242.

George FW and Wilson JD (1978). Estrogen formation in the early rabbit embryo. Science 199, 200-201.

Head RB, Perry JS and Challis JRC (1973). The hormonal maintenance of pregnancy. In: Endocrinology of the female reproductive system. Handbook of Physiology (Greep RO, Astwood EB, Geiger SR, eds), American Physiological Society, Washington DC, pp. 217-260.

King RJB and Mainwaring WIP (1974). Steroid cell interactions. Butterworths, London.

Milgrom E, Atger M, Perrot M and Baulieu EE (1972). Progesterone in uterus and plasma: uterine progesterone receptors during the estrus cycle and implantation in the guinea pig. Endocrinology 90, 1071-1078.

Milgrom E, Luu Thi M, Atger M and Baulieu EE (1973). Mechanisms regulating the concentration and the conformation of progesterone receptor(s) in the uterus. J Biol Chem 248, 6366-6374.

Psychoyos A (1973). Hormonal control of ovoimplantation. Vitam Horm 31, 201-256.

Scatchard G (1949). The attraction of proteins for small molecules and ions. Ann NY Acad Sci 51, 660-672.

Vu Hai MT, Logeat F, Warembourg M and Milgrom E (1977). Hormonal control of progesterone receptors. Ann NY Acad Sci 286, 199-209.

Vu Hai MT and Milgrom E (1978a). Characterization and assay of the progesterone receptor in rat uterine cytosol. J Endocrinol 76, 21-31.

Vu Hai MT and Milgrom E (1978b). Characterization and assay of the progesterone receptor in rat uterine nuclei. J Endocrinol 76, 33-41.

Vu Hai MT, Logeat F and Milgrom E (1978). Progesterone receptors in the rat uterus: variations in cytosol and nuclei during the oestrous cycle and pregnancy. J Endocrinol 76, 43-48.

DISCUSSION

FINN: You were rather vague about the species in which uteroglobin has been shown. Could you please be a little more specific and tell us in which species it has actually been looked for thoroughly and not shown.

MILGROM: The two questions are linked and difficult to answer. They are: 1) the biological role of uteroglobin and 2) its species distribution. Since the role of this protein is not clearly understood, the search for it in other species has involved methods which are not very satisfactory: for instance gel electrophoresis followed by staining. The putative proteins homologous to rabbit uteroglobin being supposed to have the same electrophoretic mobility and be present in similary high concentration. Alternatively some authors have developed antibodies against rabbit uteroglobin and have looked for immunological cross reactivity in other species. In human endometrial washings these experiments have led to conflicting results. In my opinion it will be very difficult to obtain a clear answer on this issue as long as the function of uteroglobin is not known and we cannot search for this protein through its functional properties.

FINN: The reason you usually get asked these questions is because they are important, and satisfactory answers aren't forthcoming. How happy are you about extrapolating from results using a marker in one species to others if you are not sure that marker is present in those species. The reason I ask is that I am a little worried about work on the rabbit. Progesterone does have rather different events in the rabbit than it has in other species studied. For instance, in most species that we have looked at, progesterone, instead of stimulating gland proliferation as it does in the rabbit, has the reverse effect and stops it. Furthermore, the rabbit requires a very much smaller dose of progesterone to affect the endometrium. How happy are you about extrapolating from the rabbit?

MILGROM: We have not extrapolated anything up to now. Uteroglobin and its messenger RNA may be used as convenient markers of progesterone action in the rabbit endometrium (Atger and Milgrom, 1977, Atger et al, 1980). As the methods are improving, other markers, technically more difficult to characterize and isolate will probably be described in the rabbit and in other species in the near future.

Only comparison of results obtained through the use of different markers in various species will show us the generality of the results obtained. May I remark that the rabbit endometrium has been widely used in pharmacological tests to characterize progestins.

MOULTON: In your experiment in which you implanted a thread to determine whether the blastocyst was contributing steroids to the receptor translocation, I was wondering if you were seeing a general effect or if trauma in one horn affected the other horn? Secondly, I was wondering if you had thought of using oil introduced through the cervix as a stimulus for only one horn, perhaps minimizing possible surgical trauma?

MILGROM: In the experiments using pseudopregnant rats there was no difference between the decidualized and nondecidualized horns in terms of receptor concentration or distribution.

MOULTON: Well, could the surgical activity in the one horn have affected the other horn to raise receptor numbers in both of them equally.

MILGROM: You are right. There are differences in total receptors concentrations between the endometria of pregnant and pseudopregnant rats.

MOULTON: The oil stimulus would be a way around that because you could do it in just that one horn without possible general trauma.

MILGROM: I do not think that the trauma was effective in both horns since one horn was decidualized and the other was not.

KENNEDY: I was intrigued by your data which indicated that the concentrations of the receptors are elevated within the implantation site and wondered if you know, or would care to speculate on the functional significance of these findings. Presumably, these elevated concentrations are not essential for decidualization since it is possible to get decidualization in response to artificial stimuli without this apparent increase in nuclear receptors.

MILGROM: Our results show an increase in nuclear transfer of receptor in the endometrium adjacent to the blastocyst. The most likely but not the only explanation for these results is local delivery of steroids from blastocyst to the endometrium. I do not care to speculate any further about this result and I may refer you to the review by Dickman (1976).

GERSCHENSON: I mentioned before to Dr. Milgrom some data from my lab on the role of blastokinin. Dr. James Murai in our lab started looking at the possible function of blastokinin or uteroglobin using a different approach. As we have cultures of rabbit uterine epithelium, we have added blastokinin to culture medium. The hypothesis was that since progesterone induces blastokinin, blastokinin may be an intermediate or messenger effector of progesterone. We found that it works in the opposite way. Blastokinin was found to be a proliferation factor for cultured rabbit uterine epithelium, even at very low concentrations, and what is most interesting is that it appears that blastokinin is increasing the levels of $PGF_2\alpha$, which is the real growth factor. This effect was not found on cultures of 3T3 cells which suggests that the blastokinin affects not the blastocysts but the endometrium.

MILGROM: Your results are very interesting. There is no consensus to date on the biological role of uteroglobin.

GLASSER: I guess many of you who have not yet entered the receptor field realize that the bloom is off the rose. From here on productive work will get increasingly difficult. Many simplicities that we generated to help us at very early stages are now falling to the force of new data. I think the pervasiveness of Dr. Milgrom's work on rabbit uteroglobin is that it clearly opens up the possibility of post-translational control as a mechanism of action for steroid hormones. This evidence has not been easy to obtain. Dr. Milgrom's data now make this a valid working hypothesis for many of the effects that we don't understand. I would like to suggest a procedural mechanism for the induction of decidualization that might bring more profit.

We know that if we use a thread or a needle as a deciduogenic stimulus the oil decidualization people will always discount the data by arguing that we have potentially wounded or traumatized the stimulated horn. We have opted to use Hank's solution as the deciduogenic agent. It is as effective as oil in the rat and does not persist in the lumen for long periods of time. It is also an excellent diluent for a large number of possible modulations.

If, in place of your cotton thread, we place 0.1 ml Hank's with nanogram quantities of progesterone in the lumen of the right uterine horn and instil Hank's without progesterone in the contralateral horn we induce decidualization in both cornua. After induction, in the horn injected with progesterone, the estradiol receptor concentration largely limited to the antimesometrial side will decrease. This is the type of change noted in a pregnant uterus. The contralateral horn, not exposed to progesterone, does not lose estradiol receptors. This is typical of a sterile, pseudopregnant horn.

The use of Hank's solution containing hormones, antibiotics, etc., has been a very effective probe with which to study the induction of deciduogenesis (Glasser, 1972; Glasser and Clark, 1975).

Additional circumstantial evidence supports a role for steroids in the implantation process. In vitro culture demonstrates that trophectoderm cells synthesize and secrete gonadal steroids. The chronology of this secretion would argue that in rat and mouse these steroid effects do not appear to be products of the free floating uterine blastocysts, nor do they seem to be involved in the attachment of the blastocyst to luminal epithelium. After blastocysts hatch, they attach either plastic or epithelial stromal or myometrium monolayers. It is not until this point when in natural gestation (using the rat as an example) the trophectoderm is penetrating the basal lamina underlying the luminal epithelium that appreciable steroid secretion by trophectoderm can be detected. At this time the dynamics of decidual steroid receptors change; probably in response to trophectoderm steroid secretion.

FINN: I would like to suggest a third possibility related to cell numbers to explain the difference between the implantation sites and the nonimplantation sites. At the site of implanting blastocyst there is a local cell proliferation by multiplication of the stromal cells confined to that area. If the nuclear receptors were more abundant in the stromal cells, and the cell number was increasing while in the other tissues, for example the myometrium and the glands, they were not: this would also change the distribution of receptors. Possibly at the same time the stromal cells in nonimplanting areas might be dying off. (There is evidence that if stromal cells aren't decidualized then many die.) You might get a big change during the implantation in the proportion of stromal cells to other cells between the implantation and nonimplantation sites. If your second experiment used artificially decidualized horns then this explanation probably isn't valid. However, as a general principle, I think that when you are measuring receptors, you should take into account cell numbers and changes in the relative populations in the various tissues of the uterus.

MILGROM: Differences in receptor concentrations in various physiological states always have two possible explanations: either the cellular concentration of receptor has changed or the cell types (containing different amounts of receptor) have changed. During the estrous cycle autoradiography clearly shows that cellular concentration of progesterone receptor has changed. However, in the experiments on implantation sites which I have presented, the difference is not in receptor concentrations but in receptor distribution between cytosol and nuclei. This is even more difficult to explain in terms of changes in cell populations. This difference in concentration must be produced by some factor(s) which promotes transfer of estrogen and progesterone receptors to the nucleus and which apparently comes from the blastocyst. One possibility is that this factor is simply the steroid which binds to the receptor.

FINN: But the hormone may be shifted to the nucleus more easily in some cells than in others, this would give an apparent change in hormone distribution due to a change in cell population.

MILGROM: Yes. This is another explanation if for some reason there are differences between cells in terms of subcellular distribution of receptor.

LOBL: I was wondering if you could explain in more detail how the autoradiography was done. Progesterone is a freely diffusible molecule. When you talk about 6 months to a year for autoradiographic development, I was wondering how you handled that.

MILGROM: The autoradiography experiments (Warembourg and Milgrom, 1977) have been done by the technique initially described by Stumpf. There is no fixation, and autoradiography is done on freeze dried sections. Hormone is not redistributed in these conditions.

FINN: What were you actually counting?

MILGROM: The dots per cell. You count a hundred cells in different sections.

BAZER: Certainly in the pig, the sequence seems to start out the same way you describe for the rabbit, where you have estrogen and then progesterone. We use the purple protein uteroferrin secreted by the pig endometrium in our studies. The blastocysts produce estrogen in the pig with one peak occurring from about day 12 to day 30. During that period uteroferrin secretion is shut off; and then when estrogen drops, uteroferrin secretion increases markedly; and with the second estrogen peak, from about 75 days to term, the uteroferrin secretion declines again. So in the pig, this particular marker seems to be secreted when progesterone is high relative to estrogen, i.e., it is somewhat similar to the rabbit. We have data in the horse which show the same sort of sequence. But in the sheep and the cow, as in experiments done with Dr. Barron, it seems that in addition to progesteorne, as Dixon and Gibbons (1979) reported in the cow with estrogen, you can get a certain amount of secretion. In addition to progesterone and estrogen there may be a need for some placental factors, whatever they might be. The time of appearance of maximum secretory activity happens to correspond with the time of large increases in plasma lactogen. Whether that is the actual hormone of importance or not I don't know. I suspect it contributes to species difference. In the large animals I think you need a high progesterone background to elicit the initial secretory response anyway, and this may be modified by other steroid and/or protein hormones.

DEY: You observe higher nuclear progesterone and estrogen receptors in the endometrial cells at the implantation site as opposed to interimplantation sites. I wonder whether you removed the blastocysts before you processed the endometrium for determination of these receptors.

MILGROM: Yes.

References:

Atger, M and Milgrom, E (1977). A progesterone-induced messenger RNA. Translation, purification and preliminary characterization of uteroglobin mRNA. J Biol Chem 252: 5412-5418.

Atger, M, Mornon, JP, Savouret, JF, Loosfelt, H, Fridlansky, F and Milgrom, E (1980). Uteroglobin: a model for the study of the mechanism of action of steroid hormones. In: Steroid Induced Uterine Proteins (Beato, Ed) Elsevier/North Holland, Amsterday. (In press.)

Dickman, Z, Dey, SK and Gupta, JS (1976). A new concept: Control of early pregnancy by steroid hormones originating in the preimplantation embryo. Vitam Horm 34: 215-242.

Dixon, SN and Gibbons, RA (1979). Proteins in the uterine secretions of the cow. J Reprod Fertil 56: 119-127.

Glasser, SR (1972). The uterine environment in implantation and decidualization. In: Reproductive Biology (HA Balen and SR Glasser, eds), Excerpta Medica Foundation, Amsterdam. p 776-883.

Glasser, SR and Clark, JH (1975). A determinant role for progesterone in the development of uterine sensitivity to decidualization and ovo-implantation. In: The Developmental Biology of Reproduction (Markert, C and Papaconstantinou, J, eds), Academic Press, New York. p 311-345.

Warembourg, M and Milgrom, E (1977). Radioautography of the uterus and vagina after [^{3}H]Progesterone injection into guinea pigs at various periods of the estrous cycle. Endocrinology 100: 175-181.

8

Hormone Production by Rat Blastocysts and Mid-Gestation Trophoblast in Vitro

Shirley A. McCormack
Stanley R. Glasser

I. Introduction

The trophoblast is a specialized tissue unique to mammals that has evolved in response to the demands of viviparity. Its overall function is that of an interface between the developing embryo and its mother. Most of our detailed knowledge of this tissue has been gained from the study of a few species, notably mouse, rat, rabbit and pig. Because the functions of the trophoblast, including hormone production, are inextricably tied to its cellular associations at any particular time during development, the following brief review of trophoblast development is given. Most of this work has been carried out in the mouse. The rat blastocyst is similar in most respects. Where other species have been used, they will be noted.

A. Differentiation and Development

"Trophoblast" is a general term applied to a variety of cell types which are derived by direct descent from the cells of the outer wall of trophectoderm of the blastocyst. These cells, probably determined as trophoblast between the 8- and 16-cell stage, are the major cell population of the zygote during the peri-implantation period (Gardner and Rossant, 1976). Their name implies a nutritive function, which, though only one of their many capabilities, emphasizes that they do not contribute to the formation of the embryo itself.

The variety of cell types included by the word "trophoblast" includes the mural trophoblast (cells forming the abembryonic wall of the blastocyst) and the polar trophoblast (cells overlying the inner cell mass or ICM). Cells of the mural trophoblast differentiate into the primary giant cells while cells of the polar trophoblast form the ectoplacental cone and the secondary giant cells (Snell and Stevens, 1966). Mural trophoblast cells are terminally differentiated and do not divide further, but polar trophoblast cells retain their ability to differentiate and divide as long as they maintain their association with the ICM (Gardner and Rossant, 1976).

At the time of implantation (day 3 of pregnancy) the mouse blastocyst consists of approximately 64 cells of which about 13 are enclosed inner cells which will become the embryo and its membranes, and the remainder are flat, tightly joined cells facing the external environment (Graham, 1971). The polar trophoblast cells form the ectoplacental cone which is the most potent invasive area of the trophoblast (Kirby, 1962, 1965) and, further, maintains the reserve of diploid cells which provide the highly differentiated cells of the definitive placenta. The first of these are the wandering giant cells which, actively phagocytic for the first 10 days of gestation, open up the maternal blood vessels which they contact, thereby creating the hemochorial state. The trophoblastic trabeculae persist as tubules carrying maternal blood. Fetal mesoderm inserts itself between the tubules as dividing septa into which the fetal blood vessels grow. The septa eventually interlace to form a labyrinth and thus establish the labyrinthine type of placental internal structure (Ramsey, p. 134, 1975). The trophoblast in the definitive rat placenta is trilaminar (Davies and Glasser, 1968) consisting of an outer layer (layer 1) of cytotrophoblast and an intermediate (layer 2) and deep layer (layer 3) thought to be syncytial (Bjorkman, 1970) although proof of this is lacking (Wynn, 1975). The cellular sheets of layer 1 are fenestrated allowing layer 2 to protrude into the maternal blood space. The cells in layer 1 occassionally undergo giant cell transformation even in late pregnancy (Davies and Glasser, 1968).

In the development of the human blastocyst, trophoblastic cells can be distinguished from ICM cells by the 58-cell stage (96 hours) at which time 53 cells are trophoblastic and 5 are ICM cells. The first contact with the mother is made by the polar trophectoderm shortly after the blastocyst enters the uterus between days 6 and 7, but implantation is not complete until the end of day 9 (Hertig and Rock, 1954). The trophoblast penetrates the lumina of the utero-placental arteries during the early implantation stages and further penetration is achieved by individual wandering giant cells. Progressively, the trophoblast of the early trophoblastic trabeculae differentiates into cyto- and syncytiotrophoblast. The trabeculae are coverted into definitive villi by the ingrowth of mesoderm, and blood vessels (derived from the rudimentary stalk of the allantosis) appear in the mesodermal cores of the villi. Thus, both cytotrophoblast and syncytiotrophoblast form the basal trophoblastic shell which constitutes the junction between maternal and fetal tissues. Unlike the rat and mouse, it is primarily the syncytiotrophoblast which is in contact with maternal blood in the human. The cytotrophoblast continues to serve throughout pregnancy as a source of syncytiotrophoblast when regeneration is required to replace damaged cells (Ramsey, 1975).

B. Functions

Various functions of the trophoblast have been deduced from these anatomical and morphological relationships. Some, but not all, have proved amenable to observation and experimentation. Although the specific mechanisms employed may differ widely between species, all of the known functions of the trophoblast are directed toward providing the support and protection necessary to maintain the developing embryo within the uterus. These functions are nutrition, implantation, proliferation, communication and immune defense. They are accomplished through the agency of a battery of hormones, steroid and protein, and possibly other factors thus far unidentified which are able to influence, directly or indirectly, the uterus, ovary, mammary gland and pituitary. Other functions not directly related to hormone production include the selection and exchange of molecules for early nutrition and waste removal via the blastocoel and later the establishment of the fetal-maternal circulatory system. In different species the trophoblast has varying degrees of invasive, phagocytotic and angiogenic capability in order to provide for the initial contact of the embryo with the uterus and for its retention and establishment there. Some of the trophoblast cells (initially those under the direct influence of the ICM) continue to proliferate. Other, pushed farther and farther from the immediate vicinity of the ICM, cease dividing, become polyploid, and carry out the major part of the hormone production. In the human, cytotrophoblast in the villi have immense and longlasting proliferative ability because they must provide an elaborate and extensive cellular support structure for the embryo as well as keep this structure functioning and repaired throughout the entire gestation period. It is not inconceivable that this proliferative ability is related to the trophoblast's capability to provide itself with a mitotically permissive environment of estrogen in some species.

It is clear that the possible production of hormones by the trophoblast as well as its susceptibility to regulation by them are important questions in the elucidation of the actual mechanisms by which the synchrony (Chang, 1950, Noyes et al, 1963; Psychoyos, 1973; Glasser and Clark, 1975) and biological accomodation of the fetal and maternal organisms are accomplished.

In the past valuable clues to the presence of enzyme systems necessary for steriodogenic pathways have been gained by histochemical means, but in vitro systems are obviously required for the actual measurement of hormone production by the trophoblast if overwhelming dilution by maternal hormones is to be avoided. Data obtained from in vitro systems are limited, as is well known, in that they can only imply what is possible rather than what actually happens in vivo. Furthermore, because of deficiencies either impossible to remedy (such as physical relationships) or not yet known to us in supplying the proper conditions, in vitro systems may many times fail even to indicate what is possible. Nevertheless, the ability to separate maternal from fetal factors is a valuable tool for obtaining information which can be used in the context of other facts gotten in vivo. In the following we will review primarily recent literature on the production of hormones by trophoblast, contrast in vivo with in vitro production where possible, and discuss some of our recent findings in this area.

II. Hormone production

A. Steroids

Although in some species the ovary is the primary source of the estrogen and progesterone required to condition the uterus for the establishment and maintenance of pregnancy, the conceptus may also be able to contribute these hormones to varying degrees to modulate its environment. Intriguing contrasts exist between species in this regard.

1. Rodents

The rodent placenta possesses enzyme systems which are required for steroidogenesis. One of these, Δ^5-3β-hydroxysteroid dehydrogenase (HSD) converts pregnenolone to progesterone (P) and has been demonstrated histochemically (Deane et al, 1962; Ferguson and Christie, 1967; Botte et al, 1968) in the rodent placenta as well as biochemically (Weiner, 1974; Chan and Leathem, 1975). Using a histochemical technic modified from Deane et al, (1972), Dickmann and Dey (1974) reported the presence of HSD in peri-implantation blastocysts (as young as the 8-cell stage) and of estradiol-17β-hydroxysteroid dehydrogenase (17 β-HSD) as early as day 4 (Dey and Dickmann, 1974). Sherman and co-workers have confirmed the presence of HSD by means of the conversion of labelled pregnenolone to P (Marcal et al. , 1975) in the rat trophoblast and have measured the production of P by mouse blastocysts and mid-gestation trophoblast in culture (Salomon and Sherman, 1975: Sherman and Atienza, 1977). But even under the most favorable conditions and with an exquisitely sensitive P assay they were never able to demonstrate the production of P by the blastocyst before or during implantation stages. Marcal et al (1975) found the HSD first detectable on day 11 in the rat and Chew and Sherman (1975) found the enzyme on day 9 in the mouse. Later, under slightly different conditions, P production by the mouse blastocysts was detected between equivalent gestation day (EGD) 6 and 7 (starting with 2-cell embryos). (Equivalent gestation day = day of pregnancy embryos are collected plus the number of days in culture, i.e. 2 + 4 = 6.) In 6 out of 7 incubation experiments using EGD 5 and 6 blastocysts, no androstenedione could be detected after incubation with dehydroepiandrosterone (DHEA) as substrate. Post blastocysts cultures, however, were able to convert significant amounts of DHEA into androstenedione as well as to metabolize the androstenedione futher (Sherman and Atienza, 1977). Neither laboratory could find evidence of the regulation of P production by gonadotropins whether of pituitary or placental origin (Dickmann and Day, 1974; Salomon and Sherman, 1975).

The trophoblast giant cells have been consistently the site of localization of the HSD. Chew and Sherman (1975) separated EDG 10 trophoblastic tissue into 3 fractions on the basis of nuclear size. The specific activity of the HSD in the giant cell fraction was 3 times greater than that in the intermediate cell fraction and 15 times that of the small cell fraction, in agreement with earlier histochemical localization of the enzyme (Deane et al, 1962; Ferguson and

Christie, 1967; Botte et al, 1968). The embryo, the yolk sac, and the decidua had very low levels of HSD activity. An apparent disparity in the localization of HSD activity between these studies and those of Sheth et al (1978) in which HSD activity is reported to reside primarily in the parietal yolk sac is, in reality, a matter of terminology and dissection technic. Dissections made by Sherman and co-workers (Marcal et al, 1975; Salomon and Sherman, 1975) did not attempt to separate the yolk sac (presumably viseral and parietal) from the trophoblast on days 8 and 9. From late on day 9 through day 12, the embryo and the yolk sac (presumably the viseral yolk sac) were removed from the trophoblast (Sherman, 1971). The dissection made by Sheth et al (1978) were done on day 11 and separated the visceral from the parietal yolk sac as well as from the chorioallantoic placenta which they assayed separately. The visceral yolk sac consists of extraembryonic endoderm and mesoderm. The parietal yolk sac, on the other hand, consists of extraembryonic endoderm, Reichert's membrane, and trophoblast giant cells (next to the maternal dicedua). The remnant of the yolk sac cavity divides the viseral from the parietal yolk sac wall. When Sheth et al, (1978) divided the parietal yolk sac between Reichert's membrane and the extraembryonic endoderm, they found most of the HSD activity in the trophoblast giant cells of the parietal yolk sac. Sherman's group had also found the HSD activity in the trophoblast giant cells which they considered under "trophoblast" rather than "yolk sac". Both groups found maximal specific activity of HSD on day 13 with maximal total production of P per conceptus occurring later: 4.3 ± 1.5 nmoles/min/conceptus on day 15 (Marcal et al, 1975) and 1.3 nmoles/min/conceptus on day 17 (Sheth et al, 1978).

This production of P from pregnenolone measured in homogenates of fresh tissue is many times the maximum measured in the medium from mouse blastocysts cultured to similar EGD in the presence of pregnenolone and collected and expressed on a 24-hour basis. In the latter case, concentrations of 0.5 to 0.8 pmoles/24 h/blastocyst were achieved by cultured mouse blastocysts of EGD 10-11 (Sherman and Atienza, 1977). When the same investigators cultured blastocysts singly on EGD 10-11, they obtained an average of 2.5 pmoles P/blastocyst/24 h produced from added pregnenolone. They found that the maximal amounts of P measured in the cultured mouse blastocysts varied from 0.5 to 5 pmoles/day. They attributed the variation to further metabolism of the P by variable amounts of surviving ICM derivatives. The capability to synthesize androstenedione from DHEA has been demonstrated in the mouse placenta. 5α-reduced metabolites result from the further metabolism of androstenedione. The presence of 3β-HSD, 17β-HSD and 5α-reductase was shown at day 15 but at day 10, 17β-HSD was lacking. No testosterone (T), dihydrotestosterone or estrogen was detected (Okker-Reitsma, 1976).

2. Others

Enzyme systems capable of synthesizing cholesterol and pregnenolone from acetate have been demonstrated in the 6-day rabbit blastocyst (Huff and Eik-Nes, 1966). Furthermore, the enzyme systems HSD and 17β-HSD, responsible for the conversion of pregnenolone to P, androstenedione to T, and estrone to estradiol-17β (E) have also been demonstrated histochemically in the 6-day rabbit blastocyst (Dickmann et al, 1975). These findings have led to the suspicion that pre-implantation rabbit blastocysts may synthesize steroids which are involved in the process of implantation. On the other hand, there is evidence that the significant concentrations of P present in the pre-implantation rabbit blastocyst may have come from the P which is present in rabbit uterine fluid and originates from the ovary (Seamark and Lutwak-Mann, 1972; Fujimoto and Sundaram, 1978; Angle and Mead, 1979). Furthermore, extensive metabolism of the P takes place in the rabbit blastocyst, but the end products are inactive metabolities of P (5β-pregnanedione and 5β-pregnanolone) and not further steroids on the pathway to estrogens (Singh and Booth, 1978). The latter investigators suggested that, since they were unable to find any evidence of E synthesis by blastocysts from either P or androgens, since high levels of E were found in blastocysts from super-ovulated rabbits, and since the injection of tritiated E resulted in its appearance in uterine tissue, uterine flushings and blastocysts, that the E present in rabbit blastocysts was, at least partly, of maternal origin.

The porcine and bovine blastocyst do appear to be capable of steroidogenesis. In the pig and the cow, implantation is superficial (non-invasive), no decidual reaction occurs, an early yolk sac is functional but the definitive placenta is chorioallantoic and the placental membrane is epitheliochorial. In the cow, attachment occurs between 30 and 35 days of pregnancy and gestation lasts 280 days. In the pig, attachment occurs between days 14 and 18 following and concommittant with elongation of the blastocyst on days 13-15. Gestation continues to 112-115 days (Ramsey, 1975). These blastocysts contain many more cells at implantation stages than do mouse and rat blastocysts.

Definitive evidence for the synthesis of estrone and E from pregnenolone by the pig blastocyst by day 12 of pregnancy has been reported by Gadsby and co-workers (1976). The presence of the necessary enzyme systems had been demonstrated earlier (Perry et al, 1975). Peak levels of estrone and E occur in the blastocysts at day 12-13. The estrogen concentrations suggest a gradient from blastocyst to uterine endometrium. The pig blastocyst, though capable of synthesizing P, probably does so as a precursor to E. The P present in the pig blastocyst is likely to have come from the maternal ovaries since its maximum in blastocysts and in maternal peripheral plasma occur at the same time (days 12-13 of pregnancy) (Flint et al, 1979).

Steroidogenesis by the bovine blastocyst has been studied by Shemesh and co-workers (1979) by comparing the accumulation of steroids in medium from cultured blastocysts with medium from blastocysts frozen immediately upon placing them in medium. These authors found P production beginning with day 13 and continuing on days 15 and 16. No T was found on day 13 but T was found on days 15 and 16. E was detected in some but not in all blastocysts. It was suggested that the E might be present because of the binding of this hormone by a protein. The bovine placenta is known to have a high sulfurylating ability (Holcenberg, 1965) and estrogen sulphotransferase has been isolated, purified, and characterized from bovine placenta (Adams and Low, 1974).

The capability of the primate or human preimplantation blastocyst to make steroids is unknown, but steroidogenesis by the feto-placental-maternal unit has bene extensively studied and documented. The steroidogenic steps carried out by these various compartments are complementary (Diczfalusy, 1970).

In several species of non-human primates (baboon, rhesus, squirrel, and cynomologus monkeys) the placentas have been shown to be capable of converting androstenedione to estrogens and pregnenolone to P and to be further capable of metabolizing P to 20α-dihydroxyprogesterone, 6β-hydroxyprogesterone and to 5α ring A saturated compounds (Ainsworth & Ryan, 1969). In this respect, they do not resemble the human placenta which does not metabolize P further to any significant extent (Solomon, 1966). The orangutan placenta, however, resembles the human much more closely in that it converts androstenedione to estrone and E, efficiently converts pregnenolone to P, and does not metabolize P further (Ainsworth & Ryan, 1969).

B. Gonadotropins

In general, the placenta secretes two kinds of peptide hormones during pregnancy. These are the chorionic gonadrotropins (CG) and the placental lactogens (PL) or somatomammotropins. In those eutherian species in which the gestation time exceeds the length of the reproductive cycle, at least one of these hormones is a part of the luteotropic complex that supports the corpus luteum in its production of P beyond the time of its normal cyclic regression.

1. Rodents

Evidence for rat PL (rPL) was first reported by Astwood and Greep in the late 1930's (1938, 1939). The tissue source of rPL as well as its luteo-mammotropic actions were conclusively demonstrated by Lyons and co-workers (1950, 1955). rPL reaches a maximum in rat serum on day 12 of pregnancy (Matthies, 1967; Kelly et al, 1973) and in placental tissue between days 15 and 17. rPL has been isolated and characterized from late pregnancy rat placenta (Robertson & Friesen, 1975). Using an RRA in which ovine prolactin (oPRL) was used as the standard and particulate rabbit mammary gland receptor bound labelled oPRL, Kelly et al, (1973a,b) found that day 12 pregnant rat serum contained up to 1.6 μg oPRL-like activity/ml and day 12 placenta contained < 1 μg/placenta. Rat blastocysts placed under the kidney capsule have been shown to produce luteotropin. Cyclic mice bearing ectopic rat blastocysts enter pseudopregnancy and both rats and mice go into prolonged pseudopregnancy following ectopic blastocyst transplantation at the time of normal implantation (Zeilmaker and Verhamme, 1978).

Evidence for a rat CG (rCG) is accumulating although its existence is still not entirely unequivocal. Some investigators have found evidence of rCG (Astwood et al, 1938; Linkie and Niswender, 1973; Haour et al, 1976; Blank et al, 1979). Others have been unable to detect rCG (Jost and Millot, 1953; Chowdhury and Steinberger, 1976). Wide and Hobson (1978) fractionated acetone-ether extracts of rat, mouse and hamster placenta by molecular sieve chromatography on Sephadex G-200. The fractions were tested for immunoreactivity to hCG, and its α and β subunits and the elution profiles were compared. The results indicated a CG in the placentas of all 3 rodents structurally similar to hCG and composed of α and β subunits. Bambra and Gombe (1978) treated rats for 5 days from days 6, 11, or 16 of pregnancy with anti-PMSG and anti-hCG and found variable necrosis of trophoblastic cells from the outer chorionic cells to the inner layers. Fetal death and resorption was 100% at the very high dose level of 10 mg/day in early and mid-pregnancy. In late pregnancy, some litters went to term. Immunofluorescence with conjugates of anti-hCG and anti-pregnant mare serum gonadotropin (PMSG) showed sharp localization in the giant and secondary trophoblast cell layers at the fetomaternal junction.
These authors concluded that an hCG or PMSG-like substance is produced by rat chorionic cells and that it plays an immunosuppresive role during pregnancy by complexing with cell membrane receptors of the outermost trophoblast giant cells and chorionic cells. Blank, Dufau and Friesen (1979) have recently reported a gonadotropin-like activity (GnLA) in the serum of pregnant rats measured by the rat interstitial cell T bioassay. The GnLA was detected at day 9, reached a peak on day 11 and declined to undetectable levels by day 15. Since the peak of rPL in concommittant samples occurred on days 12 and 13 of pregnancy, this discrepancy between the time course of appearance was taken as additional evidence that the GnLA was separate from rPL as well as from pituitary LH which remained low throughout pregnancy.

2. Others

In the rabbit, neither ovariectomy nor hypophysectomy are tolerated at any time during pregnancy. The luteotropic complex in this species appears to consist of prolactin along with estrogen from the ovary. Therefore, one would not expect to find sufficient production of either PL or CG by the rabbit trophoblast to materially support the pregnancy. Some investigators have, nevertheless, reported evidence for gonadotropic factors from the rabbit blastocyst. Singh and Adams (1978) reported that the rate of increase of serum P was significantly higher in pregnant than in pseudopregnant does from day 5-7 of pregnancy and that the transfer of day 4 or 5 blastocysts to synchronous pseudopregnant does caused a significant increase in P levels in comparison to pseudopregnant does without blastocysts. Others have reported high levels of an hCG/LH-like material in rabbit morulae (Asch et al, 1978) and blastocysts (Varma et al, 1979) as determined by immunofluorescence.

On the other hand, Ellinwood and co-workers (1979) could detect no difference in serum P concentration between pregnant and pseudopregnant rabbits at any time prior to implantation. They did find a factor in blastocoelic fluid which reduced the binding of ^{125}I-hCG to luteal membrane receptor sites but this factor was also present in uterine flushings from pregnant as well as pseudopregnant rabbits and had an estimated molecular weight of > 150,000. Furthermore, rabbit blastocysts collected 120 h after insemination produced no detectable large molecular weight protein after incubation with tritiated amino acids for 24 h. Thus, these data suggest that the rabbit blastocyst does not secrete an hCG/LH-like factor but may take up maternal gonadotropins from the uterine fluid.

In human pregnancy, either ovariectomy or hypophysectomy can be tolerated without loss of the fetus from very early stages. This is due to the production by the placenta of pregnancy-maintaining amounts of P. The human placenta also produces hCG from very early stages as well as hPL. Both hCG (Midgley and Pierce, 1962; Thiede and Choate, 1963; Dreskin et al, 1970) and hPL (Sciarra, 1963) have been localized to the syncytial trophoblast. In normal pregnancy in the early post-implantation period, there may be a period during which hCG secretion is directly quantitatively related to trophoblast mass. The hCG reaches a peak and rapidly declines even though trophoblast tissue continues to increase (Braunstein et al, 1973); hPL, on the other hand, progressively rises in titer parallel to placental mass continuing to term (Goldstein, 1971).

III. Experimental

A. Culture

We have cultured rat blastocysts collected on the morning of day 4 (day of finding sperm plugs = day 0 of pregnancy) and rat mid-pregnancy trophoblast dissected under low power magnification on the morning of day 10.

1. Blastocysts

Day 4 blastocysts were collected into and washed once with Hank's balanced salt solution without Ca^{++} or Mg^{++} (Hank's BBS-Ca-Mg). The blastocysts were then transferred to 35 mm plastic culture dishes 10-20 blastocysts/dish and incubated in 3 ml medium at 37° C, in air: CO_2 (95:5) for up to 10 days. The medium consisted of NCTC-135 (Gibco) containing 10% fetal calf serum (heat-inactivated), 100 units penicillin/ml and 100 μg streptomycin/ml. The usual outgrowth of these blastocysts can be seen in Fig. 1. The medium was collected, frozen, and replaced every 24 hours. The blastocysts were observed under phase microscopy and counted only if they successfully attached and outgrew.

2. Mid-pregnancy trophoblast

The entire trophoblastic shell (as far as possible) was dissected from day 10 embryos. It was washed once with Hank's BBA-Ca-Mg. In earlier experiments, the trophoblast was cultured as explants in 5 ml medium, 10 trophoblasts/dish. In later experiments, the trophoblast was dissociated with trypsin-EDTA or with the neutral protease Dispase (Boehinger Mannheim Biochemicals, Indianapolis, Indiana) and cultured in 3 ml medium at 50,000 cells/ml. The appearance of these cells in culture can be seen in Fig. 2.

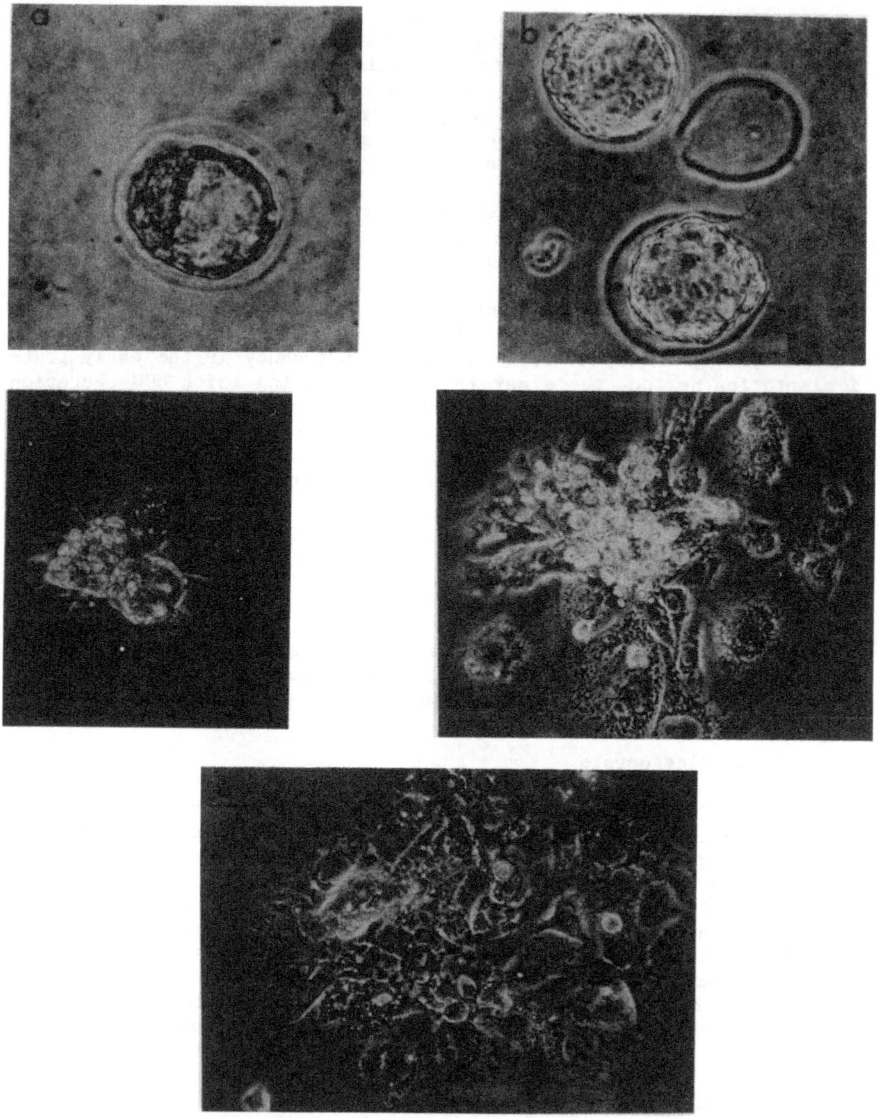

Fig. 1. a-e. Stages in the development of the rat blastocyst *in vitro*. Days 4 + 0 through 4 + 4. Blastocysts are cultured in NCTC-135 + 10% fetal calf serum (heat-inactivated) + penicillin-streptomycin (100 units-100 μg/ml) at 37° C in air: CO_2 (95:5). 200 x mag. a. The blastocyst as it is collected on the morning of day 4. b. Blastocyst expansion and shedding of the zona pellucida. c. Early outgrowth of the trophoblast cells with prominent ICM. Secretory droplets and granules can already be seen. d. Continued outgrowth of trophoblast cells. Giant cells prominent. ICM at maximum. e. Full outgrowth of trophoblast cells. ICM regressing.

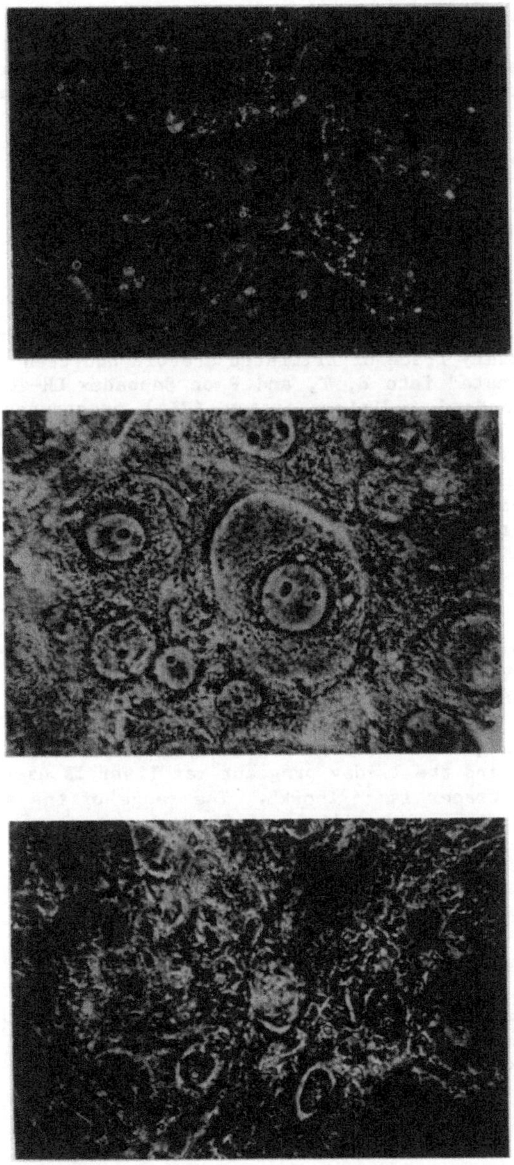

Fig. 2. a–c. Mid-pregnancy trophoblast in vitro. Trophoblast is dissected from embryos on day 10 and cultured under the same conditions as for blastocysts, Fig. 1. 200 X mag. a. Day 10 + 2. b. Day 10 + 6. Note increase in cell size. c. Day 10 + 10. Death of trophoblast cells.

Every set of blastocysts or trophoblasts included dishes of media only which were collected and changed daily along with the dishes containing cells. The highest value obtained for these controls was subtracted from the values obtained with blastocysts or trophoblasts.

B. Assays

Entire experiments were run as sets whether by RIA or RRA and compared with their own internal controls.

1. RIA

The steroids were extracted from 1 ml samples of media to which a recovery trace of tritiated steroid had been added. They were then fractionated into E, T, and P on Sephadex LH-20 columns and assayed by standard radioimmunoassay (RIA) procedures using specific antisera of known cross-reactivity with other steroids and corrected for percent recovery. The lower limits of the RIA's were; for E, 3.9; T, 7.8; P, 15.6 pg/ml. The percentage recoveries through extraction and the columns were: for E, 72.9 ± 9.4; T, 68.0 ± 11.6; P, 71.1 ± 9.9; n = 10 runs of complete experimental sets.

2. RRA

The rat placental lactogen (rPL) was asayed by radioreceptor assay (RRA) for us by Dr. Michael Blank in the laboratory of Dr. Henry Friesen. This RRA, developed and modified in Dr. Friesen's laboratory (Shiu et al, 1973) was originally designed for growth hormone. Since growth hormone and prolactin cross-react with rPL, the RRA can be adapted to assay rPL if ovine prolactin (oRPL) is used as the standard and the 17-day pregnant rat liver is used as the membrane source. The tracer is ^{125}I-oPRL. The range of the standard curve is 1-2000 ng/ml with a lower limit of 5 ng/ml.

IV. Results

A. On plates

Apparent hormone production by blastocysts from representative experiments (each a set of one collection with its media controls) is shown in Fig. 3.

Fig. 3. Hormone production by rat blastocysts <u>in vitro</u>. Blastocysts (BL) were collected from uteri on pregnancy day 4 and cultured as in Fig. 1 at a density of approximately 20 blastocysts per 35 mm plate. Media was collected and replaced in all plates every 24 hours. The various filled symbols refer to separate plates. The open circles refer to the media controls. The stippled area represents the level of the highest media control. Any production within this area is overridden by the amount of hormone in media alone. EGD = equivalent gestation day.

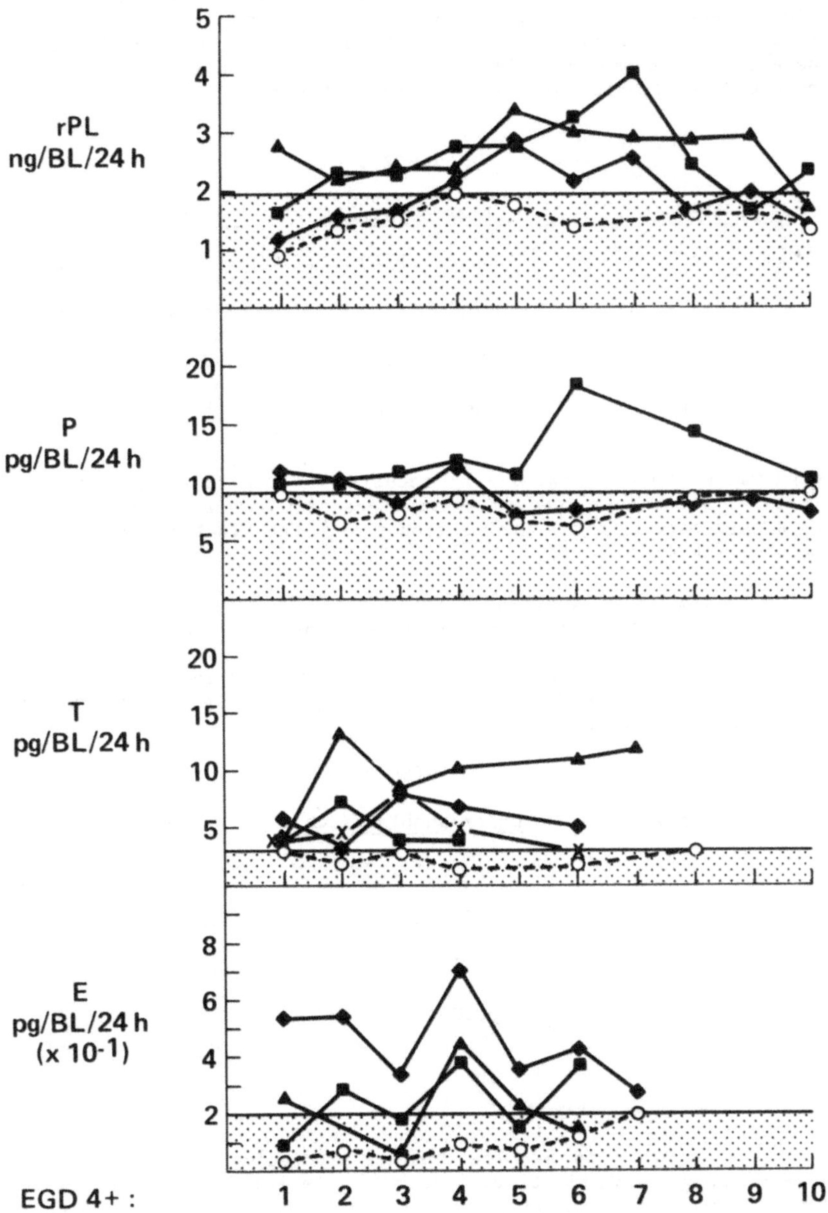

Fig. 3. See legend on facing page.

As can be seen, a great deal of variability exists between plates of blastocysts even randomly grouped. If the maxima and the EGD on which they occurred from different experiments are considered, the data can be summarized in terms of pg hormone (minus the highest control) per blastocyst per 24 hours as follows:

TABLE 1

Hormone	pg/blastocyst/24h	On EGD	n
E	44.3 ± 15.0	7-8	4
T	6.2 ± 2.1	6-14	5
P	28.4 ± 18.0	10-13	5
rPL	1820 ± 600	11-12	4

High values which occasionally occurred on the first collection day (4+1) have not been used as maxima because these may have been caused by a carryover from the uterus even though the blastocysts were washed before plating.

Similarly, apparent hormone production by mid-pregnancy trophoblast in representative experiments is shown in Fig. 4.

The maxima from different experiments, expressed as pg hormone (minus the highest media control) per trophoblast per 24 hours may be summarized as follows:

TABLE 2

Hormone	pg/trophoblast/24h	On EGD	N
E	3.5 ± 1.2	12-15	4
T	22.3 ± 7.8	12-15	6
P	250 ± 128	12-15	5
rPL	143,500 ± 615	12	2

B. On monolayers

In order to examine hormone production by blastocysts and mid-pregnancy trophoblast on separate uterine cell types we have recently adapted a method for mouse uteri (Sherman, 1978) and characterized the monolayers (McCormack & Glasser, 1980; Glasser & McCormack, this book). Epithelial, stromal, and myometrial monolayers were prepared from the uteri of immature rats which had received 2.5 μg E 24 hours previously. The uterine cell types were allowed to attach and form nearly confluent monolayers at which time (68 hours after plating) 20 blastocysts were added. Control plates consisting

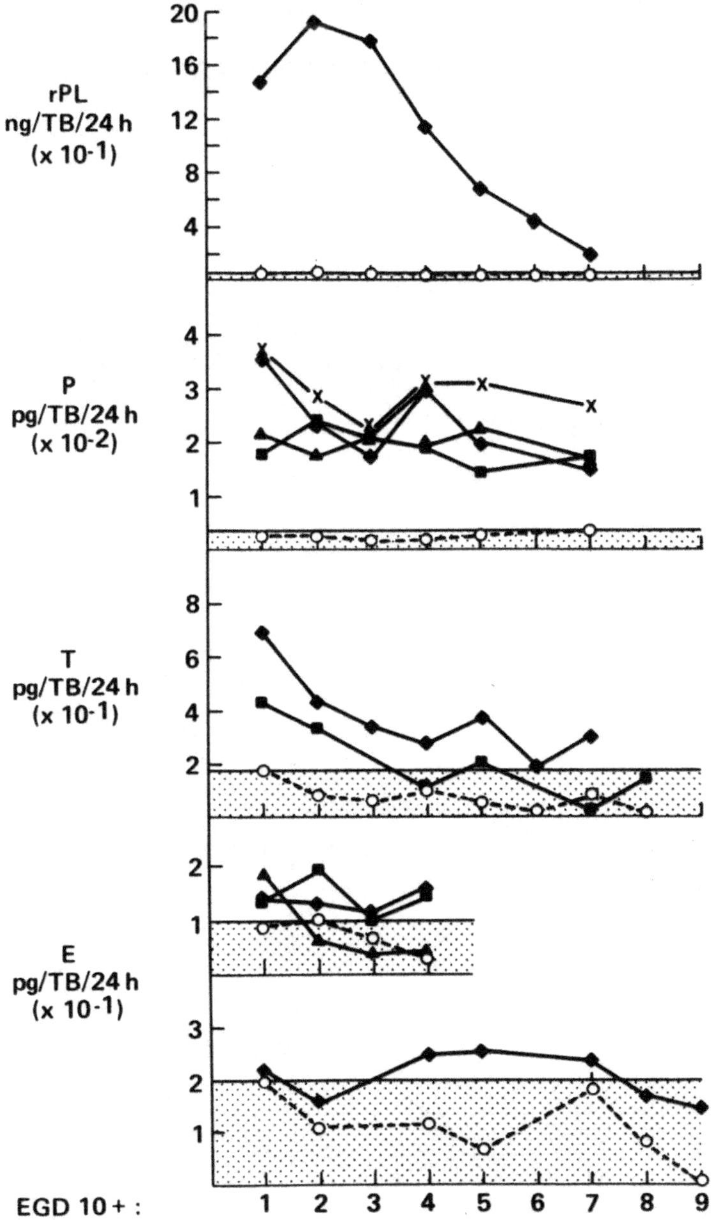

Fig. 4. Hormone production by rat trophoblast (TB) dissected from conceptuses on pregnancy day 10 and cultured similarly to blastocysts (See legend for Fig. 3.)

of media only, monolayers only, and blastocysts only were included. The results of this experiment may be seen in Figs. 5, 6, and 7.

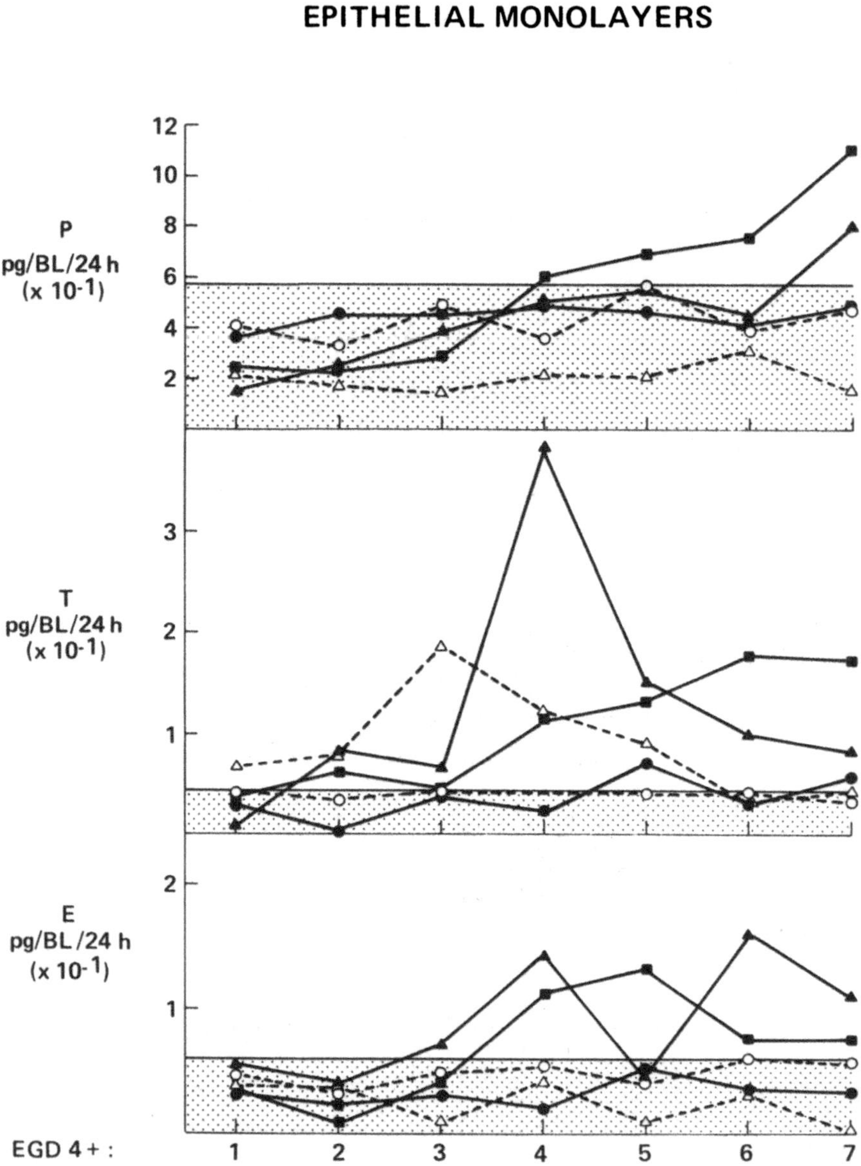

Fig. 5. Hormone production by rat blastocysts cultured on epithelial cell monolayers prepared from the uteri of immature rats injected 24 h previously with 2.5 µg estradiol-17β. The open triangles refer to blastocyst-only controls. The closed circles refer to monolayer-only controls. For further explanation see Fig. 3 and the text.

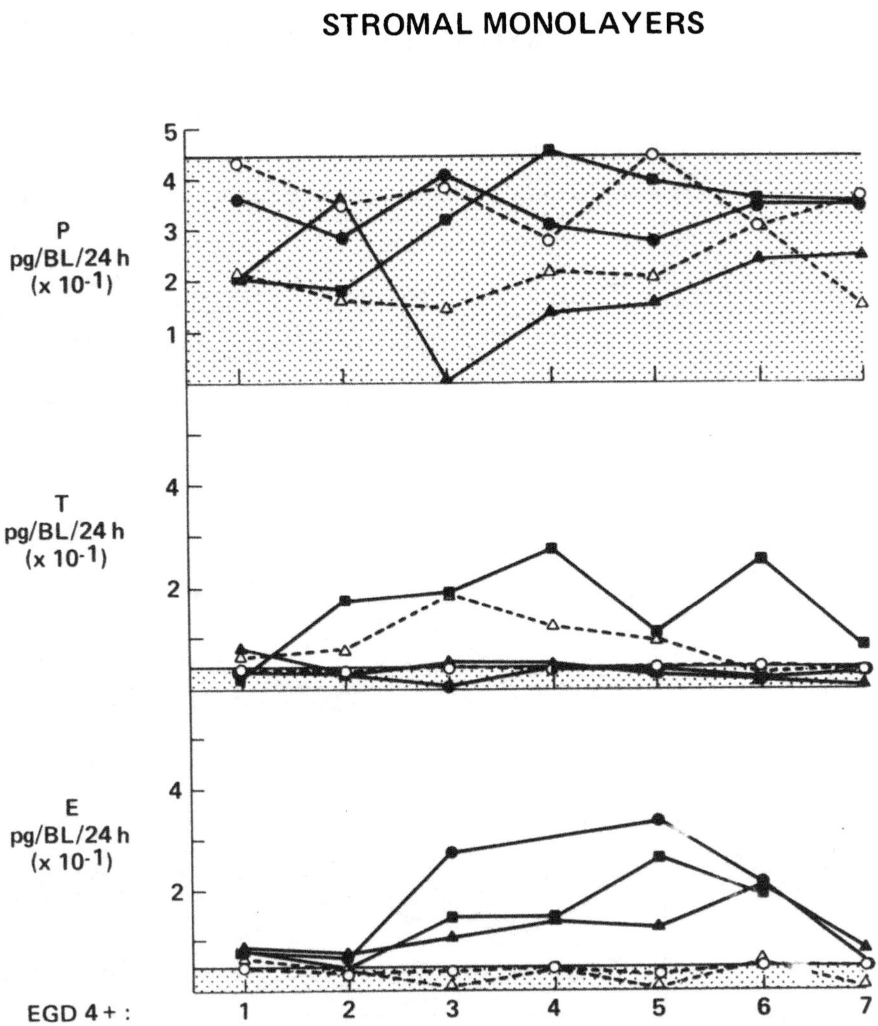

Fig. 6. Hormone production by rat blastocysts cultured on stromal cell monolayers prepared from the uteri of immature rats injected 24 h previously with 2.5 μg estradiol-17β. For further explanation see Fig. 5 and the text.

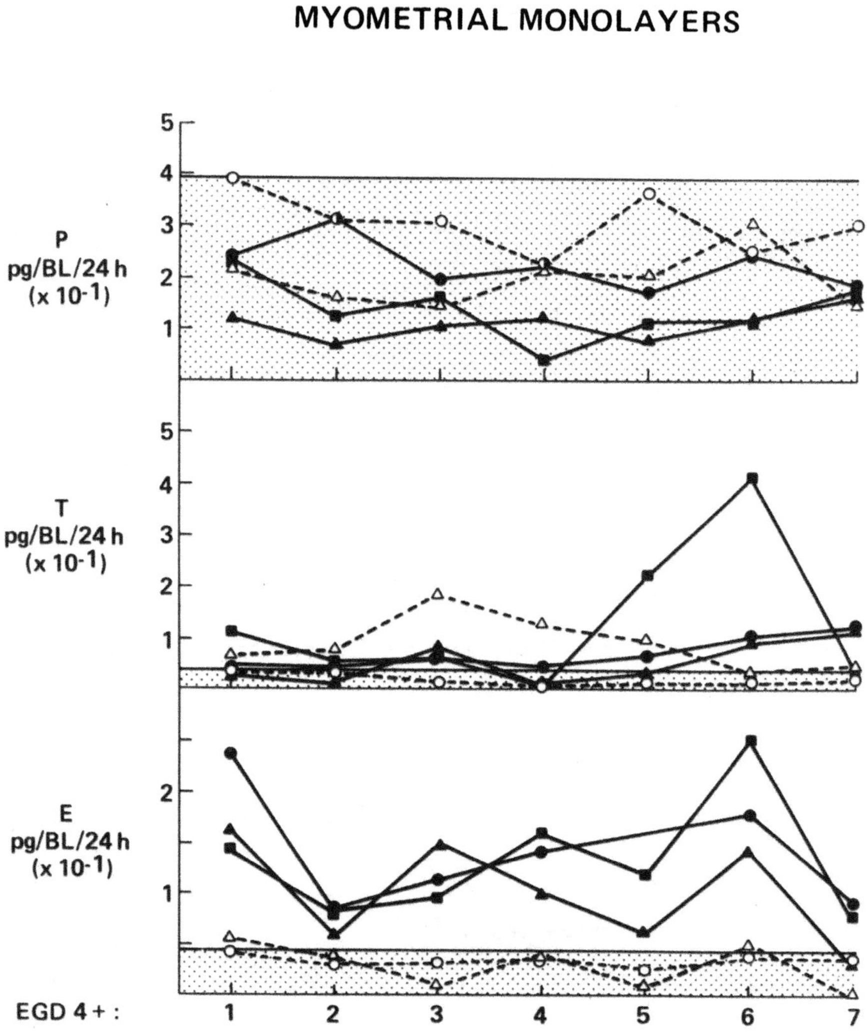

Fig. 7. Hormone production by rat blastocysts cultured on myometrial cell monolayers prepared from the uteri of immature rats injected 24 h previously with 2.5 μg estradiol-17β. For further explanation see Fig. 5 and the text.

The apparent maxima of hormone production (minus the highest media control) per blastocyst per 24 hours may be summarized as follows:

TABLE 3

PICOGRAMS/BLASTOCYST/24h

Hormone	Blastocyst Only	On EGD	Monolayer	Monolayer Only	Monolayer + Blastocysts	On EGD
E	1.1	5	Epithelial	0.9	8.9 11.5	9 10
			Stromal	29.0	26.0 20.0	9 10
			Myometrial	23.6	11.5 20.7	5 10
T	14.5	7	Epithelial	2.8	13.6 32.3	10 8
			Stromal	3.7	23.5 4.1	8 5
			Myometrial	8.0	36.9 7.2	10 11
P	<Medium Control		Epithelial	<Medium Control	47.6 22.6	11 11
			Stromal	"	<Medium Control	<Medium Control
			Myometrial	"	"	"

V. Discussion and Conclusions

Blastocysts cultured by themselves in culture dishes appear to have produced low levels of E, T, P, and rPL. However, special emphasis must be placed on the word "produced" in contradistinction to "secreted" because the conversion of labelled procursors to identified products is a minimum requirement for claiming secretion of these hormones by the blastocysts. We use the word "produce" to mean simply the appearance of hormone where cells are present by any unspecified mechanism. Obviously, where large amounts are involved after substantial lengths of time in culture, secretion is the most likely mechanism, but where small amounts are involved and which occur in the first few collections of medium, absorption, adsorption, protein binding, or contaminating vascular elements could be involved particularly where steroidogenic enzymes have not been demonstrated by others.

The production of E on EGD 7-8 is significantly above that in the concommittantly incubated media controls. It is likely, however, that this phenomenon does not represent secretion in view of the fact that

Marcal and co-workers (1975) could not detect HSD activity in the rat trophoblast before EGD 11 and that the E present in rabbit blastocysts is probably the result of uptake of maternal E (Singh and Booth, 1978). Mid-pregnancy trophoblast, on the other hand, produced very little, if any, E.

The production of T by blastocysts was very small and the days on which peak production occurred were scattered over 8 days in different cultures. For these reasons, it is doubtful that the blastocysts produced amounts of any physiological importance. Later, however, mid-pregnancy trophoblast did show T production 2 to 3 times that of the blastocysts and over a better-defined time period (EGD 12-15). However, others have not shown the production of T by blastocysts. Information on the rat trophoblast is lacking but mouse blastocysts at EGD 5 and 6 could not be shown to synthesize androstenedione, an immediate precursor of T, from DHEA (Sherman and Atienza, 1977) while blastocyst cultures at EGD 10-11 were able to do so as well as to metabolize the androstenedione further (Sherman and Atienza, 1977). However, other workers who identified the main metabolities of DHEA in the mouse placenta found androstenedione and 5α-reduced metabolites. No T, dihydrotestosterone or E was detected (Okker-Reitsma, 1976).

The production of P by rat blastocysts shows a large degree of variation between different plates of blastocysts but the timing of this maximal production is similar to that found for HSD activity in rat trophoblast (Marcal, 1975) and for mouse blastocysts (Sherman and Atienza, 1977), EGD 10-11. The extent of the production is only 10-20% of that they found, however. Later, mid-pregnancy trophoblast produced levels ten times that by the blastocysts during the time period EGD 12-15. Compared to the maximal amounts of P measured in cultured mouse blastocysts--0.5 to 5.0 pmoles/blastocyst/24 h (Sherman and Atienza, 1977)-this amounts to 0.8 pmoles/trophoblast/24 h for the rat. Thus, the rat's P production remains near the lower limits of the mouse's maximal production under our culture conditions. In this connnection it must be remembered that we are not providing pregnenolone as substrate other than that which may be present in the unstripped fetal calf serum added to the medium.

In lieu of any information on rat uterine fluid steroid concentrations, the levels of peripheral steroids on the days we removed the blastocysts and mid-pregnancy trophoblast are of interest. We have measured peripheral levels of E and P by RIA and have obtained concentrations of 9.8 ± 3.3 pg E/ml and 64.2 ± 18.9 pg P/ml (n = 15) on day 4 of pregnancy and 7.8 pg E/ml and 54.7 pg P/ml (n = 3) on day 10 (unpublished results). The P levels are very similar to those found by Morishige and co-workers (1973) which were (as estimated from a graph) 64 and 76 pg/ml on days 4 and 10, respectively. Levels of greater significance to the blastocyst or trophoblast in the uterus are those present in ovarian vein blood at these times. Concentrations of 200 ± 43 pg E/ml and 1.6 ± 0.4 ng T/ml have been reported on pregnancy day 4 in 10 minute collections of ovarian vein blood (Brodie et al, 1977).

The matter of adsorption or other uptake by the blastocysts or trophoblasts must therefore be taken into account particularly where others have not been able to show conversion of labelled immediate precursors, as in the case of E and T. However, since these maximum concentrations occurred after 2 and 10 days in culture, following the initial wash of the blastocysts or trophoblast and with changes to fresh medium every 24 hours, it seems unlikely that these maximal concentrations could be due wholly to the slow release of bound maternal steroid. Particularly in the case of P production does the release of bound steroid seem an unlikely explanation. In blastocysts a gradual rise in P concentrations occurred to a peak at 6-9 days after the blastocysts had been removed from the mother. The mid-pregnancy trophoblasts had undergone, aside from an initial wash, a subsequent dissociation step with washes, and then reached their maxima 2 to 5 days after being placed in culture.

The rPL produced by blastocysts was very low (∿1%) compared to that by mid-pregnancy trophoblast and did not reach peak levels until nearly the same EGD (11-12). The concentrations produced by trophoblast at the same time (EGD 12) were striking and matched the day on which others (Matthies, 1967; Kelly et al, 1973) have found maximal levels of rPL in rat serum.

Both P and rPL were produced by mid-pregnancy trophoblast in amounts much greater (10 and 100 times) than by blastocysts at the same EGD. An increase in the number of trophoblast cells attained in culture over those attained by blastocysts may be sufficient to explain the P difference, but for rPL this does not seem adequate and one wonders if there is step at which maternal regulation occurring between day 5 and 10 could be involved.

Hormone production by blastocysts on uterine cell monolayers showed intriguing departures from that by blastocysts incubated alone on culture dishes. Although this experiment is a preliminary one, it nevertheless illustrates the potential for supplying information that a culture system of fetal and maternal components has.

The choice of appropriate donor cells from which to prepare the monolayers must be investigated in detail. In this experiment, we used the immature rat injected 24 hours previously with 2.5 μg E. At the time the blastocysts are placed on the monolayers, 96 hours had elapsed since the E was injected. The rats were not pretreated with P, and of course, the blastocysts would not confront all 3 cell types at the same time <u>in vivo</u>. With these and other shortcomings in approximating an implantation milieu in mind, a brief comparison of the hormone production on plates vs. monolayers is as follows:

Blastocysts on epithelial monolayers produced about ¼% as much E, 2-5 times more T, and about the same amount of P as on plates alone. The E peaks occurred later on epithelial monolayers, but the T and P peaks occurred at about the same time as on plates.

Blastocysts on stromal monolayers appeared to produce about ½% as much E as on plates alone, but this result was made insignificant by the fact that the stromal monolayers by themselves had concentrations of E 5 times that of the media controls. In contrast, the stromal monolayers had T and P levels only slightly above or lower than the media controls. Blastocysts on stromal monolayers produced about 4 times more T (in one of two dishes) than on plates alone and not enough P to exceed the media control.

Blastocysts on myometrial monolayers also appeared to produce E but the level was overshadowed by the amount of E apparently produced by the monolayer control. Again, T was produced in an amount 4 times that of the monolayer control (by one of two plates) and P was found above levels in the media alone. The myometrial monolayer did not produce P levels above the media control and produced only trivial amounts of T.

A disappointing feature of this experiment was the fact that the blastocyst-only controls did not produce the amounts of hormone that they had in previous experiments. Since we had enough blastocysts for only one such plate, however, we felt it was fair to compare this experiment to the mean of previous experiments.

The apparent production of E by the stromal and myometrial monolayers was a surprise to us. It is unlikely that this E could be provided by vascular elements since the contamination of our preparations by blood is very low and, furthermore, such cells do not attach to the plate. Also, the media had been changed daily. E could perhaps have been adsorbed to the cell membranes of stromal and myometrial cells, bound by a slowly secreted protein, or released from the bodies of dead cells. Another possibility is that the E arose by the conversion of precursors made by the blastocysts with the aid of enzymes present in the stromal and myometrial cells. Experiments are in progress to confirm this result and to test these intriguing possibilities.

In conclusion, we believe that this in vitro system of blastocysts with the three main types of uterine cells will prove useful in elucidating some of the factors involved in early and mid-pregnancy communication and co-operation between the fetal and maternal components of a successful pregnancy unit. Certainly, the system will allow more controllable conditions for testing certain aspects of fetal-maternal interaction than are possible in vivo.

ACKNOWLEDGEMENTS

We gratefully acknowledge the excellent technical assistance of Mr. Robert A. May and Ms. Jo Anne Julian, the RRA's carried out by Dr. Michael Blank, and the helpful consultation of Drs. Henry Friesen, Len Martin and Michael Sherman.

REFERENCES

Adams, J.B. and Low, J. (1974). Enzymatic synthesis of steroid sulphates. X. Isolation of oestrogen sulphotransferase from bovine placenta and comparison of its properties with adrenal oestrogen sulphotransferase. Biochim. Biophys. Acta 370, 189-196.

Ainsworth, L., Daenen, M. and Ryan, K.H. (1969). Steroid hormone transformation by endocrine organs from pregnant mammals. iv. Biosynthesis and metabolism of estrogens and progesterone by primate placental preparations in vitro. Endocrinology 84, 1421-1429.

Ainsworth, L. and Ryan, K.J. (1969). Steroid hormone transformations by endocrine organs from pregnant mammals. V. The biosynthesis and metabolism of progesterone and estrogens by orangutan placental tissue in vitro. Steroids 14, 301-314.

Angle, M.J. and Mead, R.A. (1979). The source of progesterone in pre-implantation rabbit blastocysts. Steroids 33, 625-638.

Asch, R.H., Fernandez, E.O., Magnasco, L.A. and Pauerstein, C.J. (1978). Demonstration of a chorionic gonadotropin-like substance in rabbit morulae. Fertil. Steril. 29, 444.

Astwood, E.B. and Greep, R.O. (1938). A corpus luteum-stimulating substance in the rat placenta. Proc. Soc. Exptl. Biol. Med. 38, 713-716.

Astwood, E.B. and Greep, R.O. (1939). Nomenclature of gonad-stimulating hormones of placental origin. Science 89, 81.

Averill, S.C., Ray, E.W. and Lyons, W.R. (1950). Maintenance of pregnancy in hypopsectomized rats with placental implants. Proc. Soc. Exptl. Biol. Med. 75, 3-6.

Bambra, C.S. and Gombe, S. (1978). The role of placental gonadotrophins (PMSG and hCG) in pregnancy in the rat. J. Reprod. Fert. 53, 109-115.

Bjorkman, N. (1970). An Atlas of Placental Fine Structure. Williams and Wilkins, Baltimore.

Blank, M.S., Chan, J.S.D. and Friesen, H.G. (1977). Placental lactogens, new developments. J. Steroid Biochem. 8, 403-414.

Blank, M.S., Dufau, M.L. and Friesen, H.G. (1979). Demonstration of potent, gonadotropin-like biological activity in the serum of rats during midpregnancy. Science in press.

Botte, V., Tramontana, S. and Chieff, G. (1968). Histochemical distribution of some hydroxysteroid dehydrogenases in the placenta, foetal membranes and uterine mucosa of the mouse. J. Endocrinol. 40, 180-194.

Braunstein, G.D., Grodin, J.M., Vaitukaitis, J.L. and Ross, G.T. (1973). Secretory rates of HCG by normal trophoblast. Am. J. Obstet. Gynecol. 115, 447-450.

Brodie, A.M.H., Schwarzel, W.C., Shaikh, A.A. and Brodie, H.J. (1977). The effect of an aromatase inhibitor, 4-hydroxy-4-androstene-3, 17-dione, on estrogen dependent processes in reproduction and breast cancer. Endocrinology 100, 1684-1695.

Chan, S.W.C. and Leathem, J.H. (1975). Placental steroidogenesis in the rat: progesterone production by tissue of the basal zone. Endocrinology 96, 298-303.

Chang, M.C. (1950). Development and fate of transferred rabbit ova or blastocyst in relation to the ovulation time of recipients. J. Exp. Zool. 114, 197-225.

Chew, N.J. and Sherman, M.I. (1975). Biochemistry of differentiation of mouse trophoblast: $\Delta^5, \beta 3$ -hydroxysteroid dehydrogenase. Biol. Reprod. 12, 351-359.

Chowdhury, M. and Steinberger, E. (1976). Pituitary and plasma levels of gonadotrophins in foetal and newborn male and female rats. J. Endocrinol. 69, 381-384.

Davies, J. and Glasser, S.R. (1968). Histological and find structural observations on the placenta of the rat. Acta anatomica 69, 542-608.

Dean, H.W., Rubin, B.L., Driks, E.C., Lobel, B.L. and Leipsner, G. (1962). Trophoblast giant cells in placentas of rats and mice and their probable role in steroid-hormone production. Endocrinology 70, 407-419.

Dey, S. and Dickmann, Z. (1974). Estradiol-17β-hydroxysteroid dehydrogenase activity in preimplantation rat embryos. Steroids 24, 57-62.

Dickmann, Z. and Dey, S.K. (1974). Evidence that Δ^5-3β-hydroxysteroid dehydrogenase activity in rat blastocysts is autonomous. J. Endocrinol. 61, 513-514.

Dickmann, Z., Dey, S.K. (1974). Steroidogenesis in the preimplantation rat embryo and its possible influence on morula-blastocyst transformation and implantation. J. Reprod. Fert. 37, 91-93.

Dickmann, Z., Dey, S.K. and Gupta, J.S. (1975). Steroidogenesis in rabbit preimplantation embryos. Proc. Natl. Acad. Sci. USA 72, 298-300.

Diczfalusy, E. (1970). Role of the fetus, placenta and mother in steroidogenesis at midgestation. Advances in the Biosciences 6, 343-366.

Diczfalusy, E. (1974). Endocrine functions of the human fetus and placenta. (Review). Am. J. Obstet. Synecol. 119, 419-433.

Dreskin, R.B., Spicer, S.S. and Greene, W.B. (1970). Ultrastructural localization of chorionic gonadotropin in human term placenta. J. Histochem. Cytochem. 18, 862-874.

Ellinwood, W.E., Seidel, G.E., Jr., Niswender, G.D. (1979). Secretion of gonadotropin factors by the preimplantation rabbit blastocyst. Proc. Soc. Exptl. Biol. Med. 161, 136-185.

Ferguson, M.M and Christie, G.A. (1967). Distribution of hydroxysteroid dehydrogenases in the placentae and foetal membranes of various mammals. J. Endocrinol. 38, 291-306.

Flint, A.P.F., Gadsby, J.E. and Heap, R.B. (1979). Blastocyst steroids-their synthesis and action. In: Research on Steroids, v. 8, Proc. of the Serono Symposia (A. Klopper, L. Lerner, H.J. van der Molen and F. Sciarra, eds.) Academic Press, London pp. 3-10.

Fujimoto, S. and Sundaram, K. (1978). The source of progesterone in rabbit blastocysts. J. Reprod. Fert. 52, 231-233.

Gadsby, J.E., Burton, R.D., Heap, R.B. and Perry, J.S. (1976). Steroid metabolism and synthesis in early embryonic tissue of pig, sheep and cow. J. Endocrinol. 71, 45-46P.

Gardner, R.L. and Rossant, J. (1976). Determination during embryogenesis. In: Embryogenesis in Mammals, Ciba Found. Sym. 40 (new series) Elsevier, North-Holland, Amsterdam. pp. 5-18.

Glasser, S.R. and Clark, J.H. (1975). A determinant role for progesterone in the development of uterine sensitivity of decidualization and ovo-implantation. In: The Developmental Biology of Reproduction (C. Markert and J. Papaconstantinou, eds.) Academic Press, New York, pp. 311-345.

Goldstein, D.P. (1971). Serum placental lactogen activity in patients with molar pregnancy and trophoblastic tumors - a reliable index of malignancy. Am. J. Obstet. Gynecol. 110, 583-587.

Graham, C.F. (1971). The design of the mouse blastocyst. In: Control Mechanisms of Growth and Differentiation: Symposia of Soc. Exptl. Biol. No. 25 (D.D. Davies and M. Balls, eds.) Cambridge Univ. Press, Cambridge p. 371-378.

Haour, F., Tell, G. and Sanchez, P. (1976). Mise en evidence et dosage d'une gonadotrophine chorionique chez le rat (rCG). C.R. Acad. Sci. (Paris) 282, 1183.

Heap, R.B., Gadsby, J.E., Wyatt, C. and Perry, J.S. (1979). In: Monographs on Endocrinology (H.M. Beier and P. Karlson, eds.) Springer-Verlag, Berlin. in press.

Hertig, A.T., Rock, J., Adams, E.C. and Mulligan, W.J. (1954). On the preimplantation stages of the human ovum: A description of four normal and four abnormal specimens ranging from the second to the fifth day of development. Contrib. Embryol., Carnegie Inst. Washington 35, 199-220.

Hillman, N. Sherman, M.I. and Graham, C. (1972). The effect of spatial arrangement on cell determination during mouse development. J. Embryol. Exptl. Morph. 28, 263-278.

Holcenberg, J.S. and Rosen, S.W. (1965). Enzymatic sulfation of steroids by bovine tissues. Arch. Biochem. Biophys. 110, 551-556.

Huff, R.L. and Eik-Nes, K.B. (1966). Metabolism in vitro of acetate and certain steroids by six-day old rabbit blastocysts. J. Reprod. Fert. 11, 57-63.

Jost, A. and Millot, M. (1953). Homo-transplantation de placenta sur le rat male. C.R. Soc. Biol. (Paris) 147, 1738-1742.

Kelly, D.A., Shiu, R.P.C., Robertson, M.C. and Friesen, H.G. (1973). Studies of rat chorionic mamotropin by radioreceptor assay. Fed. Proc. 32, 213 (abs).

Kelly, P.A., Shiu, R.P.C., Robertson, M.C. and Friesen, H.G. (1975). Characterization of rat chorionic mammotropin. Endocrinology 96, 1187-1195.

Kirby, D.R.S. (1962b). Ability of the trophoblast to destroy cancer tissue. Nature 194, 696-697.

Kirby, D.R.S. (1965a). The "invasiveness" of the trophoblast. In: The Early Conceptus, Normal and Abnormal. (W.W. Park, ed.) University of St. Andrews Press, Edinburgh, pp. 68-74.

Linke, D.M. and Niswender, G.D. (1973). Characterization of rat placental luteotrophin. Biol. Reprod. 8, 48-57.

Lyons, W.R. (1950). Lobulo-alveolar mammary growth in the rat. In: Mechanisme Physiologique de la Secretion Lactee. Colloque International du C.N.R.S. (Strasbourg) p. 29.

Lyons, W.R., Johnson, R.E., Cole, R.D. and Li, C.H. (1955). Mammary growth and lactation in male rats. In: The Hypophyseal Growth Hormone, Nature and Actions. (R.W. Smith, O.H. Gaebler and C.N. Long, eds.) McGraw-Hill, New York. pp. 461-472.

Marcal, J.M., Chew, N.J, Salomon, D.S. and Sherman, M.I. (1975). Δ^5-3ß-hydroxysteroid dehydrogenase activities in rat trophoblast and ovary during pregnancy. Endocrinology 96, 1270-1279.

Matthies, D.L. (1967). Studies of the luteotropic and mammotropic factor found in trophoblast and maternal peripheral blood of the rat at mid-pregnancy. Anat. Rec. 159, 55-68.

McCormack, S.A. and Glasser, S.R. (1980). Differential response of individual uterine cell types from immature rats treated with estradiol. Endocrinology in press.

Midgley, A.R. and Pierce, G.B. (1962). Immunohistochemical localization of human chorionic gonadotropin. J. Exxptl. Med. 115, 289-294.

Morishige, W., Pepe, G.J. and Rothchild, I. (1973). Serum luteinizing hormone, prolactin and progesterone levels during pregnancy in the rat. Endocrinology 92, 1527-1530.

Noyes, R.W., Dickmann, Z., Doyle, L.L. and Gates, A.H. (1963). Ovum transfers, synchronous and asynchronous, in the study of implantation. In: Delayed Implantation (A.C. Enders, Ed.) Univ. of Chicago Press, Chicago, Illinois.

Okker-Reitsma, G.H. (1976). Metabolism of (^{3}H)-dehydroepiandrosterone by mouse placental tissue in vitro. Koninkl. Nederl. Akademie van Wetenschapen - Amersterdam. Proc. Series C, no. 3, 79, 290-298.

Pedersen, R.A. and Spindle, A.I. (1979). The role of the blastocoele microenvironment in early mouse embryo differentiation. Nature in press.

Pencharz, R.I. and Long, J.A. (1933). Hypophysectomy in the pregnant rat. Am. J. Anat. 53, 117-139.

Perry, J.S., Heap, R.B. and Amoroso, E.C. (1973). Steroid hormone production by pig blastocysts. Nature (London) 245,45-47.

Psychoyos, A. (1973) Hormonal control of implantation. Vitamins and Hormones 31, 201-256.

Ramsey, E.M. (1975). The Placenta of Laboratory Animals and Man. (J.D. Ebert, general ed.) Holt Rinehart and Winston, p. 134.

Robertson, M.C. and Friesen, H.G. (1975). The purification and characterization of rat placental lactogen. Endocrinology 97, 621-629.

Salomon, D.S. and Sherman, M.I. (1975). The biosynthesis of progesterone by cultured mouse midgestation trophoblast cells. Devel. Biol. 47, 394-406.

Seamark, R.F. and Lutwak-Mann, C. (1972) Progestins in rabbit blastocysts. J. Reprod. Fert. 29, 147-148.

Sciarra, J.J., Kaplan, S.L. and Grumbach, M.M. (1963). Localization of anti-human growth hormone serum within the human placenta; evidence for a human chorionic "growth hormone-prolactin". Nature (Lond.) 199, 1005-1006.

Shemesh, M., Milaguir, F., Ayalon, N. and Hansel, W. (1979). Steroidogenesis and prostaglandin synthesis by cultured bovine blastocysts. J. Reprod. Fert. 56, 181-185.

Sherman, M. (1978). Implantation of mouse blastocysts in vitro. In: Methods in Mammalian Reproduction. (J.C. Daniel, Jr., ed.) Academic Press, New York. pp. 247-257.

Sherman, M.I. (1971). The biochemistry of differentiation of mouse trophoblast: alkaline phosphatase. Devel. Biol. 27, 337-350.

Sherman, M.I. and Atienza, S.B. (1977). Production and metabolism of progesterone and androstenedione by cultured mouse blastocysts. Biol. Reprod. 16, 190-199.

Sherman, M.I. and Wudl, L.R. (1976). The implanting mouse blastocyst. In: The Cell Surface in Animal Embryogenesis and Development. (G. Poste and L. Nicolson, eds.) Elsevier, North-Holland Biomedical Press, Amsterdam. pp. 81-116.

Sheth, K., Koszalke, T.R. and Brent, R.L. (1978) Δ^5, 5β-hydroxysteroid dehydrogenase activity in the rat parietal yolk sac during pregnancy. Biol. Reprod. 19, 1024-1029.

Singh, M.M. and Adams, C.E. (1978). Luteotrophic effect of the rabbit blastocyst. J. Reprod. Fert. 53, 331-333.

Singh, M.M and Booth, W.D. (1978). Studies on the metabolism of neutral steroids by preimplantaiton rabbit blastocysts in vitro and the origin of blastocyst oestrogen. J. Reprod. Fert. 53, 197-304.

Shui, R.P.C., Kelly, P.A. and Friesen, H.G. (1973). Radioreceptor assay for prolactin and other lactogenic hormones. Science 180, 968-970.

Solomon, S. (1966). Formation and metabolism of neutral steroids in the human placenta and fetus. J. Clin. Endo. Metab. 26, 762-772.

Snell, G.D. and Stevens, L.C. (1966). Early embryology. In: Biology of the Laboratory Mouse, 2nd edition (E.L. Green, ed.) McGraw-Hill, New York pp. 205-245.

Thiede, H.A. and Choate, J.W. (1963). Chorionic gonadotropin localization in the human placenta by immunofluorescent staining. II. Demonstration of HCG in the trophoblast and amnion epithelium of immature and mature placentas. Obstet. Gynecol. 22, 433-443.

Varma, S.K., Dawood, M.Y., Haour, F., Channing,C. and Saxena, B.B. (1979). Gonadotropin-like substance in the preimplanted rabbit blastocyst. Fertl. Steril. 31, 68-75.

Weiss, T.J., Janson, P.O., Porter, K.J. and Seamark, R.F. (1978). Effects of human chorionic gonadotropin on the release of cyclic AMP and progesterone from the sheep ovary at different stages of the oestrus cycle. Acta Endocrinologica 89, 158-165.

Wide, L. and Hobson, B. (1978). Chromatographic studies on a chorionic gonadotropic activity in the placenta of the rat, mouse and hamster. Upsala J. Med. Sci. 83, 1-6.

Wiener, M. (1974). Rat placental Δ^5,3 β-HSD. I. Changes in activity with dilution and gestational age. Endocrinology 94, 967-973.

Wynn, R.M. (1975). Fine structure of the placenta. In: The Placenta and its Maternal Supply Line. (P. Gruenwald, ed.) University Park Press, Baltimore. pp. 56-79.

Zeilmaker, G.H.and Verhamme, C.M.P.M. (1978). Luteotrophic activity of ectopically developing rat blastocysts. Acta Endocrinologica 88, 589-593.

The Endometrium

9

Analysis of Hormonal Responses of the Rat Endometrium by the Use of Separated Uterine Cell Types

Stanley R. Glasser
Shirley A. McCormack

The methodology of steroid receptor analysis promised a discriminating probe which would permit the analysis of those regulatory processes involved in the interactions between the developing mamalian embryo and the uterus. This promise remains to be fully redeemed for it has become increasingly evident that no matter how sophisticated the study of whole organs, they do not provide relevant information about the functional differences between the cell subpopulations which constitute that organ.

The starkness of this observation is emphasized by studies in organs such as the uterus. The uterus presents a complex array of cell types. Each of these cell types may have very different hormone sensitivities. Thus, each cell type may represent a different and specific class of target cell with its own response pattern to a single hormone or to combinations of hormones. The ability to isolate subpopulations of cells would permit more critical analyses. These procedures would allow the design of experiments with a greater latitude of regulatory maneuvers and would also avoid generating data which reflected only the net responses of an organ.

Attempts to identify differential responses of individual cell types are not recent. They encompass a wide variety of methods and include both in situ and physical and/or chemical methods. The major approaches are outlined in Table 1, together with our appreciation of their advantages and limitations.

A METHOD TO SEPARATE UTERINE CELL TYPES

The procedure currently used in our laboratory to separate uterine, cell types is our modification of a mechanical technique taught us by Drs. Len Martin and Roger King (Imperial Cancer Research Fund, London, J.K.) and an enzymatic method made available to us by Dr. Michael Sherman of Roche Institute of Molecular Biology (1978). Modifications were made to satisfy the criteria established in our own laboratory to obtain integral, viable cells for studies of steroid hormone receptors and *in vitro* implantation.

METHODS USED TO IDENTIFY DIFFERENTIAL RESPONSES OF INDIVIDUAL UTERINE CELL TYPES		
METHODS	IN SITU	PHYSICAL
	(a) Histochemical	(a) Mechanical: Squeezing, Scraping, Shearing, Dissecting, Curetting
	(b) Autoradiographic	(b) Enzymatic: Trypsin, Collagenase Pronase, Hyaluronidase, Combinations
ADVANTAGES	o Semi-quantitative o Localization o Cell type responses	o Can separate viable cells of specific types (E,S,M) o Can perform broad range of regulatory experiments: in vivo vs in vitro, quantitative, biochemical
LIMITATIONS	o Limited biochemical approach o Fixed frame o Terminal studies	o Success relates to completeness and specificity of separation o Limited yield

Table 1. This table was prepared from the literature cited in McCormack and Glasser (1980). It represents a summary of the principal methods used to identify differential responses of individual types of uterine sub-populations, i.e., E, epithelium; S, stroma; M, myometrium (Glasser and McCormack, 1980).

The method which follows consists of four major steps during which epithelial (Step A), stromal (Step B) and myometrial cells (Step C) are consecutively separated from longitudinally slit whole uteri (Fig. 1). Step D clarifies the individual cell fractions and outlines the procedure for counting cells and the tests for viability.

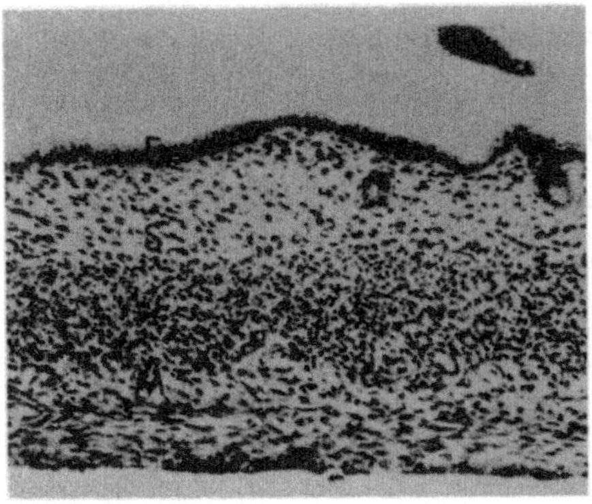

Fig. 1. Routine histological cross section through whole immature rat uterus 24 hr. after treatment with 2.5 µg E_2. A single layer of cuboidal epithelial cells (E) lines the lumen, glands may be present in the stroma (S). Myometrial (M) circular and longitudinal layers are present (X63; H and E).

STEP A:

WHOLE UTERI (SLIT LONGITUDINALLY)

Place uteri (12 immature, 6-8 mature, 350-750 mg) in 6.25 ml solution at 4°C in 20 ml capped vial

Trypsin (0.5%, Type III, bovine pancreas)

Pancreatin (2.5% in phosphate buffered saline (PBS)-Ca^{++},-Mg^{++}

4°C x 60 min

20°C x 60 min

Transfer to 15 ml conical tube, capped

Vortex (10 sec at medium speed)

Supernatant

Transfer to 15 ml capped conical tube containing 0.6 ml (1/10 vol) stripped, heated inactivated FCS

(EPITHELIAL CELLS)

Hold at 4°C

(STEP D)

Uteri

Wash 2x4.5 ml Hanks BBS-Ca^{++},-Mg^{++}

(STEP B)

Epithelial Cells

The epithelial cell fractions derived from Step A appear as plaques rather than individual cells (Fig. 2a) and contain few if any cells of any other kind. Evidence for the efficiency of this separation is provided by light microscopic examination of slit whole uteri from which epithelium has been removed (Fig. 2b), the apparent homogeniety of epithelial cell plaque suspensions under phase microscopy (Fig. 2a), the lack of fibroblastic cell colonies in epithelial cell monolayers (Fig. 2c), with significantly different uptake of ^{3}H-cytidine as compared with stromal and myometrial cells (McCormack and Glasser, 1980) and the concentration and dynamics of the estrogen receptor (RE) (Figs. 3,4); McCormack and Glasser, 1980; Glasser and McCormack, 1980).

STEP B:

UTERI (STEP A) - EPITHELIAL CELLS

↓

Suspend in 2.5 ml Trypsin (0.05%) + EDTA (0.02%) + 0.5 ml DNase (200 units) in PBS-Ca^{++},-Mg^{++}. Return to vial.
Add 6 glass beads (5 mm); Incubate 37° x 15 min
Vortex (10 sec med. speed) at 8 and 15 min

↓ (left branch)

Supernatant (turbid)
Transfer to 15 ml capped, conical tubes containing 1/10 vol. (0.3 ml) FCS
↓
(STROMAL CELLS) ←
Hold at 4°C
↓
(STEP D)

↓ (right branch)

Uteri
↓
Wash uteri 2x with 5 ml Hanks BBS-Ca^{++},-Mg^{++} → (STROMAL CELLS)
↓
(STEP C)

Stromal Cells

Stromal cell fractions (Step B) were estimated to contain approximately 10% epithelial cells. This estimate was based on histological examination of the remaining whole uterine tissue (Fig. 2E), phase microscopic appearance of stromal cell suspensions which contained single cells (Fig. 2D) and occasional tubular structures (probably glandular epithelium) but rarely any epithelial plaques. In culture, these single cell suspensions produced fibroblastic colonies (Fig. 2F). Occasional epithelial colonies which appeared probably derived from the presumed glandular epithelial structures. Stromal cells also differed from epithelial cells with respect to concentration and dynamics of the estradiol receptor (Figs. 3,4; Glasser and McCormack, 1980) and ^{3}H-cytidine uptake and incorporation (McCormack and Glasser, 1980).

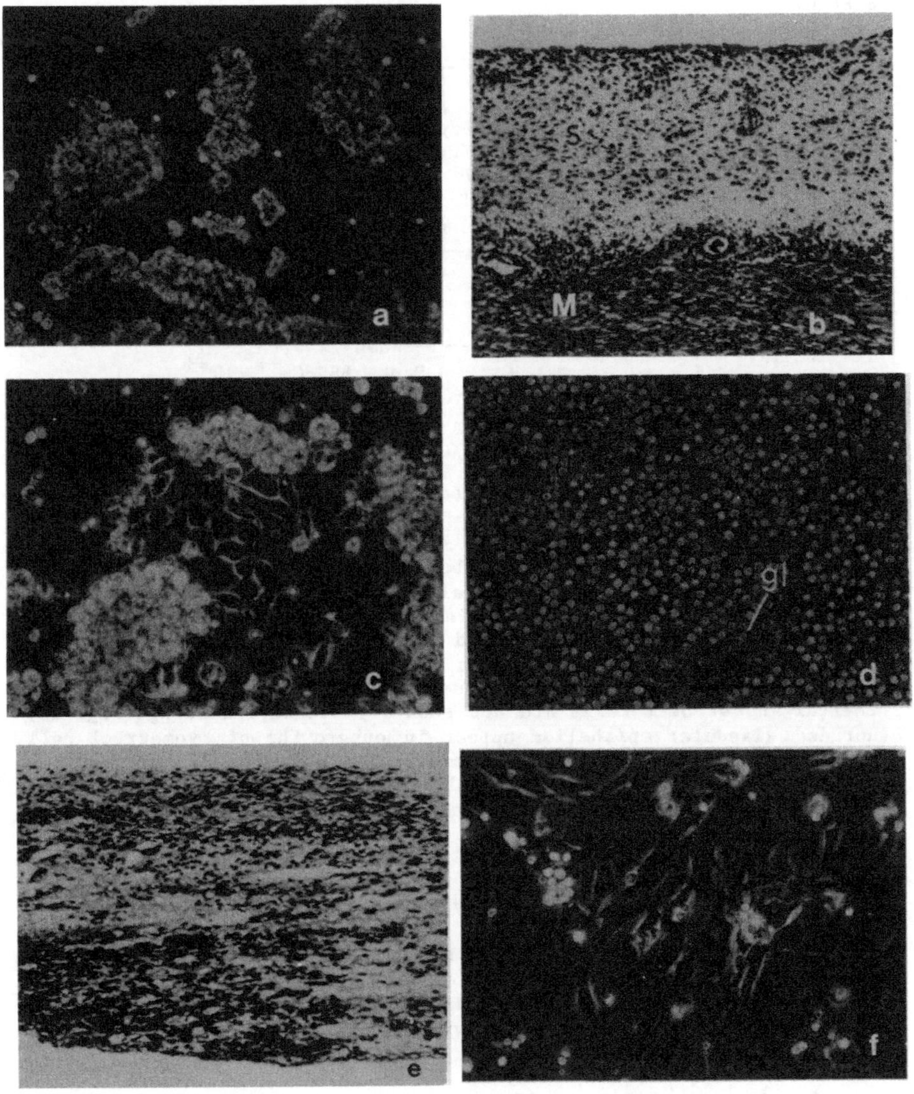

Fig. 2 (a) Typical plaque of epithelial cells still joined to each other after separation from the uterus (phase contrast, x200); (b) the uterus after removal of epithelium; stroma and myometrium still intact (X63; H and E); (c) monolayer outgrowth of epithelial cells in culture, 16 hr (phase contrast, X200); (d) a suspension of individual stromal cells after separation from myometrium, an occasional epithelial gland (gl) is present (phase contrast, X200; (e) the remaining myometrium after removal of epithelium and stromal cells (X63, H and E); (f) monolayer outgrowth of stromal cells in culture, 40 hr (phase contrast, X200).

STEP C:

UTERI (STEP B) - EPITHELIAL CELLS - STROMAL CELLS

Suspend Uteri in 2.5 ml Trypsin-EDTA + 0.5 ml DNase + 1.0 ml Collagnase (200 units, Type VI) in PBS-Ca^{++},-Mg^{++}
Return to vial. Incubate 37° x 30 min.
Vortex (10 sec at med. speed) at 15 and 30 min.

Supernatant → (MYOMETRIAL CELLS) → (STEP D)

Uteri → Wash 2x with 5 ml Hanks BBS-Ca^{++},-Mg^{++} → (MYOMETRIAL CELLS)

Myometrial Cells

Myometrial cell fractions (Step C) did not contain epithelial cell plaques but are assumed to be contaminated with stromal cells (not shown). Assessment of stromal cell contamination was difficult because deep stroma is embedded in myometrium and because separated myometrial cells appear single and rounded like stromal cells. They also produce fibroblastic colonies in culture (not shown). Histological examination of uterine tissue remaining after removal of epithelial and stromal cells did not show any stroma remaining (Fig. 2E) nor did glandular epithelium appear in outgrowths of myometrial cell suspensions (not shown). Furthermore, the uptake and incorporation of ^{3}H-cytidine by myometrial cell suspensions was different from stromal and epithelial cell preparations (McCormack and Glasser, 1980).

Viability and Yield

The viability of cells (Step D), as determined by vital dye exclusion, proves to be dependent on an individual investigator. In the best hands, we routinely obtained viability indices of 90% plus, whereas certain personnel, otherwise skilled, never produced more than 65% live cells.

Examination of fresh cell suspensions and comparable sections of uterus representing either different intervals following estradiol injection to immature female rats (McCormack and Glasser, 1980) or different times during the pre-implantation of the rat (Glasser and McCormack, 1980) demonstrated that the separate cells were intact and possessed the various characteristics of their specific type at a specific time. These data were further verified by study of whole sections and pellets prepared from individual cell suspensions for transmission and scanning electron microscopy. TEM and SEM pictures are published elsewhere (estrogen injected immature rats, McCormack and Glasser, 1980; pre-implantation uterus, Glasser and McCormack, 1980).

STEP D:

EPITHELIAL (STEP A), STROMAL (STEP B) AND MYOMETRIAL (STEP C) CELLS

Centrifuge individual cell fractions (500 x g, 5 min)

→ Discard Supernatant

↓

Wash with 15 ml Hanks BBS-Ca^{++},-Mg^{++}

→ Remove fibrous fragments

↓

Resuspend individual fractions in 5-6 drops medium (DMEM + 10% FCS [h.i.] + penicillin/streptomycin [100 units/10 ug]). Finally, take up in 10ml medium.

↓

Put through glass bead column

↓

Rinse column with 5 ml medium

↓

Resuspend gently to homogeneity

→ Remove 10 μl (Trypan blue viability test)

→ Remove 100 μl to culture (if cells are to be used fresh)

→ Remove drop to stain (permanent slide)

↓

Cells are ready to pellet and suspend in desired buffer or dilute with additional medium for plating and culture, biochemistry, receptor assay etc.

Total yield of uterine cells calculated from the sum of DNA in whole suspensions of the three cell types compared to the amount of DNA assayed in whole homogenates of intact uteri ranged from 73 to 101%. In E_2 injected immature rats, epithelial cells accounted for 1.0%; stromal cells for 3.2% and myometrial cells for 69.0% of the DNA measured in whole uteri at zero time. At 24 hours after E_2, the respective precentages were 2.7, 4.1 and 86.4 (McCormack and Glasser, 1980). The discrepancy between the sum and 100% at any one time reflects the fact that the recovery of cells from the uterus was not 100%. Most of the loss occurred in the myometrial fraction since in this study we did not carry the enzymatic digestion to complete dissolution of the uteri in order to avoid possible degradation of the estrogen receptor. Other cell loss occurred through cell breakage.

ESTROGEN RECEPTOR ASSAYS

Estrogen receptor (RE) assays served as functional evaluations of the cell separation technique. For this purpose, we chose the E_2 stimulated immature female rat to compare the estradiol (E_2) receptor dynamics in individual cell types and in the whole uterus. The immature rat uterus promised to be an excellent model because E_2 rsponses of the immature uterus are the subject of an extensive literature (O'Malley and Means, 1974; Clark et al., 1977).

We selected three post-injection periods, e.g., ½, 1 and 2 hrs, to encompass early response patterns (increased amino acid and nucleic acid uptake, stimulation of nuclear RNA polymerase activity, increase in water imbibition and uterine wet weight). Later uterine responses (sustained RNA polymerase activity, increased DNA, RNA and protein synthesis, cell hyperplasia and hypertrophy, increased uterine dry weight) were included within the experimental time periods of 8, 12, 24 and 48 hrs after the subcutaneous injection of 2.5 μg estradiol-17β (E_2).

Assay Methods

Estrogen receptor assays (RE) were carried out at 4° C, unless otherwise stated. Individual cell pellets were homogenized in conical glass-glass homogenizers in 5.5 ml of buffer (0.01M Tris, 0.0015 M EDTA (TE) and 0.1M mercaptoethanol (mer) at pH7.5. An aliquot of whole homogenate (∿0.5ml) was removed for DNA and protein analyses. The nuclear pellet was prepared by centrifugation (800xg, 10 min) of the whole homogenate.

The cytosol fraction was prepared by treating the supernatant of the whole homogenate with charcoal-dextran for 10 min with occasional mixing. Charcoal-dextran solution (1.0%:0.05%) was prepared in TE, ½ volume with respect to the supernatant volume, pelleted and drained before adding the supernatant fraction. Most of the charcoal-dextran was removed during centrifugation (2000 x g, 10 min) before recentrifugation at 105,000 x g for 60 min (rotor SW50.1; Beckman Ultracentrifuge L2-65B). Five hundred μl were removed from the supernatant for protein analysis. The remainder was used for the RE assay.

Using the original whole homogenate volume of TE-mer, the crude nuclear fraction was processed by washing the pellet from the homogenate twice and resuspending the washed pellet. Two hundred fifty μl were saved for each of the DNA and protein assays. The remainder was used in the RE assay.

The times and temperatures for maximum specific binding were determined experimentally (30° C for 30 min for cytosol and 37° C for 10 min for nuclei). These are exchange conditions which measure total receptor regardless of its occupancy by E_2 at the beginning of incubation. Scatchard analysis (1948) was carried out as previously described (McCormack and Glasser, 1976, 1978) with the following changes: the incubation mixture consisted of 250 μl cytosol or nuclear suspension, plus 20 μl tritiated E_2 and 20 μl DES or TE to make a total voume of 290 μl; the concentration range of E_2 used was 0.02 to 20 nmolar; the molar excess of DES in the non-specific binding series of tubes was 100 times that of E_2, and hydroxylapatite (HAP) was used to separate bound E_2 from free E_2 in cytosol.

The separation of bound from free E_2 with HAP was carried out as follows: at the end of the incubation period, the tubes were placed in an ice bath 500 μl of ice cold HAP (prepared as a 60:40 HAP:TE suspension) was added, the tubes were mixed every 5 minutes for 15 min and centrifuged at ~3500 x g for 10 min. The supernates were discarded and the HAP pellets washed with 1.5 ml TE-mer 3 times. To the well-drained HAP pellets, 1 ml of absolute ethanol was added and mixed well. The tubes were incubated at 30° C for 30 minutes, centrifuged at 3500 x g for 10 min and decanted into 5 ml of ACS liquid scintillation cocktail for counting.

The incubation period of nuclear suspensions was terminated by placing the tubes in an ice bath and adding 1.5 ml cold TE-mer immediately. After chilling 5 min, the tubes were centrifuged at 3500 x g for 5 min. The supernates were discarded and the pellets washed twice with 1.5 ml TE-mer. One milliliter of absolute ethanol was added; the tubes were incubated for 10 min at 30° C, mixed, chilled, and centrifuged at 3500 x g for 10 min. The supernant was then decanted into minivials containing 5 ml ACS and counted.

Separated Cell Types from Immature Rat Uterus

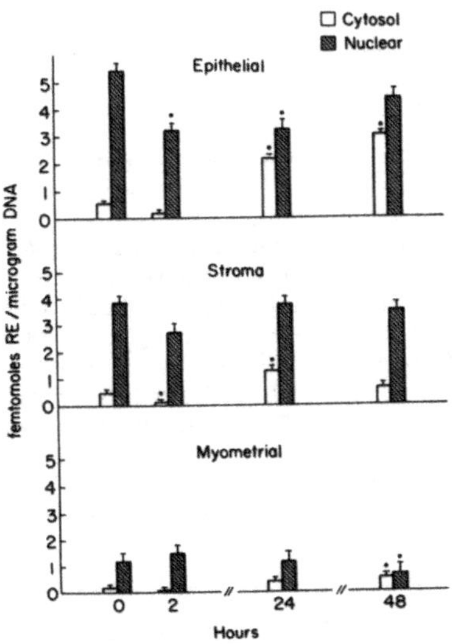

Fig. 3. Estrogen receptor concentration in high speed cytosol and nuclear fractions of cell types separated from the immature rat uterus following injection of 2.5 μg E_2. Myometrial nuclear estrogen receptor concentrations were significantly lower ($p < 0.01$) than either epithelial or stromal nuclear estrogen receptors at all times. (★) designates data significantly different ($p < 0.05$) from corresponding zero time (McCormack and Glasser, 1980)

The nuclear estrogen receptor (RnE) of epithelial cells at zero time was 5.5 fmol/μg DNA and the concentration of cytosol estrogen receptor (RcE) was 0.5 fmol/μg DNA (Fig. 3). Following E_2 stimulation, RnE concentrations in epithelial cells fell significantly to 3.2 fmol/μg DNA ($p < 0.05$) to 2.3 fmol/μg DNA 24 hr after E_2 administration. This increased the percentage of total RE in the cytoplasm to more than 65% from the pre-injection level of 10% (Table 2).

Stromal RnE was 3.8 fmol/μg DNA at zero time and did not change significantly during the 48 hrs following E_2. However, RcE responded to the hormone by increasing significantly ($p < 0.05$) from 0.4 at zero time to 1.3 fmol/μg DNA at 24 hrs thereby shifting RcE/RnE distribution from 5 to 35%. By 48 hrs, stromal cell RE concentrations were at pre-injection levels (Fig. 3, Table 3).

Table 2: Partition of the estrogen receptor between cytosol (RcE) and nucleus (RnE) in uterine cell types following sc injection of 2.5 μg E_2 in immature rats.

Percent (± SEM) of Total Cellular RE

Time (h)	Epithelial cells		Stromal cells		Myometrial cells	
	cytosol	nucleus	cytosol	nucleus	cytosol	nucleus
0	8.5	91.5 ± 3.0	11.3	88.7 ± 2.1	13.5	86.5 ± 3.0
2	4.3	95.7 ± 3.4	*4.0	96.0 ± 2.4	*1.0	99.0 ± 3.4
24	**40.0	60.0 ± 3.4	**25.3	74.7 ± 2.4	*26.0	74.0 ± 3.4
48	**41.0	59.0 ± 3.4	15.3	84.7 ± 2.4	**44.0	56.0 ± 3.4

Significantly different from corresponding 0-time,

*p < .05
**p < .01

(McCormack and Glasser, 1980)

Myometrial cells were assayed from the undissociated mince of myometrium. Prior to E_2 injection, myometrial cells contained significantly less ($p < 0.01$) RnE (1.2 fmol/μg DNA) and RcE (0.2 fmol/μg DNA) than either epithelial or stromal cells (Fig. 3). During the 48 hrs following E_2, the concentration of RnE fell significantly in the stroma ($p < 0.05$) to 0.7 fmol/μg DNA while RcE rose to 0.5 fmol/μg thereby creating essentially equal cytosol and nuclear RE compartments.

Table 3: Percent of the total uterine estrogen receptor (RE) in immature rat uterine cell types following sc injection of 2.5 μg E_2.

Time (h)	Epithelial cells ± SEM	Stromal cells ± SEM	Myometrial cells ± SEM
0	5.4 ± 0.8	10.2 ± 0.8	84.2 ± 1.9
2	3.9 ± 1.0	*7.4 ± 0.9	88.7 ± 2.2
24	5.8 ± 1.0	7.6 ± 0.9	84.0 ± 2.2
48	7.8 ± 1.0	**4.0 ± 0.9	87.7 ± 2.2

Significantly different from corresponding 0-time

*p < .05
**p < .01

(McCormack and Glasser, 1980)

Comparison With Data From Whole Immature Rat Uterus

The total RE concentrations found in separated cell types are similar in magnitude to those previously reported for the whole uterus of the immature rat (Gorski et al, 1971; Clark and Peck, 1976). The data are different with respect to the partition of RE between cytosol and nucleus. For purposes of comparison, we have converted the data of Clark et al (1979) from pmol/uterus to fmol/μg DNA (McCormack and Glasser, 1980). When compared to our data (Fig. 3), these recalculations demonstrate that the total RE concentration of the immature rat uterus is simlar whether measured in separated cells or intact whole uterus. The calculations reinforce our observation that the partition of RcE/RnE in individual cells is different from that measured in whole uterus.

Low cytosol concentrations of RE in mechanically separated uterine cell fractions have been recorded under somewhat different experimental conditions (Martel and Psychoyos, 1978). The concentration of RcE in endometrial and myometrial fractions of untreated castrate uterus were 1.0 and 0.25 fmol/μg DNA, respectively. Twenty-four hours after the last of three E_2 injections (0.25μg), the myometrial RcE concentration rose to 1.0 fmole/μg DNA. RnE was not measured.

The reason for the differential partitioning of RE to the epithelial cell nuclear compartment is not clear. Our representative zero time data (RcE, 4.02/μg DNA; RnE, 0.40 fmol/μg DNa) are similar to the zero time data of Clark et al (1979), i.e., 4.80 and 0.80 fmol/ g DNA in RcE and RnE, respectively. Thus, we reason that our RE assay methodology was not at fault. The possibility that the period of elevated temperature used in Step A to increase the yield of epithelial cells might artifactually translocate RE to the epithelial cell nucleus, even before E_2 administration, prompted us to analyze RE in epithelial cells kept at 4°C throughout the entire procedure (poor yield). An identically low RcE (0.6 fmol/μg DNA) was measured in separated epithelial cells under both sets of temperature conditions. While RnE was lowered at 4°C (2.0 fmol/μg DNA) the concentration was still three times greated than RcE.

Other factors that we have tested and found not to be responsible for the partitioning effect included: possible E_2 contamination of pancreatin, possible damage to cell and/or nuclear membranes and an increase in cell death. We continue to explore this phenomenon. It is important to note that the concentration of RcE can be increased in epithelial cells 24 and 48 hrs after the injection of E_2 (Fig. 3).

The concentration of RE in each cell type, expressed as a percent of total uterine RE (Table 3) showed that in response to E_2 (48 hrs), RE in myometrium increased 4%, decreased 6% in stroma and increased 3% in epithelium. Only the stromal increase was statistically significant ($p < 0.01$) compared with pre-treatment values of 84% total uterine RE for myometrium, 10% for stroma and 5% for epithelium.

The redistribution of RcE/RnE is recorded in Table 2. Approximately 10% of total cell RE, in all three cell types, was found in cytosol before E_2, the remainder was in the nuclear fraction. Within 2 hrs after E_2, RcE fell to less than 5% of total RE in all cell types. However, by 24 hrs, RcE had become a substantial percentage of total

RE (replenishment?). Each cell type responded individually. These shifts in RE distribution might be considered as integral to the late expressed responses to E_2. Each cell type responded individually and the changes were maintained through 48 hrs.

The apparent K_d for the cytosol and nuclear RE in the different cell types ranged from 1 to 10 x 10^{-10}M. There were no significant differences between the cell types, cytosol and nuclear RE or whole uteri in either the immature (McCormack and Glasser, 1980) or pregnant rats (Glasser and McCormack, 1980). The single exception was that epithelial cell cytosol RE ($5.6 \pm 2.9 \times 10^{-10}$M) was statistically significantly different ($p < 0.005$) than nuclear RE ($2.7 \pm 0.9 \times 10^{-10}$M by students's paired t test. Martel and Psychoyos (1978) have also reported a significant difference ($p < 0.005$) between the K_d of endometrium (epithelium + stroma) (K_d = 3×10^{-10}M) and myometrium (K_d = 6x 10^{-10}M) in ovariectomized adult rats.

Estrogen Receptors In The Whole Pre-Implantation Uterus

Previous attempts to measure the concentration of uterine RE during the period from conception to implantation have not been in agreeement (Glasser and Clark, 1975; Martel and Psychoyos, 1976; Glasser and McCormack, 1979). We have now studies RE in uterine cytosol and nuclear compartments under rigorous kinetic conditions (McCormack and Glasser, 1979) using a 12-point Scatchard analysis done under exchange conditions (Anderson et al, 1972). Pregnant rats of established cyclicity and proven fertility were used. The presence of a sperm positive vaginal smear and a copulatory plug designated day "0" of the pregnancy.

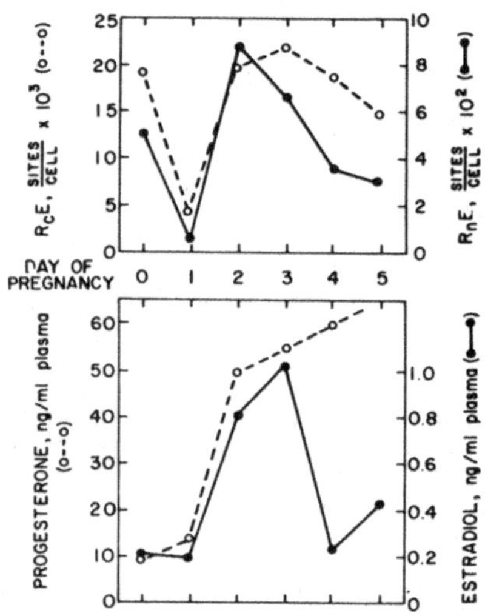

Fig. 4 (Top panel) Comparison of cytosol and nuclear receptor complexes in the uterus of pregnant rats. Day "0" of pregnancy designates presence of vaginal sperm. Data are expressed as sites per cell. (Bottom panel) Comparative plasma titers of progesterone and estradiol from the same rats. Steroid titers were measured by specific radioimmunoassay (Glasser and McCormack, 1979).

The concentrations of both the cytosolic estrogen receptor (RcE) and the nuclear estrogen receptor (RnE) on day zero (Fig. 4) reflected the receptor response to the previously elevated proestrus plasma estrogen levels. The low concentrations on day 1 were considered to represent the influence of low diestrus plasma estrogen (E). Plasma progesterone (P) was low on both days. Both plasma E and P rose markedly between gestation days 1 and 2. This change in steroid levels was paralleled by a 4-fold increase in RcE and an increase greater than 30-fold in RnE. The changes in RE were assigned to the influence of E on the synthesis, translocation and replenishment of its own receptor. We could not assign an unequivocal role to rising plasma titers of P. We made the assumption, based on the data of Hseuh et al, (1976), that the primary focus of P action was on the depression of RE replenishment. This effect of P assumed to have influenced the measured RE.

From its peak on day 2, the concentration of RnE fell to a plateau on day 4. This preceded the fall in RcE which began on day 3 after a continued rise from day 2 (Fig. 4). The basis for these changes was the resultant of the interaction of rising plasma P (diminished replenishment) and falling plasma E (depressed synthesis). We could not reasonably account for the fall in RnE while RcE was still rising. Modulating factors which we considered to be operable but not defineable included: the influence of rising plasma P on the dynamics and concentration of both RE and RP, the functional responses of uterine epithelium as differentiated from the responses of the stromal cells during the pre-implantaiton period (Tachi et al, 1972). Separate experiments designed to clarify certain issues by repeating the protocols of Martel and Psychoyos (1976) could neither confirm or deny that interesting work. Thus, the role of steroid hormone receptors in the maturation of uterine sensitivity for decidualization and receptivity for ovo-implantation remained to be defined.

Estrogen Receptors In Individual Cell Types of the Pre-Implantation Uterus

Analysis of individual cell populations did not definitively clarify the role of RE in the pre-implantation uterus. However, these studies did emphasize the limitations of whole organ analysis and delineated the specific response of each cell type. The elevated RcE and RnE concentrations described for the whole uterus (Fig. 4; Glasser and McCormack, 1979) attributed to proestrus plasma actually reflected the RE concentrations of the epithelial cells (Fig. 5). It is of interest to note that on day "0" stromal cell concentrations of RE were low and RnE > RcE (Fig. 5).

Synthesis and replenishment of RE did not appear to be a late response of epithelial cells to pre-ovulatory E. For while these cells proliferate (Martin and Finn, 1968; Martin et al, 1973; Tachi et al, 1972) the concentration of RcE and RnE fell as plasma E reached its nadir in diestrus. While there were no significant changes in the concentration of RcE during days 0-2 (Fig. 5), stromal RnE increased gradually from a level of 0.50 fmol/μg DNA on day "0" to 1.35 fmol/μg DNA on day 3 irrespective of the complex shifts in plasma P and E (Fig. 5).

It cannot be determined if the accumulation of RE by the stromal

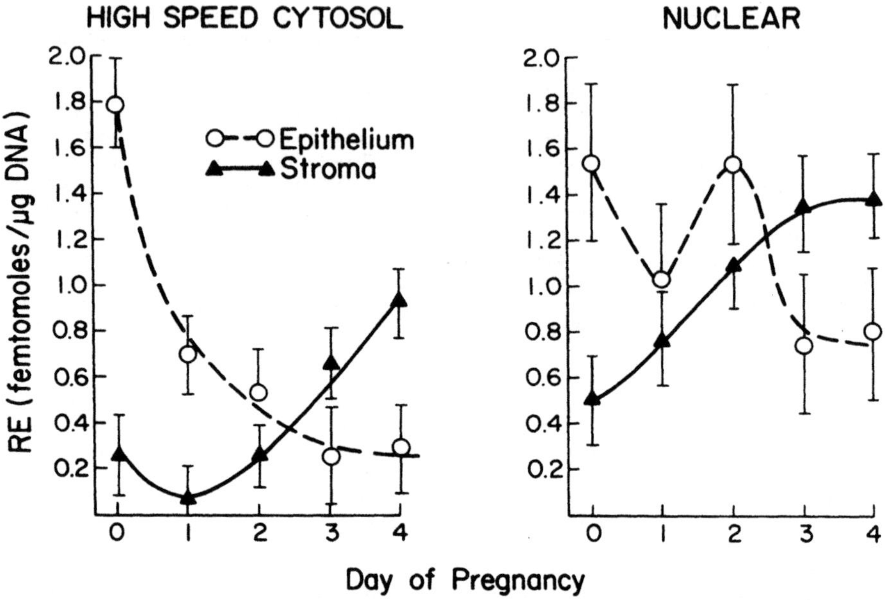

Fig. 5. Estrogen receptor concentrations in high speed cytosol and nuclear fractions of epithelial and stromal cells separated from pregnant rat uteri on various days of gestation. Data are expressed as fmol/µg DNA ± SEM. Compare these data with top panel Fig. 4. (Glasser and McCormack, 1980)

cell nucleus was due to translocation or a decrease in nuclear RE degradation. Changes in stromal cell cytosol receptor appeared to be too subtle to analyze during pre-implantation days 0-2. After day 2, RE increased significantly in the cytosol compartment in the face of markedly enlarged plasma P titers (Fig. 4) and continued to do so after the nucleus no longer accumulated RE (Fig. 5).

There are 4 evident shifts in RE concentration of uterine cell sub-populations. The nature of these altered interactions between the cells of the pre-implantation uterus and the hormones which regulate them cannot be clarified by our present understanding of how a hormone influences the ontogeny of its own receptor, the receptors of the other hormones or the interaction of different hormones in a single target cell. For these reasons, our previous interpretation of cause and effect regarding steroid hormone receptors of the pre-implantation uterus seems too simple.

Since on a physico-chemical basis (McCormack & Glasser, 1980), there are no discernible differences in the nature of RE, be it found in epithelium or stroma, cytoplasm or nucleus, the role of cell-cell communication remains to be defined,. This is fundamental if we are to attempt to explain why the same hormonal environment which will charge the stromal cell nucleus and subsequently the stromal cell cytosol with increasing RE concentrations will not sustain the RE concentration of the epithelial cells. Although these data are supportive of previous histological data (Martin and Finn, 1968; Martin et al, 1973; Tachi et al, 1972) we are still without a fair clue as to how the shift in the site of steroid hormone action is accomplished. What is the strategic advantage of this shift and of the consistent distribution of RE, in both epithelium and stroma, that favors the nuclear component.

CO-CULTURE OF BLASTOCYSTS WITH SPECIFIC UTERINE CELL TYPE MONOLAYERS

One of the purposes for which we developed these cell separation techniques was to provide specific cell monolayers with which to co-culture rat blastocysts. We appreciate that this type of co-culture or _in vitro_ implantation is not the perfect analog for _in vivo_ implantation (Enders et al, 1980). Nevertheless, that system can be used productively if the limitations of the model are recognized.

The interaction between monolayers of uterine cell types and rat blastocysts was monitored by measuring the rate and success of hatching and attachment as well as the daily steroid production by the blastocysts. In these experiments (Fig. 6) the monolayers of epithelial or stromal cells were prepared from immature rat uterus. Blastocysts were recovered from the uteri of pregnant rats on day 4 of gestation and co-cultured with the established monolayers. The conditions for successful _in vitro_ culture of peri- and post-implantation rat blastocysts are described elsewhere in this volume (McCormack and Glasser). The data from the co-culture experiments were compared with the steroid secretory patterns (progesterone, testosterone, estradiol) of blastocysts outgrowing in culture on plastic dishes.

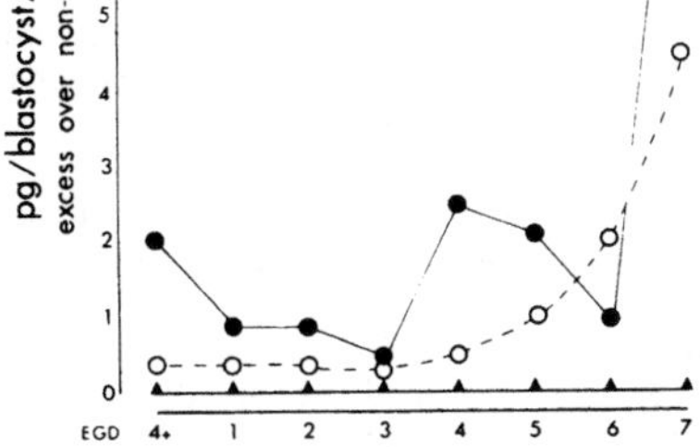

Fig. 6. Daily production of progesterone by rat blastocysts co-cultured with monolayers of epithelial or stromal cells. Monolayers were derived from cells separated from immature rat uteri. Comparison is made on equivalent gestation days (EGD) to blastocysts cultured _in vitro_ on plastic dishes. Steroid values are corrected for control measurements of incubated cell-free media.

The data in the co-cultured experiment depicted in Fig. 6 are derived by comparing P production by blastocysts at similar time periods (equivalent to their gestation days, EGD). Media were changed daily. Control values are the highest values obtained in the assay of co-incubated cell-free media. This value is subtracted from the experimental value and that data expressed as pg steroid/blastocyst/ 24 hrs in excess of the non-cellular control.

It is readily apparent that co-culture of developing blastocysts with established stromal cell monolayers suppressed the P secretory ability of the blastocyst to non-detectable levels. Growth on epithelial cell monolayers cancelled P production during EGD 4+0 to 4+7 (52% of P produced by contemporary blastocysts cultured in plastic dishes).

The data presented in this paper validate the use of viable, essentially homogeneous populations of individual cell types as effective probes in the definition of target cell responses to hormones and other regulatory agents. The use of these cell populations makes it possible to differentiate target cell responses while avoiding the indirect or retrospective relationships of function and cytology that necessarily arise from analysis of whole organs. The techniques used at the present time are not represented as complete. We continue to improve the facility and the efficiency of these methods so their usefulness as probes will be recognized by morphologists and biochemists alike and applied to a broader range of investigations.

ACKNOWLEDGEMENTS

We are indebted to Ms. Jo Anne Julian and Mr. Robert A. May for their technical assistance. We gratefully acknowledge the helpful suggestions of Dr. Len Martin (Imperial Cancer Research Fund, London, England) and Dr. Michael I. Sherman (Roche Institute of Molecular Biology, Nutley, N.J.) for helpful suggestions during the early stages of this work.

These investigations were supported by NIH grants HD-12964 as well as HD-07495 and National Cancer Institute grant CA-20853.

REFERENCES

Anderson, J.N., Clark, J.H. and Peck, E.J. (1972). The relationship between nuclear receptor estrogen binding and uterotrophic responses. Biochem. Biophys. Commun. 48, 1460-1468.

Clark, J.H. and Peck, E.J. (1976). Nuclear retention of receptor-estrogen complex and nuclear acceptor sites. Nature 260, 635-637.

Clark, J.H., Peck, E.J. and Glasser, S.R. (1977). Mechanism of action of sex steroids in the female. In: Reproduction in Domestic Animals, 3rd Ed. (H.H. Cole and P.T. Cupps, eds.) Academic Press, New York pp. 143-173.

Clark, J.H., McCormack, S.A., Padykula, H., Markaverich, B. and Hardin, J.W. (1979). Biochemical and morphological changes stimulated by the nuclear binding of the estrogen receptor. In: Effects of Drugs on the Cell Nucleus (H.A. Busch, ed.) Academic Press, New York (in press).

Enders, A.C., Chavez, D.J. and Schlafke, S. (1980). Comparison of implantation in utero and in vitro. In: Cellular and Molecular Aspects of Implantation (S.R. Glasser and D.W. Bullock, eds.) Plenum Publishing Co., New York, (in press).

Glasser, S.R. (1972). The uterine environment in implantation and decidualization. In: Reproductive Biology (H.A. Balin and S.R. Glasser, eds.) Excerpta Medica Fdn., Amsterdam, pp. 776-833.

Glasser, S.R. and Clark, J.H. (1975). A determinant role for progesterone in the development of uterine sensitivity to decidualization and ovoimplantation. In: The Developmental Biology of Reproduction (C. Markert and J. Papaconstantinou, eds.) Academic Press, New York, pp. 311-345.

Glasser, S.R. and McCormack, S.A. (1979). Cellular and molecular aspects of decidualization and implantaiton. In: Proteins and Steroids in Early Mammalian Development (H. Beier and P. Karlson, eds.) Springer-Verlag. Berlin (in press).

Glasser, S.R. and McCormack, S.A. (1980). Separated cell types as analytical tools in the study of decidualization and implantation. In: Cellular and Molecular Aspects of Implantation (S.R. Glasser and D.W. Bullock, eds.) Plenum Publishing Co., New York (in press).

Gorski, J., DeAngelo, A.B. and Barnea, A. (1971). Estrogen actions: the role of specific RNA and protein synthesis. In: The Sex Steroids (K.W. McKerns, ed.) Appleton-Century-Crofts, New York, pp. 181-195.

Hsueh, A.J.W., Peck, E.J. and Clark, J.H. (1976). Control of uterine estrogen receptor levels by progesterone. Endocrinology 98, 438-444.

Martel, D. and Psychoyos, A. (1976). Endometrial content of nuclear estrogen receptor and receptivity for ovoimplantation in the rat. Endocrinology 99, 470-475.

Martel, D. and Psychoyos, A. (1978). Progesterone-induced oestrogen receptors in the rat uterus. J. Endocrinol. 76, 145-154.

Martin, L. and Finn, C.A., (1968). Hormonal regulation of cell division in epithelial and connective tissues of the mouse uterus. J. Endocrinol. 41, 363-371.

Martin, L., Finn, C.A. and Trinder, G., (1973). Hypertrophy and hyperplasia in the mouse uterus after oestrogen treatment: an autoradiographic study. J. Endocrinol. 56, 133-144.

McCormack, S.A. and Glasser, S.R. (1976). A high affinity estrogen binding protein in rat placental trophoblast. Endocrinology 99, 701-712.

McCormack, S.A. and Glasser, S.R. (1978) Ontogeny and regulation of a rat placental estrogen receptor. Endocrinology 102, 273-280.

McCormack, S.A. and Glasser, S.R. (1980). Differential response of individual uterine cell types from immature rats treated with estradiol. Endocrinology (in press).

O'Malley, B.W. and Means, A.R. (1974). Female steroid hormones and target cell nuclei. Science 183, 610-620.

Scatchard, G. (1949). The attraction of proteins for small molecules and ions. New York Acad. Sci. Ann. 51, 660-672.

Sherman, M.I. (1978). Implantation of mouse blastocysts in vitro. In: Methods in Mammalial Reproduction (J.C. Daniel, Jr., ed.) Academic Press, New York, pp. 247-257.

Tachi, C., Tachi, S. and Lindner, H.R. (1972). Modification by progesterone of oestradiol-induced cell proliferation, RNA synthesis and oestradiol distribution in the rat uterus. J. Reprod. Fertil. 21, 59-76.

DISCUSSION

KATZENELLENBOGEN: Do the uterine epithelial or stromal cells exhibit tissue specificity? Have you used other nonuterine epithelial cells or stromal or fibroblast cells to provide monolayers?

GLASSER: We think there is information in the uterine epithelial cells that is different than that found in epithelial cells taken from other tissues.

KATZENELLENBOGEN: Have you used any other endpoint, or do you plan to use another endpoint, besides steroid production?

GLASSER: Yes, another parameter that we have used as an outgrowth characteristic is rat placental lactogen secretion. Hatching time, attachment time, attachment rate success, and invasiveness or noninvasiveness are other characteristics that are unique to the blastocyst response to individual uterine cell types.

MOULTON: I realize this is a difficult thing to check, but I wonder if your separation methods have an effect on the levels of steroid receptor that you measure.

GLASSER: There are differences in our data versus previously reported data, particularly in the cytoplasmic compartment. [This is one of the reasons we did transmission and scanning electron microscopy studies of these cells. The suggestion was that there might be injury and subsequent leakage.] Our experiments challenged work in our own department. We reviewed our data and did every experiment that was suggested or that we could think of. For instance, one of the steps that is used to increase the yield of cells is to raise the temperature to 37° during the second phase of the trypsin-pancreatin incubation. This increases the yield but opens the possibility of temperature induced translocation. Working at lower temperatures with the resulting lower cell yields, the same number of cytoplasmic receptors are obtained, so we are not dealing with a temperature translocation. We have satisfied ourselves and a large number of critics that the numbers that we see, although different from those seen in the whole uterus, may be real numbers. It may be that all the data worked out on the whole uterus may have to be redone in terms of separated cells.

We can place cytoplasmic receptors in the cell by the hormonal treatment of that animal and they don't leak out during cell separation. The heterochromatin, if we are using immature animals, stays in the nucleus. Further, high EM magnification indicates that the cell and nuclear membranes maintain integrity.

MOULTON: We have used another method of cell separation in our work in the deciduoma. It's more of an analytic technique rather than the elegant work you are doing here, where you culture the separated cells. If you have a large number of cells that have diversity in cell size, then velocity sedimentation at unit gravity enables separation according to cell size. There are unique populations of cells within the deciduoma that have different synthetic capacities, different enzyme levels and, we hope to show in the future, different levels of receptor. We have run into the problem, however, that as we digest the tissue with collagenase the estrogen receptors become quite sensitive.

GLASSER: Collagenase is probably the worst thing we have yet subjected a cell to, even in the lowest concentrations. Morphologically, collagenase treated cells look like they have been riddled. We have done initial studies using your sedimentation techniques, but more interesting and far easier is something we have derived from Dr. Gerschenson's paper. Stromal cells are put into culture, then after a short time the media are poured off. Attached stromal cells are left behind and the putative glandular epithelium is in the supernatant fraction. Differential attachment may prove to be attractive in the separation of the stroma from the glandual epithelium. There are many ways to go. The next thing that we have to do is to increase our yields so that the separate cell culture becomes more useful biochemically.

GERSCHENSON: I would like to mention something very simple. Most collagenase preparations, unless one buys chromatographically pure enzyme, are contaminated with phospholipase activity, which could explain their toxicity.

BIGGERS: As far as I am aware these are the first cultures of rat blastocysts. All the work done until now has been done with the mouse. Could you describe how the rat blastocyst behaves in more detail, and tell us whether there are differences in the way the blastocysts proliferate on different substrates, e.g., on plastic, epithelial and stromal monolayers?

GLASSER: I would be glad to. We have had success with NCTC-135 media instead of NCTC-109 used with mouse blastocysts. Day 4 rat blastocysts are recovered from the uteri and washed. The obviously defective ones are removed and the remainder are put into culture. At 20 to 28 hours there is evidence of hatching and at 28 to 36 hours the blastocysts begin to attach. The blastocyst presents a very diffuse cytoskeleton during hatching out. When it attaches there is evidence of organization of the cytoskeleton and as the trophoblast grows out on the plastic dish, you begin to see regular tubulin and stressed fiber formation. Outgrowth is rather rapid and will continue for about 14 days, then deterioration begins. The inner cell mass is not maintained very well with our culture conditions, and by 4 or 5 days in culture has begun to cavitate and disappear. The cell types that we note are primarily trophoblast giant cells. As the blastocysts grow out we monitor steroid secretion. At equivalent gestation day 11 the production of rat placental lactogen begins, and then at about equivalent gestation date 20, the cells show signs of fatigue and begin dying off. (See McCormack and Glasser, this volume).

Hormonal Regulation of Proliferation and Differentiation of Rabbit Uterine Epithelium: Cell Culture and Animal Studies

J.T. Murai
C.J. Conti
I. Gimenez-Conti
J.R. Depaoli
E.A. Conner
L.E. Gerschenson

INTRODUCTION

Beatson (1) described for the first time in 1896, that hormones could exert a strong influence in the growth of a human cancer. His observation that ovariectomy induced regression of metastatic breast cancer cannot yet be explained on cellular and/or molecular bases. Part of the difficulty, also observed in all neoplasms of endocrine tissues, has been the still-limited knowledge of the basic mechanisms of hormone action. We have recently tried to improve the general understanding of the relationship between hormones and neoplasia by studying the ovarian hormone regulation of proliferation and differentiation of rabbit endometrium.

There is strong evidence that ovarian hormones play a prevalent role in the pathogenesis of endometrial carcinoma in humans and rabbits. Estrogens have been described as having a promoting role (1-6), while progestins have the opposite effect (6,7-9). A better understanding of the effects of each ovarian steroid and their interaction on endometrial cell growth and function could provide information relevant to the study of endometrial hyperplasia and carcinoma, suggesting improved methods of treatment for these widespread gynecologic disorders and shedding some light on the role of hormones in the development of cancer.

Estrogens and progestins have a remarkable trophic effect upon endometrium, which requires continued exposure to the hormones for optimal development. The mechanisms of action of these hormones and their interactions are not very well understood. Two of the most important reasons are: the complexity of the target tissue and the difficulty of dealing with homeostatic mechanisms in whole animals.

Correspondence should be addressed to L.E. Gerschenson.

*Staff Member, Atomic Energy Commission, Argentina.

**Staff Member, National Research Council, Argentina.

***Visiting Scientist from the Institute of Cardiology, National Academy of Medicine, Argentina.

****Applied Biological Sciences Laboratory, Inc., Glendale, Calif.

We consider that the use of a cell culture experimental system and its regulation by hormones provides a relatively simpler model than the whole animal. Simplicity is an important factor, but demonstrable extrapolation to the whole animal is essential for the relevance of our studies. Therefore, in our endeavors, we try to maintain a symbiotic relationship between in vivo and in vitro research.

RESULTS AND DISCUSSION

Because this paper is meant to be a summary of the latest results obtained in our laboratory, we have not emphasized methodological details. The reader is referred to appropriate references for these methods.

Proliferation Studies Using Cultured Cells

We have developed a new model system of primary cultured rabbit endometrial epithelial cells, using chemically defined medium (10-18), which were found to respond to the addition of natural or synthetic estrogens by an increase in the initiation of DNA synthesis, measured by the fraction of labeled cells after a pulse of ^{3}H-thymidine (^{3}H-Tdr) or by an increase in cell number. Progesterone was found to antagonize the estrogenic effect.

It was surprising to find that progesterone alone did not have any mitogenic effect on the cultured cells, since this ovarian hormone has a limited proliferation effect on rabbit uterine epithelium, resulting finally in quiescent terminally differentiated cells. In our cultured cell system, we have not observed this action, but only the antagonistic effect towards estrogens also observed in whole animals (see below in section on Proliferation and Differentiation Studies in Whole Animals).

We tried then to determine if the estrogenic regulation of proliferation was elicited by controlling the number of cells entering the cell cycle or by shortening the length of the cell cycle. We found that untreated cultures have 60-80% nondividing or quiescent cells and that estrogens shifted most of these nondividing cells into the cell cycle (13).

The presence of at least two cell populations (quiescent vs. cycling cells) prompted us to ask at least two questions: Were the hormones affecting only one cell population or both? Were there any cell cooperativity phenomena involved?

To answer these questions, we developed techniques to separate and culture both cell populations. We used lethal concentrations of ^{3}H-Tdr and cytosine arabinoside (13,19) to eliminate cycling cells, and addition of colcemid, resulting in the accumulation of mitotic cells which are less strongly attached to culture dishes, to isolate cycling cells (13,20). Then the effects of estrogens, progesterone and other hormones were assayed on the proliferation of the two cell populations (13).

Table 2 shows that only the quiescent cells responded to diethylstilbestrol, but both cell populations responded to the addition of epidermal growth factor or prostaglandin $F_{2\alpha}$. Prostaglandin E_2 was found not to have any effect.

TABLE 1

Effect of Estrogens and Progesterone on Proliferation of Cultured Endometrial Cells

Hormones Added	Concentration (M)	Labeling Index Exp. A	Exp. B	Exp. C	Cell Number per Petri Dish
No Addition		33.4±5.7	26.4±6.1	17.4±4.9	135,000±16,228
Diethylstilbestrol (DES)	10^{-7}	57.2±3.7*			
Estradiol-17β (E_2)	10^{-10}		24.7±2.6		
	10^{-9}		33.1±3.6		
	10^{-8}		51.2±6.3*		
	10^{-7}	55.0±6.0*	43.0±1.3*	34.2±4.0*	195,000±13,639*
	10^{-6}		43.0±1.4*		
Estradiol-17α	10^{-7}		29.2±3.6		
Progesterone (P)	10^{-7}	32.1±3.2			
DES + P	10^{-7}-10^{-7}	34.6±5.4			
DES + E_2	10^{-7}-10^{-7}	37.8±6.1			

Labeling index is the percentage of cells with labeled nuclei per total number of epithelial cells (15). The hormones and ^{3}H-Tdr were added 24-30 hours before the determinations.

Values are means ± S.E.M. Mean = average of 5 dishes (dia. = 5 cm).

*Statistically significant when compared with No Addition group using the t test.

TABLE 2

Effect of Hormones on Different Cell Populations of Cultured Endometrial Cells

	Original Mixed Cell Culture	Quiescent Cells	Cycling Cells
No Additions	31.8 ± 3.4	4.9 ± 0.8	23.3 ± 4.8
10^{-7} M Diethylstilbestrol (DES)	46.0 ± 1.0*	18.0 ± 0.4*	13.2 ± 4.6
10^{-7} M Progesterone (P)	22.2 ± 5.5	3.5 ± 0.7	33.5 ± 4.2
DES + P	30.0 ± 2.7	17.2 ± 0.8*	24.4 ± 0.2
10^{-9} M Epidermal Growth Factor (EGF)	52.5 ± 4.8*	9.2 ± 1.2*	46.9 ± 3.0*
5 x 10^{-7} M Prostaglandin $F_{2\alpha}$ (PGF)	40.5 ± 1.1*	8.6 ± 1.2*	38.4 ± 3.3*

*Data are expressed as in Table 1.

We also found that estrogens and progesterone do not regulate the proliferation of the cell line, BALB/3T3, widely used for this type of study, pointing out a specific effect of these hormones on our cultured endometrial cells. The specificity of the progesterone inhibitory effect upon estrogenic stimulation of growth is shown by the fact that progesterone was found not to antagonize the effects of either epidermal growth factor or prostaglandin $F_{2\alpha}$ on the proliferation of endometrial mixed cell cultures.

A puzzling finding was that only a fraction of the quiescent cells responded to the estrogenic stimulus, although the response was very high. Possible explanations considered were poor cell viability or different cell densities; both were found unsatisfactory. However, our recent in vivo work described below suggests the existence of two quiescent cell populations in the rabbit uterine epithelium, one of them luminal and the other one glandular. The proliferation of the latter appeared to be the only one regulated by estrogen administration. Therefore, it is possible that in our cultures, two quiescent cell populations coexist, but only one of them would show an estrogenic response, explaining in this way the above described finding.

Table 2 shows also that progesterone did not inhibit the effect of diethylstilbestrol on the quiescent cells. We considered the possibility that the cycling cells could metabolize progesterone to an active compound or that progesterone could induce the dividing cells to synthesize and/or secrete a factor which could be inhibiting the estrogenic effect. The experiment summarized in Table 3 supports strongly the hypothesis described above. Culture media with or without progesterone was incubated for 2 days with either quiescent cells or a mixed cell population (quiescent plus cycling cells). The conditioned media was then assayed for biological activity on quiescent cells.

TABLE 3

Effect of Conditioning Media on the Estrogenic Effect on Quiescent Cells

	Medium Conditioned with Mixed Cell Cultures		Medium Conditioned with Quiescent Cells	
	With 10^{-7} M Progesterone	Without Progesterone	With 10^{-7} M Progesterone	Without Progesterone
No Additions	2.7 ± 0.4	2.7 ± 0.1	2.9 ± 0.3	3.2 ± 0.1
10^{-7} M Diethylstilbestrol (DES)	3.0 ± 0.5	17.1 ± 0.8*	18.4 ± 1.1	19.0 ± 1.2*
10^{-7} M Progesterone (P)	4.0 ± 0.2	3.0 ± 0.2	3.4 ± 0.2	4.0 ± 0.3
10^{-7} M DES + 10^{-7} M P	2.6 ± 0.2	16.0 ± 0.1*	17.9 ± 0.8*	18.1 ± 0.9*

Data are expressed as in Table 1.

The data obtained showed that an inhibitor of the estrogenic effect on proliferation is present in the medium, as a result of the interaction between a mixed cell culture and progesterone. Since the same effect was not observed using media conditioned with quiescent cells, we believe that a progesterone-induced estrogen inhibitor results from the interaction between cycling cells and the ovarian hormone.

When two other progestins, 17,21-dimethyl-19-nor-pregna-4,9-diene-3,20-ione (R5020) and 20 α-hydroxy-pregn-4-en-3-one, were assayed for estrogen-inhibitory effect as above, no biological effect was detected, suggesting a strong progesterone specificity.

We have found recently that rabbit endometrial cells, when plated at higher density, will not respond to estrogens by an increased proliferation. After studying several possible explanations, we found that as in low density cultures treated with progesterone, high density cultures produce an estrogen inhibitor factor, which appears to be an acidic protein, difficult to precipitate with ammonium sulphate and of an approximate M.W. of 20,000. We believe this protein is probably similar to the one produced under progesterone influence by low density cultures. We have also detected during purification of the estrogen-inhibitor factor, another substance, probably of protein nature, since it precipitates at high ammonium sulphate concentration with an approximate M.W. of 1,000, but this factor produces a several-fold stimulation in the proliferative effect of estrogens (21).

The production of factors by cultured cells which promote or inhibit proliferation of cultured cells has been described (22) as well as the existence of many growth factors for cultured cells (23). However, the possible occurrence of molecules involved in the regulation of ovarian steroid hormones is a novel concept.

Sirbasku (24) suggested that estrogen-related growth factor activities can be identified in normal estrogen target tissues of rodents and that these activities are specific for hormone-responsive cells. Sonnenschein and Soto (25) proposed that α-fetoprotein could play a role in the growth regulation of estrogen-sensitive tumor cells.

Kano-Sueoka et al. (26) have identified phosphoethanolamine as a pituitary-derived growth-promoting substance that specifically stimulates a rat mammary carcinoma cell line.

We believe that the mechanisms of action through which ovarian hormones regulate endometrium proliferation are more complex than foreseen. They probably include ovarian hormone-dependent factors which could play a key role either as triggers or regulators.

The presence of a progesterone-induced estrogen inhibitor factor as well as an estrogen-stimulating factor in endometrium could open up new research and therapeutic avenues and might suggest that endometrial hyperplasia and carcinoma might be metabolic diseases of a sort, in which the production of these factors might be altered due to hereditary, nutritional or hormonal causes.

Proliferation Studies Using Animals and Differentiation

The rabbit endometrium consists of a luminal epithelium made up of columnar cells and a stroma riddled with tubular glands or crypts which are also composed of columnar cells. The glands open into the lumen to form a continuous layer of columnar cells and the cells of both the luminal and glandular epithelium have been shown to be morphologically similar by light and electron microscopy (28,29). As we mentioned above, we described in primary cell cultures of rabbit endometrium at least two cell populations, resting and dividing, which respond in different ways to estrogens and progestins (3). This heterogeneity of epithelial cell types could be attributed in part to the fact that the cells may have originated from either the luminal and/or glandular epithelium. To examine whether the heterogeneity of epithelial cells was due to the isolation of cells originating from different parts of the epithelium, in vivo proliferation experiments were performed to assess the possibility of observing the existence of specific target cells for different ovarian hormones.

We developed a method to measure cellular proliferation in small sections of uteri from rabbits that were not injected with hormones. It consists of a short-term in vitro incubation of the uterine sections in chemically defined Ham's F-12 medium (10) containing ^{3}H-thymidine to measure DNA synthesis by determination of the labeling index. The incubation was carried out at 37°C with rapid shaking and the length of the incubation varied between 1-18 hours.

Using this technique, we studied the proliferative effects of the ovarian hormones on the different areas of the uterine epithelium (17). Table 4 shows labeling indexes in control and estradiol-treated rabbits in both luminal and glandular uterine epithelium. Estradiol decreased labeling indexes in the luminal cells but increased labeling indexes of the glandular cells. Progesterone-treated rabbits were studied at 24 and 48 hours post-treatment. This hormone increased the labeling index of the luminal cells. The effect at 48 hours was higher than at 24 hours. In the same table, we show the effect of progesterone on glandular cells, which was similar to the effect of the same hormone in luminal cells. However, it took longer for the increase in glandular cell proliferation to be expressed. Administration of estradiol-17β for up to 5 days had the same effect as the one shown here and it did not show increased labeling of glandular cells.

TABLE 4

Effect of Estradiol-17β and Progesterone on the Labeling Index of Rabbit Uterine Epithelium

	Luminal Cells	Glandular Cells
Control (Oil)	1.58 ± 0.57	4.10 ± 0.20
Estradiol-17β/24 hours	0.65 ± 0.05	8.85 ± 0.44*
Progesterone/24 hours	5.99 ± 0.55*	5.72 ± 1.12
Progesterone/48 hours	43.54 ± 1.12*	48.52 ± 10.05*

Values are means ± S.E.M. of percentage of epithelial cells with labeled nuclei per total number of epithelial cells. Mean: average of 2-4 rabbits.

*Statistically significant when compared with control group using the t test.

Hormone dose, s.c.: Estradiol-17β, 1 mg/kg/day. Progesterone, 5 mg/kg/day.

Tissue sections were incubated for 3 hours in medium plus ^{3}H-thymidine.

Table 5 shows the results of an experiment in which both estradiol and progesterone were injected into the same animal. The labeling indexes are lower than in control rabbits, indicating that under these conditions, estradiol and progesterone inhibited each other and paradoxically decreased the normal epithelial cell proliferation.

TABLE 5

Effect of Simultaneous Administration of Estradiol-17β and Progesterone on the Labeling Index of Rabbit Uterine Epithelium

	Luminal Cells	Glandular Cells
Control (Oil)	1.06 ± 0.31	2.82 ± 0.78
Estradiol-17β + progesterone/24 hr	0.12 ± 0.05*	0.40 ± 0.26*

Mean: Average of 3-6 rabbits. Data are expressed as in Table 4.

An interesting result of our in vivo proliferation studies was the observation of structures which resembled various stages of gland or crypt formation. These structures consistently appeared only in rabbits treated with progesterone for short periods of time and may represent the initiation of arborization from the uterine lumen. Labeling indexes of the cells in those precursor structures indicate that they are foci of increased cellular proliferation which is consistent with our hypothesis of new gland or crypt formation from luminal epithelium. The mechanisms by which rabbit endometrial arborization takes place during pregnancy or pseudopregnancy are not very well understood. However, the most recent hypothesis have suggested that folding of the epithelium could play a major role (27). The older and more classical explanation is that arborization is due to gland formation (29). Our data are more consistent with the latter hypothesis.

Another interesting observation which resulted from our in vivo proliferation studies was that changes in basement membrane and cell cytoskeleton might play a role in gland formation by changing the degree of epithelial cell anchorage. We observed that progesterone induced a marked thickening of epithelial basement membrane and that microfilaments appear to go from the epithelial cell to and through the basement membrane (17).

To study basement membrane formation, we utilized an immunohistochemical technique to monitor rabbit basement membrane synthesis. Antibody to basement membrane was produced in sheep using basement membrane isolated from rabbit lens capsules. Using the indirect antibody technique, rabbit anti-sheep γ-globulin coupled to horseradish peroxidase was reacted to sheep antibodies and horseradish peroxidase allowed to oxidase a chromogen, diaminobenzidine, which produces a stable, colored product visible by light microscopy.

The increased cell proliferation induced by progestins, coupled with the possible increased anchorage could reasonably explain the arborization induced by progestins. Several authors have suggested that basement membrane could play a role in epithelial development (30-32). Our contention is that the possible main role of endometrial basement membrane resides in epithelial cell anchorage and contributes to the development of secretory endometrium.

Hormonal Receptor Studies

As described above, we have shown that the ovarian hormones are involved in the regulation of cellular proliferation (10-15). The basic question we then decided to answer was how the ovarian hormones were exerting their effects to control cell proliferation. To answer this question, the parameter we decided to examine was how the hormone receptor levels varied with different hormonal treatments since the effects of the hormones were believed to be elicited through the action of hormone receptors.

To begin our studies, we developed an assay to measure estrogen receptor levels in our cultured rabbit endometrial cells (16). The technique is a whole cell assay and measures total receptor populations; that is, the assay cannot differentiate between cytoplasmic and nuclear receptors. Using the assay, we characterized the nature

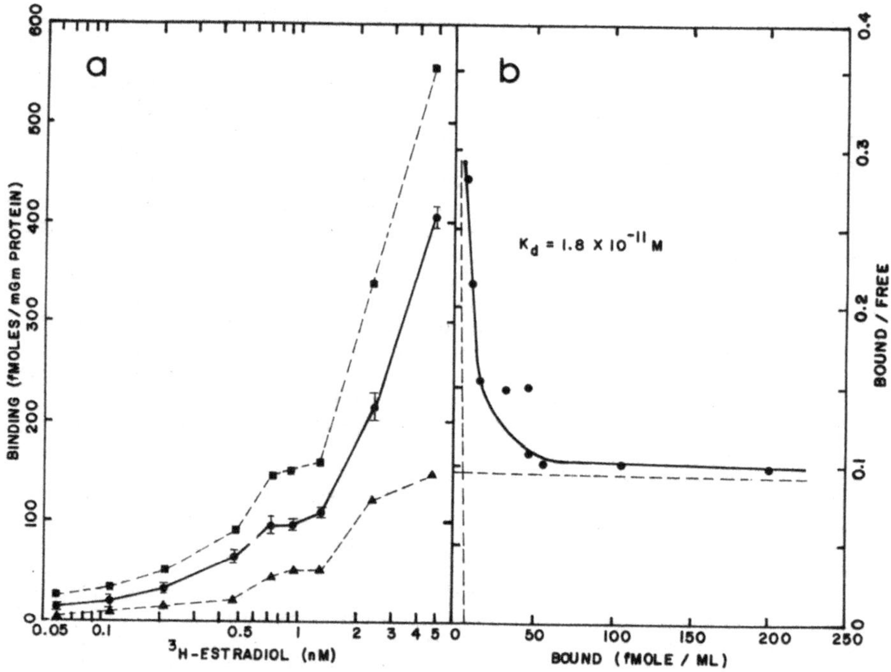

FIGURE 1

Estradiol Saturation Curve and Scatchard Plot. Each point represents the mean of 5 plates $\pm$ S.E.M. Since the number of cells varied slightly from plate to plate, the total counts were normalized to cpm/mg protein. Figure 1a is an estradiol saturation curve. (□), represents total estradiol binding; (Δ), represents nonspecific estradiol binding; (O), represents specific estradiol binding. Figure 1b is a Scatchard plot of the same data. The two components of the curve were estimated by the method of Rosenthal (33). Corrections were made for ^{3}H-estradiol binding to the plastic dishes nonspecifically.

of the estradiol binding to ensure we were measuring specific estrogen receptors. Figures 1a and 1b shows the saturation kinetics of the estradiol binding and a Scatchard plot of the same data to measure the binding constants. From the figures, it appears that two populations of receptors are present in our system. One population shows a limited number of binding sites with high affinity (1.8 x 10^{-11} M), which one would expect if one were measuring specific estrogen receptors, while the second binding component has low affinity but very high capacity. However, this second component appears in such extremely large numbers that whether they are relevant to steroid action in our system is not known at this time.

Another characteristic of the estrogen receptor was its steroid specificity (Table 6). The binding was fairly specific for estradiol, although progesterone appears to interfere slightly with the binding; however, this decrease may not be due to progesterone binding to the estrogen receptor, but rather to a rapid decrease in the estrogen receptor levels induced by progesterone.

TABLE 6

Steroid Specificity of Estradiol Binding

Hormone (10^{-7} M)	^{3}H-Estradiol Bound (cpm/mgm protein x 10^{-3}) $\bar{x} \pm$ S.E.M. n = 5	% of Control
Control	9.15 ± 0.39	100
Estradiol-17β	4.47 ± 0.47	48.8
Diethylstilbestrol	5.97 ± 0.36	65.2
Progesterone	7.07 ± 0.33	77.2
Testosterone	8.16 ± 0.19	89.1
Hydrocortisone	8.77 ± 0.33	95.8

Cells were plated at 1.5 x 10^{6} cells per 60 mm culture dish and washed twice one day later to remove unattached cells. The steroid specificity of the estradiol binding was examined by adding competing steroid hormones to the estradiol receptor assay. ^{3}H-estradiol plus a 100-fold excess of unlabeled competing hormone was added and incubated for one hour at 37°C. The excess ^{3}H-estradiol was washed out with cold 0.9% saline and the cells dissolved in NaOH and receptor levels measured. The concentrations of the ^{3}H-estradiol used in the binding assay was 1 x 10^{-9} M.

We examined how pretreatment of the cells with ovarian hormones affected the estradiol receptor levels (Table 7). In the experiment, the cells were pretreated for 24 hours with the hormones listed in the Table, the hormones washed out, any bound hormones allowed to egress from the cell and estrogen receptor levels measured.

It was found that progesterone pretreatment for 24 hours decreased the number of estogen receptors, as was expected since progesterone has been reported to antagonize the stimulatory effect of estradiol, probably by decreasing the estradiol receptor levels <u>in vivo</u> (34-38). Contrary to our expectations, estradiol pretreatment also was found to decrease the estrogen receptor levels. This was a surprise, since estrogen administration in vivo has been reported to increase the estrogen receptor levels in ovariectomized animals (36-39) or at least replenish the receptor levels to their original levels (40-42). However, in support of our observation, previous investigators have shown in vivo and in culture that upon treatment with estradiol, nuclear estrogen receptors decreased and appear not to be replenished (43-44).

TABLE 7

Effect of Hormones on Estradiol Receptor Levels

Hormone Treatment (10^{-7} M each)	^{3}H-Estradiol Bound (cpm/mgm protein x 10^{-3}) $\bar{x} \pm$ S.E.M. n = 5
Control	5.24 ± 0.21
Estradiol-17β	3.01 ± 0.22
Progesterone	2.43 ± 0.09
Estradiol-17β + Progesterone	1.99 ± 0.21

Cells were plated at 1.5 x 10^6 cells per 60 mm culture dish and washed twice one day later to remove unattached cells. Control medium or medium containing unlabeled hormones were added and incubated for 24 hours. After the incubation period, cells were washed 5 times to remove hormones and control medium was added to the cells to allow the bound hormones to egress from the cells. After a 4-hour egress period (with a change of medium at 2 hours), the cells were assayed for receptors. The concentration of ^{3}H-estradiol used in the binding assay was 1 x 10^{-9} M. Each point in each of the parallel assays represents an average of 5 culture dishes.

Further studies of the decrease in the estrogen receptors after pretreatment with estradiol and progesterone show that this decrease in estrogen receptors only occurs with these two hormones; that is, pretreatment with other hormones such as testosterone or hydrocortisone does not affect the estrogen receptor levels. Thus, it appears that the decrease in estrogen receptors is steroid specific with only progesterone or estradiol being able to regulate the estrogen receptor levels. Kinetic studies on the decrease of the estrogen receptor showed that the two hormones appear to reduce the estrogen receptor levels by different mechanisms of action. Our results show that progesterone decreases estrogen receptors slowly and linearly suggesting that progesterone is probably inhibiting selectively the synthesis of the estrogen receptor; on the other hand, estradiol decreases estrogen receptors rapidly and maintains receptor levels at a low level suggesting that estradiol is decreasing receptors by utilizing available estrogen receptors and not replenishing them. Finally, it appears that the decrease in estrogen receptors caused by pretreatment with the two hormones is reversible; that is, once the hormones are removed, the estrogen receptor levels recover to their original levels.

We have also been studying hormone receptors in vivo. We have established that there are specific receptors in rabbit uterine homogenates. The rabbit uterine cytosol estradiol receptor has a K_d of approximately 3×10^{-10} M, is extremely specific for estradiol, sediments at approximately 7-8S in sucrose density gradients and behaves as a classical estradiol receptor. The rabbit uterine cytoplasmic progesterone receptor has a K_d of approximately 3×10^{-9} M, is fairly specific for progesterone, and sediments at approximately 6-7S in sucrose density gradients.

Experiments were carried out using ovariectomized rabbits to examine how ovarian hormone pretreatment affected hormone receptor levels. Results showed that, as in our tissue culture experiments, both progesterone and estradiol were able to decrease the estrogen receptor levels (unpublished results). Thus, our in vivo studies confirmed the results obtained in culture that both progesterone and estradiol pretreatment decrease the estrogen receptor levels.

The significance of the decrease in estrogen receptor levels caused by estradiol pretreatment is unknown; however, the decrease may be related to refractoriness exhibited by many target tissues to prolonged stimulation by its respective hormone. Desensitization or refractoriness is a well known physiological response of a tissue to a specific stimulus. Many peptide hormones, as well as the catecholamines, have been shown to produce a desensitization response in the target tissue for that particular hormone (45-49, 54-61). Mouse and rat uteri have also been reported to become refractory to prolonged estrogenic stimulation (50-53). One mechanism suggested for a refractory response of a tissue is the down regulation of the receptors for that hormone in the target tissue (54-61). Thus, it may be possible that the decrease in estrogen receptors that we observe on estrogen administration may be associated with the refractory response exhibited by mouse and rat uteri to constant estrogenic stimulation.

Studies on the Function of Uteroglobin (or Blastokinin)

Uteroglobin (or blastokinin) is a low molecular weight protein (MW 15,000) that is secreted maximally in adult rabbit uteri 5 days after coitus or when pseudopregnancy is induced. The function of uteroglobin is unknown although several authors have suggested that its function may be related to the fact that uteroglobin binds progesterone (62-65).

Originally, we were interested in uteroglobin as a biochemical marker to monitor tissue specific functions of uterine cell lines we have isolated. However, more recently we have been interested in uteroglobin since we found it to be an effective mitogen for our cultured uterine epithelial cells. The stimulatory activity of uteroglobin appears to be specific for uterine cells since uteroglobin had no effect on BALB/3T3 cells (18).

As a result of a basic experiment carried out to show that uteroglobin was the direct cause of increased cellular proliferation in our endometrial cells, an interesting observation was made that suggested that uteroglobin action could be mediated through another compound. We had been studying several mitogens for our endometrial cells: 17β-estradiol, epithelial growth factor, prostaglandin $F_{2\alpha}$ ($PGF_{2\alpha}$) and uteroglobin. In the experiment, the growth factors were tested for mitogenic activity on the endometrial cells in the presence and absence of antibodies to the corresponding growth factors (Table 8). Results showed that in the absence of the antibodies, the factors stimulated proliferation; however, in the presence of the corresponding antibodies which bound the factors, there was no increase in proliferation indicating that these factors were responsible for the increased proliferation. An unexpected result appeared when we added different combinations of mitogens and antibodies as a control to show that only the corresponding antibody could inhibit the stimulatory effect of their respective mitogens. When we tested for stimulation of cell proliferation by uteroglobin in the presence of $PGF_{2\alpha}$ antibody, the $PGF_{2\alpha}$ antibody inhibited the uteroglobin stimulatory effect suggesting that uteroglobin may be stimulating cell proliferation by modulating $PGF_{2\alpha}$ synthesis. In a latter study, we found that not only could the antibody to $PGF_{2\alpha}$ inhibit increased proliferation by uteroglobin, but also the presence of indomethacin could also inhibit stimulation of proliferation by uteroglobin further suggesting that uteroglobin action may be mediated through $PGF_{2\alpha}$ synthesis.

TABLE 8

Uteroglobin Growth Promoting effect

Addition	Labeling Index
Control	43.2 ± 5.3
$PGF_{2\alpha}$ (5×10^{-7} M)	61.3 ± 4.6*
$PGF_{2\alpha}$ Ab	50.5 ± 3.0
$PGF_{2\alpha}$ + $PGF_{2\alpha}$ Ab	44.6 ± 4.1
UG (1×10^{-7} M)	70.0 ± 5.6*
UG Ab	40.6 ± 6.7
UG + UG Ab	39.1 ± 2.6
UG + $PGF_{2\alpha}$ Ab	54.4 ± 7.4

$PGF_{2\alpha}$, prostaglandin $F_{2\alpha}$; UG, uteroglobulin. The growth factors assayed were incubated in the presence or absence of antibodies to the factors. The antibodies were added to the cultures before the factors. See Table 1 footnote for more information.

We have carried out a preliminary experiment using whole animals, which shows the possible involvement of $PGF_{2\alpha}$ in stimulating proliferation of the uterine epithelial cells. We injected rabbits with oil (control), indomethacin, progesterone or indomethacin plus progesterone and 24 hours later the rabbits were sacrificed. Since progesterone induces uteroglobin synthesis, we were interested in examining whether indomethacin was effective in inhibiting the stimulation of cell proliferation in vivo. We found that indomethacin alone had no effect upon proliferation; however, when injected in combination with progesterone, indomethacin was able to inhibit stimulation of cell proliferation caused by progesterone treatment. More precisely, indomethacin inhibited stimulation of cell proliferation only in the glandular epithelial cells and had no effect on the luminal epithelial cells. Thus, in vivo indomethacin can inhibit stimulation of cell proliferation in support of our culture data; and solidifying our hypothesis of the possible involvement of $PGF_{2\alpha}$ in progesterone and uteroglobin action.

We are presently carrying out experiments to measure $PGF_{2\alpha}$ levels directly to examine whether $PGF_{2\alpha}$ levels do fluctuate in relationship to uteroglobin presence and increased cell proliferation. We hope to show some direct evidence that $PGF_{2\alpha}$ is involved with uteroglobin stimulation of cell proliferation.

In summary, we have indirect evidence that stimulation of cell proliferation induced by progesterone administration may be related to uteroglobin synthesis which, in turn, may be related to prostaglandin $F_{2\alpha}$ synthesis; and $PGF_{2\alpha}$ may be the final mitogen in progesterone action. Although direct proof of this is yet to be obtained, experiments are under way to demonstrate if such a relationship exists. In support of this idea, it is well documented that progesterone induces the uterus to undergo decidualization (66). Associated with the decidual response, is increased arborization of the uterine lumen possibly precipitated by increased cell proliferation resulting in gland formation (17). Prostaglandin $F_{2\alpha}$ has also been found to induce the decidual response in mice (67), thus it may be that the decidual response induced by progesterone may actually be mediated through prostaglandin $F_{2\alpha}$.

CONCLUSIONS AND SUMMARY

We described and discussed several aspects of hormonal regulation of rabbit uterine epithelium. They give us a picture of a very complex biological system where the ovarian hormones trigger explosive architectural and biochemical changes.

It appears that estrogens and progestins act on different target cells. Some of these cells produce substances that can inhibit or increase the proliferative effect of estrogens. Progesterone induces the secretion of a protein, uteroglobin which appears to promote epithelial cell proliferation through an increase of prostaglandins. Progesterone also induces a dramatic increase in basement membrane, suggesting that this structure plays an important role in endometrial arborization.

Both estradiol and progesterone were found to decrease in cultured cells or animals the total number of estrogen receptors, probably by different mechanisms. The progesterone effect explains its antagonism to estradiol, however the estradiol effect in down-regulating its own receptor is still difficult to understand because of its positive effect on proliferation in the same experimental conditions. However, as we pointed out previously, "the presence of heterogeneous cell populations, in terms of hormone responsiveness or differentiation, is important to the concept of hormonal receptor regulation. It suggests that the interpretation of experiments showing sex steroid hormonal regulation of hormonal receptors should include the possibility that the effects could be mediated through hormone-directed cytodifferentiation. This phenomenon would result in unexpected changes of a heterogeneous cell population adding a higher level of complexity to the experimental model" (13).

The demonstration of other regulatory mechanisms, rather than only the direct action of the ovarian hormones, appears to make more difficult our understanding of the biology and pathology of endometrium, but should eventually help us to reach a level of knowledge resulting in successful preventive and therapeutic measures directed towards endometrial diseases.

ACKNOWLEDGEMENTS

These studies were supported by grants from the USPHS (CA 12536, CA 25365, F32 HD 05529), The American Cancer Society (BC-326) and R.J. Reynolds Industries, Inc. We would like to thank Ms. M. Andersson, J. Young, D. English, R. Lieberman and D. Kercheville for their expert help. We would also like to thank the publishers of Life Sciences and Endocrine Research Communications for the permission to reproduce Tables 2, 3, 6, 7 and Figure 1.

REFERENCES

1. Beatson, G.T., Lancet 2 (1896) 104.
2. Speert, H., Cancer 2 (1949) 597.
3. Gusberg, S.B., Obstet. Gynecol. 30 (1967) 287.
4. Siiteri, P.K., Cancer Res. 38 (1978) 4360.
5. Baba, N. and Von Haam, E., Progr. Exp. Tumor Res. 9 (1967) 192.
6. Griffiths, C.T., Craig, J.M., Kistner, R.W., Rothman, K.T., Steiner, G.J. and Tomic, M., Gynecol. Oncol. 3 (1975) 259.
7. Kistner, R.W., Int. J. Gynecol. Obstet. 8 (1970) 561.
8. Bonte, J., Acta Obstet. Gynecol. Scand. Suppl. 19 (1972) 21.
9. Wait, R.B., Obstet. Gynecol. 41 (1973) 129.
10. Gerschenson, L.E., Berliner, J.A. and Yang, J., Cancer Res. 34 (1974) 2873.
11. Gerschenson, L.E. and Berliner, J.A., J. Steroid Biochem. 7 (1976) 159.
12. Berliner, J.A. and Gerschenson, L.E., J. Steroid Biochem. 7 (1976) 153.
13. Gerschenson, L.E., Conner, E.A. and Murai, J.T., Endocrinology 100 (1977) 1468.
14. Murai, J.T., Conner, E.A., Yang, J., Andersson, M., Berliner, J. and Gerschenson, L.E., J. Toxicol. Environ. Health 4 (1978) 449.
15. Gerschenson, L.E., Conner, E.A., Yang, J. and Andersson, M., Life Sci. 24 (1979) 1337.
16. Murai, J.T., Lieberman, R.C., Yang, J. and Gerschenson, L.E., Endocr. Res. Comm. 6 (1979) in press.
17. Conti, C.J., Gimenez-Conti, I.B., Conner, E.A. and Gerschenson, L.E., J. Cell Biol. 83 (1979) 253a.
18. Murai, J.T., Conti, C.J. and Gerschenson, L.E., J. Cell Biol. 83 (1979) 110a.

19. Thompson, L.H., Mankovitz, R., Baker, R.M., Till, J.E., Siminovitch, L. and Whitmore, G.F., Proc. Nat. Acad. Sci. USA 66 (1970) 377.
20. Petersen, D.F., Anderson, E.C. and Tobey, R.A., Methods Cell Physiol. 3 (1968) 347.
21. Depaoli, J.R. and Gerschenson, L.E., manuscript in preparation.
22. Lozzio, B.B., Lozzio, C.B., Bamberger, E.G. and Lair, S.V., in "International Review of Cytology" (G.H. Browne and J.F. Danielli, eds.) pp. 1-47, Academic Press, New York (1975).
23. Baserga, R., "Multiplication and Division in Mammalian Cells," Marcel Dekker, New York (1976).
24. Sirbasku, D.A., Proc. Nat. Acad. Sci. USA 75 (1978) 3786.
25. Sonnenschein, C. and Soto, A.M., J. Nat. Cancer Inst. 63 (1979) 835.
26. Kano-Sueoka, T., Cohen, D.M., Yamaizumi, Z., Nishimura, S., Mori, M. and Fujiki, H., Proc. Nat. Acad. Sci. USA 76 (1979) in press.
27. Davies, J. and Hoffman, L.H., Amer. J. Anat. 137 (1973) 423.
28. Davies, J. and Hoffman, L.H., Amer. J. Anat. 142 (1975) 335.
29. McPhail, M.K., J. Physiol. 83 (1934) 145.
30. Bernfield, M.R., Cohn, R.H. and Banerjee, S.D., Amer. Zool. 13 (1973) 1067.
31. Meier, S., Anat. Rec. 191 (1978) 447.
32. Vracko, R., Amer. J. Pathol. 77 (1974) 314.
33. Rosenthal, H.E., Anal. Biochem. 20 (1967) 525.
34. Leung, B.S. and Sasaki, G.H., Biochem. Biophys. Res. Comm. 55 (1973) 1180.
35. Brenner, R.M., Resko, J.A. and West, N.B., Endocrinology 95 (1974) 1094.
36. Mester, J., Martel, D., Psychoyos, A. and Baulieu, E.E., Nature 250 (1974) 776.
37. Hsueh, A.J.W., Peck, E.J., Jr. and Clark, J.H., Endocrinology 98 (1976) 438.
38. West, N.B., Verhage, H.G. and Brenner, R.M., Endocrinology 99 (1976) 1010.
39. Pavlik, E.J. and Coulson, P.B., J. Steroid Biochem. 7 (1976) 369.
40. Sarff, M. and Gorski, J., Biochemistry 10 (1971) 2557.
41. Cidlowski, J.A. and Muldoon, T.G., Endocrinology 95 (1974) 1621.
42. Mester, J. and Baulieu, E.E., Biochem. J. 146 (1975) 617.
43. Anderson, J., Clark, J. and Peck, E.J., Jr., Biochem. J. 126 (1972) 561.
44. Howitz, K.B. and McGuire, W.L., J. Biol. Chem. 253 (1978) 8185.
45. Kakuichi, S. and Rall, T.W., Mol. Pharmacol. 4 (1968) 367.
46. Makman, M.H., Proc. Nat. Acad. Sci. USA 68 (1971) 885.
47. Ho, R.J. and Sutherland, W.W., J. Biol. Chem. 246 (1971) 6822.
48. Remold-O'Donnell, E., J. Biol. Chem. 249 (1974) 3615.
49. Hunzicker-Dunn, M. and Birnbaumer, L., Endocrinology 99 (1976) 185.
50. Epifanova, O.I. and Smolenskaya, I.N., Bull. Exp. Biol. Med. USSR 56 (1963) 1278.
51. Finn, C.A., Martin, L. and Carter, J., J. Endocrinol. 44 (1969) 121.
52. Lee, A.E., J. Endocrinol. 55 (1972) 507.

53. Stormshak, F., Leake, R., Wertz, N. and Gorski, J., Endocrinology 99 (1976) 1501.
54. Kahn, C.R., Neville, D.M., Jr. and Roth, J., J. Biol. Chem. 248 (1973) 244.
55. Gavin, J.R., Roth, J., Neville, D.M., Jr., DeMeyts, P. and Buell, D.N., Proc. Nat. Acad. Sci. USA 71 (1974) 84.
56. Mukherjee, C., Caron, M.G. and Lefkowitz, R.J., Proc. Nat. Acad. Sci. USA 72 (1975) 1945.
57. Kababian, J.W., Zatz, M., Romero, J.A. and Axelrod, J., Proc. Nat. Acad. Sci. USA 72 (1975) 3735.
58. Mickey, J., Tate, R. and Lefkowitz, R.J., J. Biol. Chem. 250 (1975) 5727.
59. Lesniak, M.A. and Roth, J., J. Biol. Chem. 251 (1976) 3720.
60. Hinkle, P.M. and Tashjian, A.H., Jr., Biochemistry 14 (1976) 3845.
61. Conti, M., Harwood, J.P., Hsueh, A.J.W., Dufau, M.L. and Catt, K.J., J. Biol. Chem. 251 (1976) 7729.
62. Garcea, N., Campo, S., Caruso, A., Milano, L. and Bompiani, A., Int. J. Fert. 19 (1974) 197.
63. Beato, M. and Baier, R., Biochim. Biophys. Acta 392 (1975) 346.
64. Rahman, S.S., Velayo, N., Domres, P. and Billiar, R.B., Fert. Ster. 26 (1975) 991.
65. Fridlansky, F. and Milgrom, E., Endocrinology 99 (1976) 1244.
66. O'Malley, B.W., Means, A.R. and Sherman, M.R., in "The Sex Steroids" (K.W. McKerns, ed.), Appleton-Century-Crofts, New York, p. 315 (1971).
67. Sananes, N., Baulieu, E.E. and LeGoascogne, C., Molec. Cell. Endocrin. 6 (1976) 153.

PART III
UTERINE ENZYME REGULATION

The Endometrium

11

Cyclic Change of Estradiol Metabolic Enzymes in Human Endometrium During the Menstrual Cycle

Linda Tseng
James Mazella

ABSTRACT

Estradiol dehydrogenase (E_2DH), estrogen sulfatase and sulfotransferase are the three major estrogen metabolic enzymes found to be present in the human endometrium. The activities of these enzymes were compared in a group of normal endometrial specimens at various stages of the menstrual cycle. The average value of E_2DH activity estimated from the rate of conversion of tritiated estradiol (E_2) to estrone (E_1), in the presence of an excess amount of NAD, was 2.8 nmol of E_1 formed/mg protein/h in proliferative endometrium and 22 in secretory endometrium. The estrogen sulfatase activity was estimated by measuring the rate of conversion of [^{3}H]-estrone sulfate (E_1S) to E_1. The average value was 1.6 nmol/mg protein/h with no significant change in activity during the menstrual cycle. The sulfotransferase activity, estimated from the rate of conversion of [^{3}H]-E_1 to [^{3}H]-E_1S, in the presence of an excess amount of adenosine 3'-phosphate 5'-phosphosulfate (PAPS) had an average value of 0.03 nmol/mg protein/h in the secretory endometrium but was not detectable in the proliferative phase.

Studies of subcellular distribution of these metabolic enzymes indicated that the activities of E_2DH and sulfatase were found to be membrane bound to various particulates in both epithelial glands and stromal cells, while sulfotransferase activity was found only in the soluble fraction of the epithelial glands of the secretory endometrium. The K_m value of E_2DH and sulfatase are in the order of 10^{-6} M while sulfotransferase is 5×10^{-9} M. The relatively small K_m value of sulfotransferase indicates that this enzyme may effectively compete the binding of estrogen to its receptor protein in the glandular epithelial cells of the secretory endometrium.

The estradiol metabolism in endometrial specimens was further analyzed at a low E_2 concentration in a superfusion system. It was found that intracellular E_2 concentration at the steady state of superfusion is inversely proportional to the summation of the rate of release of the metabolites, E_1, E_1S and estradiol-3-sulfate. This result indicates that the rate of metabolism in tissue will be the major regulating factor for the intracellular E_2 concentration.

INTRODUCTION

Previous studies of estradiol (E_2) metabolism in vitro from several groups of investigators can be summarized as follows: When endometrial specimens were incubated or superfused with E_2 at a concentration equivalent to plasma levels, the formation of estrone (E_1) is active throughout the menstrual cycle, and the formation of estrogen sulfate is active only in the secretory endometrium (Gabb and Stone, 1974; Buirchell and Hahnel, 1975; Pack et al., 1979; Liu and Tseng, 1979). Estrone rather than estrogen sulfate is the predominant product since the cell capacity for oxidation is much higher than sulfation.

Estradiol dehydrogenase (E_2DH), estrogen sulfatase and sulfotransferase are the three major enzymes regulating the metabolism of estrogen in human endometrium. Estradiol dehydrogenase interconverts E_1 and E_2 and the favored direction in the intact endometrial cells is towards the oxidation of E_2. The capacity for the oxidation was significantly increased in secretory endometrium. This was first noticed in the double isotope superfusion system. In this system it was found that when endometrium was superfused with E_2, the retention of E_2 in the tissue changes during the menstrual cycle. The intracellular E_2 concentration obtained at the steady state of superfusion is lower in secretory endometrium than in proliferative endometrium (Tseng and Gurpide, 1972). The estrogen sulfatase hydrolyzes the sulfates in endometrial tissue which enhances the utilization of circulating estrogen sulfate. The sulfotransferase catalyzes the reverse reaction of sulfatase; it sulfurylates the free intracellular estrogen to form estrogen sulfate. The formation of estrogen sulfate facilitates the expulsion of estrogen from this target tissue.

The endometrial sulfotransferase was investigated in the present study. The relative activities and kinetic constants of three estrogen metabolic enzymes were compared in a group of normal endometrial specimens at various stages of the menstrual cycle. In addition, the subcellular distribution and localization of these enzyme activities were determined in glandular epithelial and stromal cells. These analyses enhance the understanding of the overall metabolic pattern of estrogen observed in intact cells.

MATERIALS AND METHODS

Endometrial Tissue, Epithelial Glands and Stromal Cells

Human endometrial specimens used for this study were obtained from patients who had been subjected to curettage or hysterectomy for a variety of medical reasons. Results presented in this article were from specimens diagnosed as normal endometrium. Epithelial glands and stromal cells were separated by digesting the endometrial tissue fragments with 1 mg/ml of collagenase solution followed by sequential sedimentation and filtration. The detailed description of the procedure has been reported in the previous publication (Liu and Tseng, 1979).

Reagents

[6,7-^{3}H]E_2 (SA, 48 Ci/mmol), [6,7-^{3}H]E_1 (SA, 58.3 Ci/mmol), [6,7-^{3}H] estrone sulfate (E_1S) (SA, 53 Ci/mmol), [4-^{14}C]E_2 (SA, 55.7 mCi/mmol), and [4-^{14}C]E_1 (SA, 50 mCi/mmol) were purchased from New England Nuclear Corp. (Boston, Mass). [4-^{14}C]-E_1S was prepared based on the method by Levitz (1963). The [4-^{14}C] estradiol-3-sulfate (E_2S) was prepared by the reduction of [^{14}C]-E_1S with sodium borohydride (10 mg/ml). The reduction was conducted in ethanol overnight at room temperature. The purity of the tracers was checked before use by a thin layer chromatography. Adenosine 3'-phosphate 5'-phosphosulfate (PAPS) was purchased from P-L Biochemical, Inc. (Milwaukee, Wisc.). Crystalline E_1, E_2, E_2-3,17β-disulfate were purchased from Steraloids, Inc. (Wilton, N.H.). Estrone sulfate and E_2S were kindly supplied by Ayerst Research Laboratory (Montreal, P.Q., Canada).

Enzymes Assay

The activities of E_2DH and sulfatase were measured by the methods described previously (Tseng, 1978; and Gurpide et al, 1976). The enzyme assay mixture for E_2DH contained NAD^+ (1.4 umol),[^{3}H]-E_2 (20 nmol; SA 10^6 dpm/nmol) and approximately 1 mg protein of the tissue homogenate in 1 ml of Tris buffer (0.05 M, pH 8). The sulfatase activity was measured in Tris buffer (0.05 M, pH 7.0) containing [^{3}H]-E_1S (10 nmol/ml; SA 1.5×10^6 dpm/nmol) and approximately 0.5 mg of protein/ml of the tissue homogenate.

The estrogen sulfotransferase activity was measured by the modified procedure of Rozhin et al. (1974). The final assay solution contained 100,000xg cytosol of the tissue homogenate (equivalent to 0.5 mg tissue protein/ml), 50 nmol/ml of PAPS and various concentrations of [^{3}H]-E_1 or [^{3}H]-E_2 (0.001 to 1 nmol/ml) in Tris buffer (0.05 M, pH 8) with 10 mM $MgCl_2$ and 0.5 mM dithioerythritol. Reaction was initiated by addition of [^{3}H]-E_1 in ethanol solution (1% v/v final concentration of ethanol) to the assay mixture prewarmed at 37 C. The reaction was stopped by extracting the substrate from the aqueous solution with ethylacetate. The initial rate of the formation of the product, E_1 for E_2DH or sulfatase and E_1S or E_2S for sulfotransferase was used to estimate the enzyme activity. The isolation of estrogens was achieved using experimental procedure described in the previous publication (Liu and Tseng, 1979). A known amount of [^{14}C]-E_1, [^{14}C]-E_1S or [^{14}C]-E_2S was added to each sample to serve as an internal standard for the quantitation of the respective product formed. Protein content in each sample was determined by Bio Rad protein assay (Bradford, 1977). The enzyme activities were expressed as nmol of product formed/mg of tissue protein/h.

Superfusion of Endometrial Tissue Fragments with [^{3}H]-E_2

Human endometrial specimen obtained from curettage was cut into small pieces, rinsed with saline and placed in the superfusion chamber described in the previous publication (Tseng et al., 1972). Earl's balance salt solution (EBSS) containing 0.8 pmol/ml of [^3H]-E_2 was pumped to the chamber with a constant flow rate (15 ml or 18 ml/h). The outflow was collected into several fractions at various superfusion intervals. The radioactive estrogens in the superfusate and the tissue were analyzed at the steady state of superfusion. This occurs when the rate of [^3H]-E_2 entering the cells equals the rate of [^3H]-E_2 and its metabolites leaving the cells, and the concentration [^3H]-E_2 and other metabolites in the tissue remain constant (Gurpide and Welch, 1969).

RESULTS

Estrogen Sulfotransferase Activity at Various [^3H]-E_1 or [^3H]-E_2 Concentrations

The estrogen sulfotransferase activity was determined at various [^3H]-E_1 or [^3H]-E_2 concentrations (0.01 to 200 nM) in a secretory endometrial cytosol. Fig. 1 shows the initial velocity of formation of E_1S and E_2S in the presence of an excess amount of PAPS. The rate

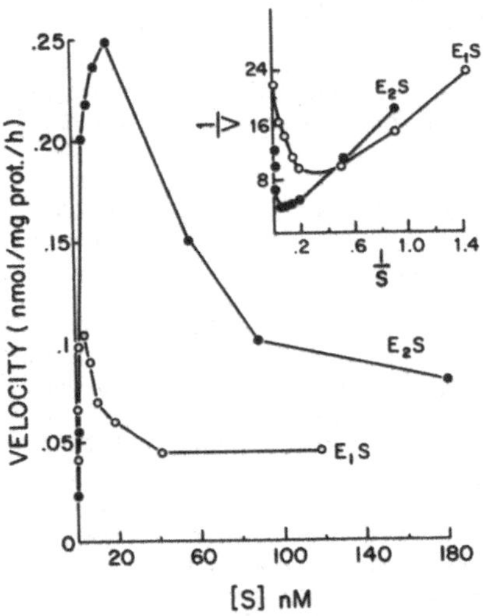

Fig. 1. Initial velocities of the formation of E_1S or E_2S at various E_1 or E_2 concentrations measured in a secretory endometrial cytosol with PAPS (50 uM) in Tris buffer (0.05 M pH 8, $MgCl_2$ 10 mM, and dithioerythritol 0.5 mM) at 37 C.

of formation of estrogen sulfate changes at various substrate concentration, with E_2 being more active than E_1. No significant amount of E_2 disulfate was found in the reaction mixture. The initial velocity of the formation of both E_1S and E_2S was inhibited at high substrate concentration. The apparent K_m estimated from the first part of the curve is 5 nM for E_1 and 25 nM for E_2.

Variations in cytosol protein concentration in the assay mixture within the range of 0.07 to 1 mg of tissue protein/ml did not affect the specific activity of sulfotransferase when 10 nM of $[^3H]$-E_1 was used for the substrate.

Subcellular Distribution of Estrogen Sulfatase and Sulfotransferase Activities

The subcellular distribution of estrogen sulfatase activity was examined in particulates (microsomes, mitochondria, and nuclei) and 100,000xg cytosolic fractions of the tissue homogenate. The sulfatase activity was found in the mitochondrial and microsomal fractions but was not in the soluble fraction.

The sulfotransferase activity was present in both tissue homogenate and cytosol but not detectable in particulates. The initial rate of formation of E_1S was compared in a secretory endometrium using tissue homogenate and 100,000xg cytosol (Fig. 2). The rate of formation of E_1S was slower in the homogenate than in the cytosol at various incubation time. The slower rate observed in tissue homogenate is probably due to the partial hydrolysis of E_1S by sulfatase present in particulate fractions. Therefore, the sulfotransferase activity was measured using cytosol of the tissue homogenate to avoid the interference of the sulfatase.

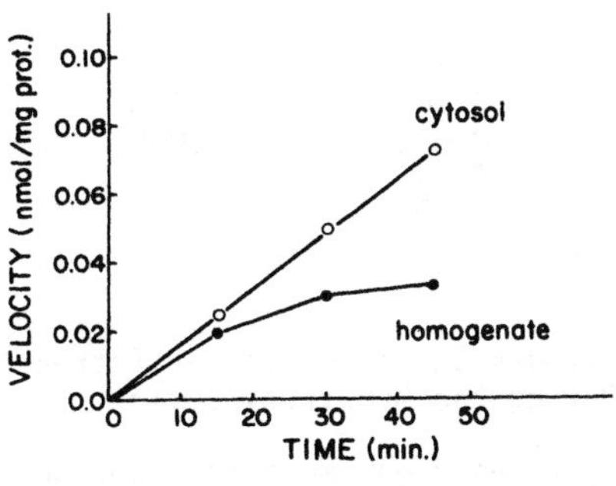

Fig. 2. Rate of conversion of E_1 to E_1S during incubation of homogenate and 100,000xg supernatant of a secretory endometrium, PAPS (50 uM) and E_1 (0.8 uM) in Tris buffer (0.05 M, pH 8, $MgCl_2$ 10 mM, dithioerythritol 0.5 mM) at 37 C.

Distribution of Estrogen Sulfatase and Sulfotransferase Activities in Endometrial Glands and Stroma

The activities of sulfatase and sulfotransferase were measured in tissue, isolated epithelial glands and stromal cells. Table 1 shows the comparison of these enzyme activities. Estrogen sulfatase was present in both types of cells while sulfotransferase was localized only in the glandular epithelial cells. The sulfotransferase was measured at the substrate concentration ($[^3H]$-E_1, 5 nM) which shows the highest initial velocity (Fig. 1). There is tremendous variation in the rate from tissue to tissue. The same type of variation occurs to the activity in glands. No significant amount of activity was found in stromal cells. These data are consistent with the previous publication (Liu and Tseng, 1979) that estrogen sulfates were not formed in the stromal cells. These findings indicate that sulfotransferase is a specific enzyme which is present only in the glandular epithelial cells of the endometrium.

TABLE 1. DISTRIBUTION OF ESTROGEN SULFATASE AND SULFOTRANSFERASE ACTIVITIES IN EPITHELIAL GLANDS AND STROMAL CELLS

Type of Enzyme	Tissue	Glands	Stroma
	(nmol/mg prot./h)		
Sulfatase	2.1	0.63	0.60
Sulfotransferase	0.11	0.31	
	0.004	0.005	
	0.013	0.035	n.d.*
	0.092	0.12	.0006
	0.081	0.10	.0012

* n.d. not detectable

Comparison of E_2DH, Estrogen Sulfatase and Sulfotransferase Activities in Human Endometrium During the Menstrual Cycle

The activities of E_2DH, estrogen sulfatase and sulfotransferase were compared in a group of human endometrial specimens (Table 2). Estradiol dehydrogenase and sulfatase activities were measured in tissue homogenate with an excess amount of substrate. The sulfotransferase activities were measured in cytosol with $[^3H]$-E_1 at a concentration 200 nM which shows an activity of approximately one-half the maximum rate.

TABLE 2. COMPARISON OF E_2DH, ESTROGEN SULFATASE AND SULFOTRANSFERASE ACTIVITIES IN HUMAN ENDOMETRIUM

Type of Tissue	E_2DH	Sulfatase	Sulfotransferase
		($\frac{\text{nmol product}}{\text{mg prot./h}}$)	
prol.	1.6	1.1	n.d*
prol.	3.4	1.8	n.d.
prol.	3.8	1.4	n.d.
prol.	2.5	1.8	n.d.
$\bar{X}$	2.8	1.5	
early sec.	25	1.4	0.045
early sec.	19	1.9	0.020
mid sec.	32	1.3	0.026
mid sec.	23		0.020
sec.	13	2.7	0.024
sec.	17	1.0	0.040
$\bar{X}$	22	1.7	0.029
K_m	1uM	2uM	5nM

* not detectable, prol. = proliferative, sec. = secretory

The value of E_2DH and sulfatase activities in this group of specimens were similar to the previous published results (Tseng and Gurpide, 1975; and Gurpide et al., 1976). Approximately a ten fold increase in E_2DH activity was observed during the secretory phase. The average value of sulfatase activity is 1.6 nmol/mg prot./h with no significant change during the menstrual cycle. The sulfotransferase activity was not detectable in proliferative phase under the assay condition. The average value in secretory phase is about 0.03 nmol E_1S formed/mg prot./h.

The sulfotransferase activities were also measured in secretory endometrial specimens at the substrate concentration ([^{3}H]-E_1, 5 nM) which exhibits the maximum enzyme rate. The average value determined in eighteen specimens is 0.05$\pm$ 0.04 ($\bar{X}\pm$SD) nmol/mg prot./h. It is evident that the capacity of E_2DH and sulfatase greatly exceeds that of sulfotransferase (E_2DH : sulfatase : sulfotransferase; 500-1000 : 50-100 : 1). The apparent K_m value of E_2DH and sulfatase are 1 and 2 uM respectively and the sulfotransferase is approximately 5 nM.

Effect of E_2 Metabolism on the Intracellular Concentration of E_2 in a Superfusion System

In order to determine whether the metabolism in endometrium can influence the intracellular E_2 concentration, the endometrial tissue fragments were superfused with [^{3}H]-E_2 in EBSS buffer solution. Table 3 and Fig. 3 show the rate of various estrogens released from tissue and the intracellular concentration of [^{3}H]-E_2 measured at the steady state of superfusion. In each of these experiments about 80 mg of endometrium tissue fragments was used. The estradiol concentration in the superfusion medium were similar to the plasma level, 0.8 pmol/ml. The estimated rate of entry of E_2 was about 2 to 3 pmol/hr. (Tseng, Stolee and Gurpide, 1972). The rate of release of E_1, E_1S and E_2S reflects the rate of the conversion of E_2 to these compounds in the tissue. A higher rate of conversion results in a lower intracellular E_2 concentration. The relationship between the rate of release of metabolites and intracellular E_2 concentration of four different endometrial specimens is indicated in Fig. 3. The summation of the rate of release of these metabolites was inversely proportional to the intracellular E_2 concentration. These data indicate that the rate of intracellular metabolism is the major factor that determines the intracellular E_2 concentration.

TABLE 3. SUPERFUSION OF HUMAN ENDOMETRIUM WITH [^{3}H]-E_2 (0.8 pmol/ml)

(Rate of Superfusion 18 ml/h (prol.) 15 ml/h (sec.))

Type of Tissue	Rate of Estrogens Release from Tissue (pmol/g_{tissue} /h)			Intracellular Concentration (pmol/g_{tissue})
	E_1	E_1S	E_2S	E_2
E.prol.	5.6	n.d.	n.d.	9.2
L.prol.	17.0	n.d.	n.d.	4.0
E.sec.	7.5	6.1	3.5	3.2
Sec.	8.6	10.0	3.0	0.8

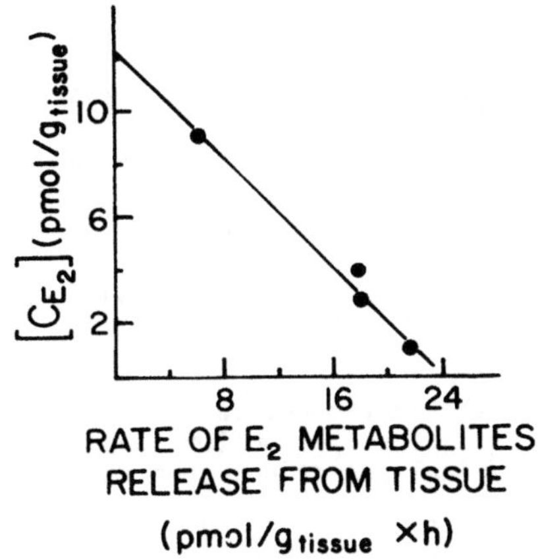

Fig. 3. Intracellular E_2 concentrations, of four different endometrial specimens shown in Table 3, obtained at the steady state of superfusion vs rate of E_2 metabolites (E_1, E_1S and E_2S) release from tissue.

DISCUSSION

The initial velocity of formation of E_1S and E_2S shown in Fig. 1 clearly indicates that estrogen sulfotransferase activity in human endometrium is different from the adrenal sulfotransferase studied by Adams (1967) and Rozhin et al., (1977). The apparent K_m value of the endometrial enzyme estimated from Fig. 1 is about one-hundred times less than the adrenal enzyme. Inhibition of the initial velocity occurred with both E_1 and E_2 in the endometrial cytosol while the adrenal sulfotransferase exhibited the substrate inhibition only with E_2 (Adams 1967). It is not clear what causes the inhibition at high substrate concentration, but it was found that inhibition was not caused by sulfatase. If the substrate inhibition is of the dead-end type (Cleland 1970), the inhibition constant, K_i, estimated from the reciprocal plot shown in Fig. 1 is 2 nM for E_1 and 10 nM for E_2. The extremely low K_m or K_i values indicate that the sulfotransferase has a high affinity for E_1 or E_2 which is almost in the same order of the affinity constant of estrogen to its receptor protein.

The possible interference of the binding of E_2 to its receptor (R) by sulfotransferase (Sulf) is illustrated in the following equations:

$$E_2 + R \rightleftharpoons E_2R \qquad K_d\ (10^{-9}\ M)$$

$$E_2 + Sulf \rightleftharpoons E_2Sulf \longrightarrow Product \qquad K_m\ (10^{-8} - 10^{-9}\ M)$$

$$[E_2][R] = K_d[E_2R] \qquad (1)$$

$$[E_2][Sulf] = (K_m + [E_2])[E_2\ Sulf] \qquad (2)$$

In cytosol, E_2 can bind to receptor or to enzyme at the steady state. If equation (1) is combined with equation (2), the following relationship is obtained.

$$\frac{[E_2R]}{[R]} = \frac{[E_2Sulf]}{[Sulf]} \times \frac{K_m + [E_2]}{K_d} \qquad (3)$$

When the apparent K_m of the enzyme complex is close to the value of the dissociation constant K_d of the E_2R complex, and E_2 is present at a low level as in the physiological condition, then equation 3 reduces to:

$$\frac{[E_2R]}{[R]} = \frac{[E_2Sulf]}{[Sulf]}$$

Thus the sulfotransferase, even at a concentration as low as the receptor level, can effectively alter the binding of E_2 to its receptor. The sulfotransferase acts as a competitor and a deactivator by converting E_2 to estrogen sulfate which does not have the binding affinity to the receptor. Although the capacity of sulfotransferase is very small, it synergistically deactivates the E_2 with E_2DH in the epithelial glands in the secretory phase. Therefore, the probability that the receptor will bind to the hormone may become nil. This hypothesis may explain the phenomenon observed in endometrium, that the biologic function of E_2 in terms of cell proliferation, the mitoses, stops during the early secretory phase.

Table 3 indicates that the capacity of sulfatase surpasses the sulfotransferase in secretory endometrium. However, these two enzymes are localized in different subcellular fractions, and the very high affinity of sulfotransferase to estrogen enables the sulfation to occur readily in intact cells.

In stromal cells, the E_2DH is the major metabolic enzyme. It converts E_2 to the less active E_1 which readily difuses out from cells. Also, when the endometrium is exposed to a pharmological dose of estrogen, sulfotransferase is not effective due to its small capacity and the E_2DH is responsible for removal of the excessive estrogens.

Since progesterone stimulates E_2DH (Tseng and Gurpide 1975, and Tseng 1978), it therefore serves as a protective agent in the endometrium, a tissue which is known to be susceptible to neoplastic transformation by chronic stimulation of estrogen. However, this protection through the mechanism of metabolism is selective to those estrogens which can serve as a substrate of the dehydrogenase but not compounds such as DES, mestranol and ethynlestradiol.

Fig. 3 indicates that the summation of the rate of release of these metabolites was inversely proportional to the intracellular E_2 concentration. In the absence of metabolic enzymes, it would be expected that the intracellular hormone concentration to be equivalent to or larger than its receptor level at the steady state condition. The concentrations obtained in these experiments were smaller than the expected E_2 receptor level in either proliferative or secretory endometrium although enough E_2 was supplied to saturate the receptor during the superfusion. These findings were consistent with the endogenous E_2 level found in endometrium, which is lower than the E_2 receptor level either in the proliferative or secretory phase determined by several groups of investigators. (Proliferative phase: E_2R = 20-30 pmol/g tissue; E_2 = 4 pmol/g tissue; secretory phase: E_2R = 7, E_2 = 1.8 Gurrero, et al., 1975; Batra, et al., 1977; Pack, et al., 1979; Bayard, et al., 1978; Tseng, et al., 1977; Crooker, et al., 1974). Therefore the estrogen metabolism in tissue will be the major regulating factor for the intracellular E_2 concentration.

In general, the physiological significance of estrogen metabolism in human endometrium may be visualized as follows: There are three estrogen metabolic enzymes and a receptor protein that regulate the estrogenic actions in human endometrium. The estradiol receptor concentration is in excess to the hormone; therefore, change in the intracellular levels of E_2 regulated by the metabolic enzymes can be the rate limiting factor of its action.

Estrogen sulfatase is a tonic ingredient for the endometrium to utilize the conjugate estrogens. Estradiol dehydrogenase is the major deactivating enzyme for E_2 in this target tissue. It regulates the intracellular E_2 concentration in endometrium during the entire menstrual cycle in conjunction with the blood borne circulating estrogens. The sulfotransferase present in the epithelial glands of the secretory phase intensifies the removal of the estradiol from the cells.

ACKNOWLEDGEMENTS

This work was supported by grants from the NIH HD-10933 and NYSHRC 1197 and 1522.

REFERENCES

Adams, J.B. (1967). Enzyme synthesis of steroid sulphates. Biochemica ET Biophysica Acta. 146, 522-528.

Batra, S., Grundsell, H. and Sjoberg, N.O. (1977). Estradiol-17β and progesterone concentrations in human endometrium during the menstrual cycle. Contraception. 16:2, 217-224.

Bayard, F., Damilano, S., Robel, P. and Baulieu, E.E. (1978). Estradiol and progesterone receptors in human endometrium. J. Clin. Endocrinol. Metab. 46, 635-648.

Bradford, M.M. (1976). A rapid and sensitive method for the quantitation of microgram quantity of protein utilizing the principle of protein dye binding. Anal. Biochem. 72, 248-254.

Buirchell, B.J. and Hahnel, R. (1975). Metabolism of estradiol-17β in human endometrium during the menstrual cycle. J. Steroid. Biochem. 6, 1489-1494.

Cleland, W.W. (1970). Steady state kinetics. in "The Enzyme." (Boyer, P., ed.). Vol. 2, Kinetics and Mechanisms. New York, Academic Press. P. 1-61.

Crocker, S.G., Milton, P.J.D. and King, R.J.B. (1974). Uptake of 6, 7-^{3}H oestradiol-17β by normal and abnormal human endometrium. J. Endocr. 62, 145-152.
Dallenback-Hellweg (1977). The normal histology of the endometrium. in "Histopathology of the Endometrium." Springer-Verlag, New York, Heidelberg, Berlin. P. 22-82.
Gabb, R.G. and Stone, G.M. (1974). Uptake and metabolism of tritiated oestradiol and oestrone by human endometrial and myometrial tissue in vitro. J. Endocrinol. 62, 109-123.
Guerrero, R., Landgren, B.M., Monteil, R., Cekan, Z. and Diczfalusy, E. (1975). Unconjugated steroids in the human endometrium. Contraception. 11:2, 169-177.
Gurpide, E., Gusberg, S.B. and Tseng, L. (1976). Estradiol binding and metabolism in human endometrial hyperplasia and adenocarcinoma. J. Steroid Biochem. 7, 891.
Gurpide, E. and Welch, M. (1969). Dynamics of uptake of estrogens and androgens by human endometrium. 244, 5159-5169.
Levitz, M. (1963). Synthesis of estrone-6,7-^{3}H sulfate-^{35}S. Steroids. 1, 117-120.
Liu, H.C. and Tseng, L. (1979). Estradiol metabolism in isolated human endometrial epithelial glands and stromal cells. Endocrinology. 104:6, 1674-1680.
Pack, B., Tovar, R., Booth, E. and Brooks S. (1979). The cyclic relationship of estrogen sulfurylation to the nuclear receptor level in human endometrial curettings. J. Clin. Endocrinol. and Metab. 48, 420-424.
Rozhin, J., Huo, A., Zemlicka, J. and Brooks, S.C. (1977). Studies on bovine adrenal estrogen sulfotransferase. J. Biol. Chem. 252, 7214-7220.
Tseng, L. and Gurpide, E. (1972). Changes in the in vitro metabolism of estradiol by human endometrium during the menstrual cycle. Am. J. Obs.Gyn. 114, 1002-1008.
Tseng, L., Stolee, A. and Gurpide, E. (1972). Quantitative studies on the uptake and metabolism of estrogens and progesterone by human endometrium. Endocrinology. 90, 390-404.
Tseng, L. and Gurpide, E. (1975). Induction of human endometrial estradiol dehydrogenase by progestins. Endocrinology. 97, 825-833.
Tseng, L., Gusberg, S.B. and Gurpide, E. (1977). Estradiol Receptor and 17β dehydrogenase in normal and abnormal human endometrium. Ann. N.Y. Acad. of Sci. 286, 190-198.
Tseng, L. (1978). Steroids specificity of the induction of estradiol dehydrogenase in human endometrium. Endocrinology. 120, 1398-1403.

DISCUSSION

DESOMBRE: Linda, in your presentation you spoke about glandular epithelia. Do you have any information as to whether there are any differences in estradiol dehydrogenase levels between luminal and glandular epithelium?

TSENG: We tend to distinguish epithelial cells from stromal in our preparation. I assume most of the epithelial cells we have isolated are glandular epithelial cells. I can't definitely tell the population of luminal epithelial cells in this preparation. In the stromal cell suspension there must be some lymphocytes or other kinds of cells which we cannot distinguish either. We can only remove red blood cells.

MILGROM: I would like to ask you about the equilibrium between estrone and estradiol. You told us you found that the reaction goes from estradiol to estrone in the cells based on Km evaluation. Is this correct?

TSENG: Yes. In addition to the apparent Km and Vmax analysis, if the tissue is incubated or superfused with estradiol or estrone, most of estrogen found in tissue or in medium is estrone.

MILGROM: Could you comment on the NAD^+/NADH ratio in the cells as a control element of this equilibrium?

TSENG: Yes. It would influence a lot the shifting of the reaction equilibrium. I mentioned that the steroid metabolic pattern in the uterus varies from species to species. In rabbit, we have seen the opposite direction of interconversion between E_1 and E_2. I don't have data for the NAD^+ and the NADH distribution in human endometrium.

MILGROM: My second question was exactly about that, how does it work in other species?

TSENG: I think that Dr. Brooks will talk about the comparison studies in pig and human uterus, where it is quite similar. In rabbit uterus, the favored direction is toward the reduction. If one incubates rabbit uterus with estradiol, 80 to 90% of E_2 remains as such. On the other hand, 80-90% of incubated estrone will be converted to estradiol.

BAULIEU: Two questions. One, are there any data showing that estradiol or estrone sulfate are secreted out from the endometrium in vivo?

TSENG: No.

BAULIEU: Besides progestogens, corticosterone and deoxy-corticosterone induced estradiol dehydrogenase and cortisol did not. What about synthetic corticosteroids such as dexamethasone?

TSENG: Corticosterone and deoxycorticosterone were studied to see the effect of these compounds, which have additional hydroxyl groups on the 11β and 21 carbon positions, in comparison to progesterone, on endometrial stimulation.

GREENBLATT: We know that mitosis ceases in the epithelial glands and the stroma in the secretory phase, in general, but is very active in the proliferative phase. You imply that progesterone limited the proliferative activity of the epithelium, but then you went on to say that it did not have this effect with DES, ethinyl estradiol or mestranol. Why not?

TSENG: Neither ethinyl estradiol or DES are substrates of the E_2 dehydrogenase, thus, these compounds accumulate in endometrium and are not removed through the mechanism of metabolism as is estradiol.

GREENBLATT: If you administer, say, large doses of ethinyl estradiol to a patient with an adenomatous hyperplasia, you can give 10 mg of Provera for 10 to 15 days and change that into a secretory endometrium.

TSENG: Right, progesterone can reduce the estrogen receptor but not the intracellular ethinyl estradiol or DES concentration.

KATZENELLENBOGEN: Linda, I have two short questions. You mentioned that the estradiol dehydrogenase generally converts estradiol to estrone in the human. My question is, in the postmenopausal woman, where the major estrogen is estrone, is there sufficient estradiol dehydrogenase activity in the uterus to cause the conversion of estrone to estradiol?

TSENG: Yes. The estradiol dehydrogenase activity in most of the postmenopausal endometrial specimens that we have studied were similar to the activity in proliferative endometrium.

KATZENELLENBOGEN: In the literature one sees much discussion of the fact that the dehydrogenase tends to convert estrogens from potent to weak forms. I think that in the postmenopausal women it may, in fact, be the reverse.

TSENG: The estrogen metabolic pattern of postmenopausal endometrium studied in vitro is not different from the normal proliferative endometrium.

KATZENELLENBOGEN: You discussed the relationship between levels of estrogen receptor and intracellular tissue concentrations of estradiol, and you found considerably more receptor than estradiol. I wondered, in secretory tissue in particular, whether you are measuring total estrogen receptors, since much of the receptor population is presumably occupied by hormone. How much of the estrogen in the tissue is estrone, for example? Does that account for the difference in levels between intracellular hormone and receptor levels?

TSENG: The estradiol receptor level I have indicated on the slide is the average value of total receptor concentrations, occupied and unoccupied, from four different groups of investigators. The receptor level is higher than the endogenous estradiol. Estrone concentration in endometrium is less than that of estradiol.

LOBL: Could you speculate on the nature of the change in the dehydrogenase activity. Has anyone looked at the changes in dehydrogenase activity and correlated it with estrogen induced cancers? Additionally, is it your hypothesis that certain compounds are potentially more carcinogenic because these compounds cannot be acted on by the steroid dehydrogenase?

TSENG: I am not sure anyone has studied the correlation of dehydrogenase activity with cancer. Roger King and his co-workers studied hyperplastic endometrium from postmenopausal subjects. Sequential treatment with estradiol and progesterone resulted in a twenty-fold increase in the E_2 dehydrogenase activity.

BAULIEU: In the endometrial cancer of postmenopausal women we do not find very much difference from the values of estradiol dehydrogenase you found in the normal proliferative phase in normal cycles. There is no significant difference between the well and the poorly differentiated tumors, although it tended to be higher in well differentiated ones. When you challenge the receptor binding curves with antiestrogen (tamoxifin) we do not see very much change; if anything sometimes we see a decrease (Montel et al, in preparation).

BROOKS: I just want to add to Etienne's comments. Buirchell and Hahnel have published data relating to the activity of these two enzymes in endometrial hyperplasia and cancer. Both of these abnormal endometria resemble proliferative tissue in their enzyme profile, i.e. estradiol dehydrogenase activity was present but there was evidence of estrogen sulfotransferase.

DESOMBRE: Did you say that the antibody to the placental dehydrogenase is non-crossreactive with the endometrial enzyme?

TSENG: We have had difficulty solubilizing the membrane bound enzyme and once it is solubilized it is not stable. It is slightly different with the placental microsomal enzyme, which can be solubilized by phospholipase and still maintain a certain amount of activity to show the cross reactivity with the antibody. Phospholipase destroys the endometrial enzyme. That is the difficulty. We are still trying.

Mechanisms of Regulation of Uterine Enzyme Levels by Estradiol

Kenneth L. Barker

Estradiol induces a dramatic increase in the activity of a variety of events which support or lead to uterine hypertrophy and hyperplasia. Notably, uterine permeability to the exogenous substrates required for growth and development and the synthesis of RNA, protein and lipid are early events which increase in cells of this tissue in response to the hormone. These and subsequent events require the participation of a variety of enzymes and it is not surprising that the amounts and activity of many such proteins are increased as the uterine response to estradiol progresses. The focus of this discussion will center on identification of a variety of estrogen related cellular events which participate in regulation of an estrogen inducible uterine enzyme and the cellular mechanisms through which these events function to cause the levels of this enzyme to increase and/or decrease. The enzyme system to be described is that of glucose-6-phosphate dehydrogenase (G6PD) which is the first enzyme in the hexose monophosphate (HMP) or pentose phosphate pathway which is an alternate pathway for glucose metabolism in most tissues. G6PD catalyzes the oxidation of D-glucose-6-phosphate to 6-phospho-D-gluconolactone with the simultaneous reduction of NADP to NADPH. The HMP pathway functions: a) to produce pentose phosphates which are used for nucleotide and nucleic acid synthesis, b) to produce reducing equivalents in the form of NADPH (2 molecules for each molecule of glucose-6-phosphate which enters the pathway) for use in biosynthetic reductive reactions including fatty acid synthesis, steroid reductions, and hydroxylation reactions and c) to provide an alternative pathway for glucose utilization under conditions where the glycolytic pathway might be rate limiting at a point prior to formation of glyceraldehyde-3-phosphate.

G6PD has been purified and characterized from the cytosol of several mammalian species and/or tissues including human erythrocytes, rat mammary gland, rat and mouse liver, and bovine adrenal cortex (1,2). In general, the enzymes prepared from these mammalian sources are "similar" and are composed of subunits which by immunological and molecular weight criteria may be identical proteins within species. The monomeric subunits have a molecular weight of about 60,000 based on their rate of migration on SDS-polyacrylamide gels. The monomers are catalytically inactive, however in the presence of NADP, the inactive monomers form a catalytically active dimer containing one or perhaps two moles of NADP per mole of dimer. At reduced ionic strength and pH and in the presence of Mg^{++}, the dimers aggregate to form tetramers and hexamers. Using standard polyacrylamide gel electrophoretic methods, one to four isozymes of G6PD activity can be separated. These have been identified to be aggregates of the active dimer based on: a) their relative molecular weights, b) their immunological cross reactivity and c) their ability to generate all four "isozymes" from the purified dimer by changing ionic conditions (3). The amino acid compositions of rat liver, bovine adrenal, human erythrocyte and mouse liver G6PD are known and all have a similar composition. A particularly striking feature of the molecule is the presence of pyroglutamate on the amino terminus of the monomer of the human erythrocyte, bovine adrenal, rat liver and rat uterine enzymes (4-6). Genetic variants of the enzyme are found in some tissues (best studied in human erythrocytes) and the genes for cytosol hepatic and erythrocyte G6PD are controlled and likely located on the X-chromosome. The cytosol G6PD or another protein with G6PD-like activity is frequently found in association with microsomes and evidence exists for the presence and functional activity of the oxidative portion of the HMP pathway in association with isolated microsomes from a variety of tissues including the rat uterus (7).

REGULATION OF UTERINE G6PD LEVELS AND THE ACTIVITY OF THE HMP PATHWAY BY ESTRADIOL

The relationship between uterine G6PD activity and the proportion of glucose which is metabolized through the HMP pathway relative to the glycolytic pathway has been evaluated during the first 24 hours of the <u>in vivo</u> response of the uterus from the ovariectomized mature rat to a single intravenous injection of estradiol (8). Uterine tissue from rats given 5 µg of estradiol for various intervals of time were assayed for cytosol G6PD activity, for the relative ability of tissue slices from each uterus to produce $^{14}CO_2$ from either (1-^{14}C) glucose or (6-^{14}C) glucose and for the rate of incorporation of (6-^{14}C) glucose into (^{14}C) uterine lipids. The ratio of formation of $^{14}CO_2$ from the C-1/ C-6 positions of glucose was used as an index of the relative proportion of glucose which was metabolized through the HMP pathway, since during the conversion of glucose-6-phosphate to pentose phosphates by this pathway, carbon 1 but not carbon 6 is removed as CO_2. Since carbon 6 is ultimately released as CO_2 by the tricarboxylic acid cycle from a common derivative (glyceraldehyde-3-phosphate) which is produced from glucose after it passes through either of the HMP or the glycolytic pathways, the amount of $^{14}CO_2$ derived from this carbon estimates the sum of utilization of both pathways. The entry of carbon 6 from glucose into lipid is unaffected by the pathway of utilization of the glucose since again, the acetyl CoA precursor is subsequently derived from glyceraldehyde-3-phosphate which is a common product of both pathways and the rate of incorporation of ^{14}C from the C-6 position of glucose into total uterine lipid was used as an index of the relative rate of uterine lipid synthesis.

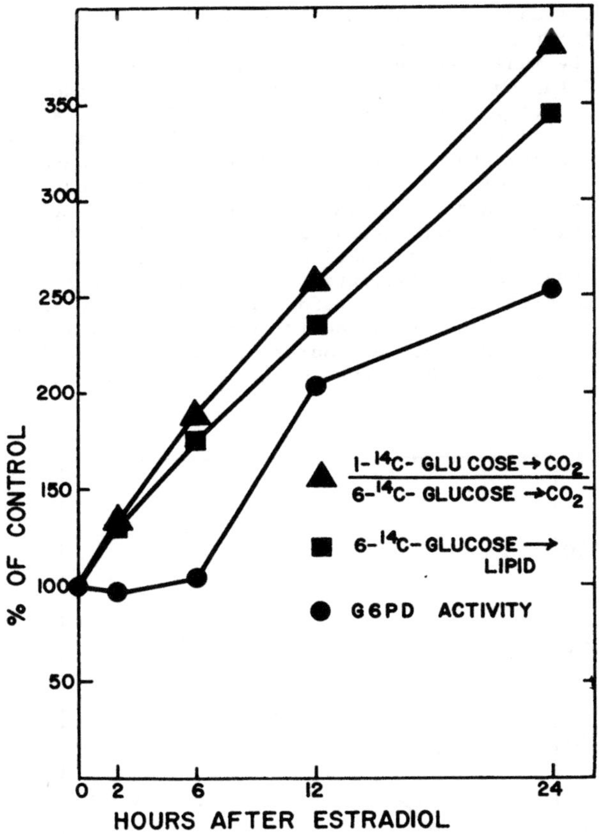

Fig. 1. Effect of estradiol on the total relative levels of glucose-6-phosphate deydrogenase (G6PD) in the rat uterus, the relative rate of incorporation of (6-^{14}C) glucose into the total uterine lipid fraction and the relative change in the ratio of $^{14}CO_2$ produced per uterus from (1-^{14}C) glucose/(6-^{14}C) glucose by uterine segments incubated in vitro for 2 hours. Data from Barker and Warren (8).

A summary of these results is given in Fig.1. It can be seen that the level of uterine G6PD activity remains constant for the first 6 hours after estradiol administration after which it increases 2-fold by the 12th hour. In subsequent studies it was found that the activity of the enzyme continues to increase through the 36th hour of the response after which it gradually decreases to control levels by day 6 (9). Interestingly, the utilization of the HMP pathway was significantly increased by the 6th hour ($P < 0.01$) and was increased in a linear manner ($P < 0.01$) throughout the first 24 hours of the response. The synthesis of lipid was similarly increased in a linear manner during the entire 24 hour period. A most significant point to be made from these observations is that the increased utilization of the HMP pathway precedes the estrogen induction of uterine G6PD activity by 4-6 hours indicating that regulation of the pathway must occur first by increasing the availability of substrate or cofactor for the enzyme and that the estrogen induction of the activity of this enzyme may occur, at least in part, indirectly from some component which is produced by the increased utilization of the HMP pathway. A correlation plot of the indexes of lipid synthesis and HMP pathway utilization reveals that lipid synthesis is coupled to HMP pathway utilization (Fig. 2). Since fatty acid synthesis is coupled to the conversion of NADPH to NADP and since NADP is required for the forward activity of the two oxidative steps of the HMP pathway, these results suggest that uterine lipid synthesis may drive the HMP pathway by increasing the NADP/NADPH

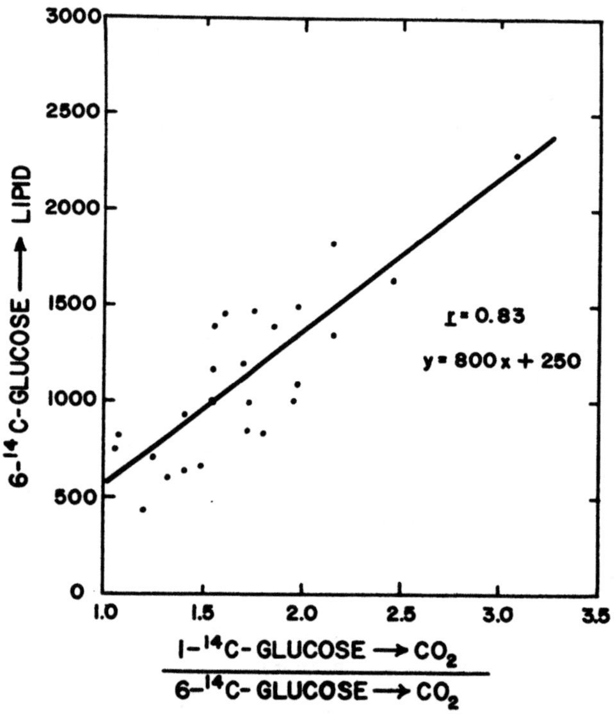

Fig. 2. Correlation plot of the relationship between the rate of lipid synthesis and the utilization of the hexose monophosphate pathway by uterine segments from control and estradiol-treated rats. Individual valves for the last two parameters given in Fig. 1 are plotted as indicated.

ratio of the uterine cytosol. Measurement of the NADP/NADPH ratios reveals that in fact, this parameter does increase during the first 6 hours (10) and in addition after 4 hours (2 hours before G6PD activity begins to increase) there is a significant net increase in the amount of the coenzyme, NADP, required to activate the new G6PD apoenzyme (Fig. 3). The utilization of NADPH by uterine lipid synthesis may also be responsible for inducing de novo NADP synthesis from nicotinic acid in the uterus since NADPH is a powerful inhibitor of NAD kinase (11). These observations clearly indicate that the amount of uterine G6PD activity, which is the first enzyme in the HMP pathway, is not rate limiting for the utilization of this pathway and that the subsequent change in G6PD activity may be due to a combination of the direct stimulation of uterine G6PD mRNA synthesis by estradiol, and adaptive changes in uterine G6PD synthesis which indirectly, occur due to estrogen induced increases in HMP pathway utilization in the tissue and increased uterine NADP levels. These results also suggest that the estrogen induced increase in uterine lipid synthesis which was first recognized by Aizawa and Mueller (12) may be a primary site of estrogen action in the uterus which has received little attention in recent years.

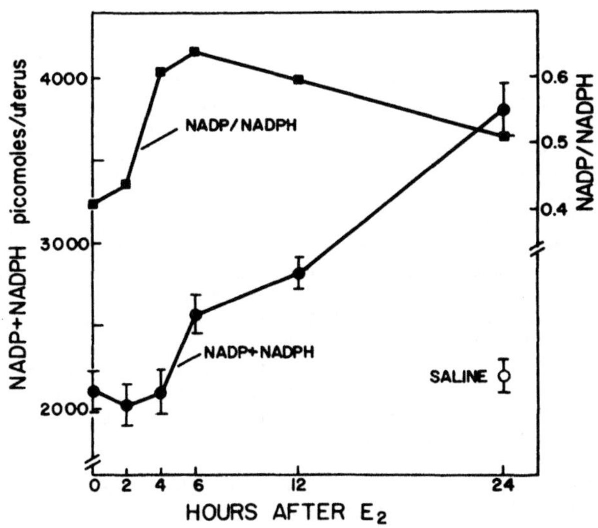

Fig. 3. Effect of estradiol on the amount and ratio of NADP and NADPH in the uterus of the ovariectomized mature rat. Data from O'Dorisio and Barker (10).

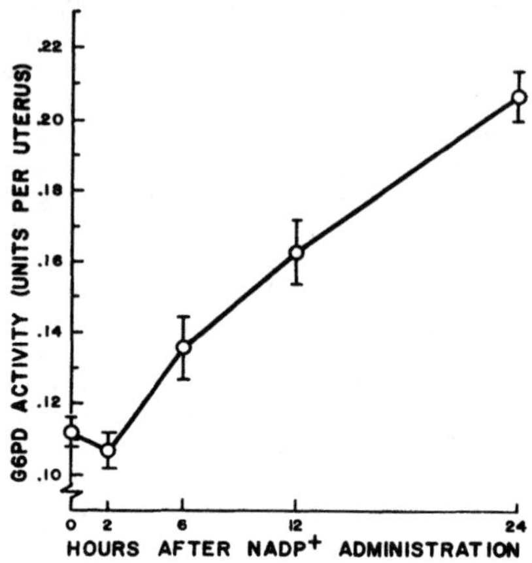

Fig. 4. Effect of intrauterine application of 5 μmoles of NADP on the activity of uterine glucose-6-phosphate dehydrogenase in the ovariectomized mature rat. Data from Barker (13).

INDUCTION OF UTERINE G6PD LEVELS BY ESTROGEN-INDEPENDENT INCREASES IN UTERINE NADP LEVELS AND HMP PATHWAY UTILIZATION

Techniques have been developed to increase the uterine levels of NADP and HMP pathway utilization to evaluate the direct effects of these actions on the activity of G6PD in uterine cytosols. Uterine NADP levels were increased by the direct intrauterine administration of 5 μmoles of NADP (13) and uterine HMP pathway utilization was increased by the intrauterine administration of 50 μmoles of NaF (14). Fluoride causes an increase in HMP pathway utilization by blocking the glycolytic pathway at the enolase catalyzed reaction due to the presence on this enzyme of a tightly bound magnesium ion which readily complexes with fluoride ion. The effects of NADP on the activity of uterine G6PD are given in Fig. 4. Clearly NADP administration increases the activity of uterine G6PD and it is noteworthy that this response exhibits a minimum 2 hour lag before increases in enzyme are observed. These results are consistent with the possibility that estradiol induced increases in NADP levels could participate in part, as an intermediate step in the regulation of uterine G6PD levels by the hormone.

The results given in Fig. 5 indicate that NaF induces an increase in HMP pathway utilization within 2 hours after NaF administration and after a lag of at least 4 hours, uterine G6PD activity is then increased. Results given in the lower panel of Fig. 5 indicate that fluoride did not cause an increase in overall glucose uptake since the production of $^{14}CO_2$ from carbon 6 of glucose is constant. Results of other studies (14) indicated that NaF is not acting on this enzyme by stimulating cAMP production through its effect on

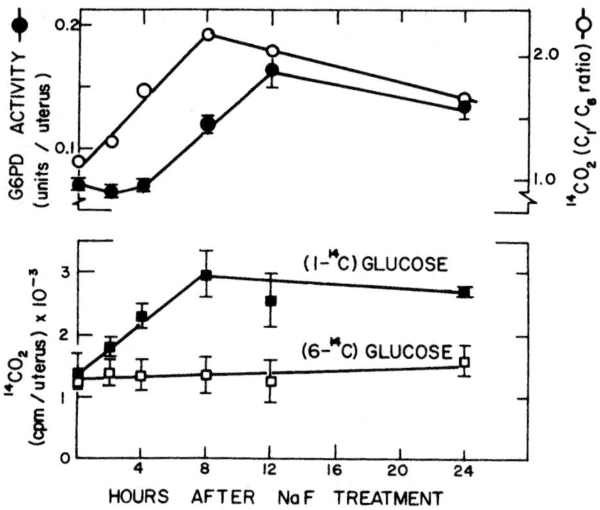

Fig. 5. Effect of intrauterine application of 50 µmoles of NaF on the activity of uterine glucose-6-phosphate dehydrogenase and the relative rate and ratio of $^{14}CO_2$ production during a 2 hour incubation from (1-^{14}C) glucose and (6-^{14}C) glucose by uterine segments from ovariectomized mature rats. Data from Smith and Barker (14).

adenylyl cyclase (which is stimulated by fluoride in broken cell preparations) since theophylline could not potentiate the fluoride response and since intrauterine administration of cAMP could not induce the activity of uterine G6PD. These results suggest that increased NADP levels and HMP pathway utilization can induce uterine G6PD activity in the absence of stimulation of the uterus by estradiol.

The relationship between estradiol, NADP and NaF treatments was further evaluated by determining the sensitivity of each response to actinomycin D and cycloheximide treatments (13, 14). The results summarized in Table 1 indicate that the estradiol but not the NADP or NaF induced increases in uterine G6PD levels are sensitive to the actions of actinomycin D while all three responses were sensitive to the actions of cycloheximide. These results indicate that the estrogen response is dependent on synthesis of RNA while the NADP and NaF responses occur at a post-transcriptional level of protein synthesis. Since cycloheximide blocked the actions of all three

Table 1

Effect of actinomycin D and cycloheximide on the estradiol, NADP and NaF induced increases in uterine glucose-6-phosphate dehydrogenase G6PD activity

Treatment	G6PD Activity (units/uterus)		
	Saline (0.3M)	Actinomycin D (5 μg/rat)	Cycloheximide (500 μg/rat)
Saline (0.15M)	0.115±0.006(8)	0.125±0.004(6)	0.112±0.008(4)
Estradiol (5 μg/rat)	0.171±0.004(7)**	0.109±0.007(4)	0.112±0.008(4)
NADP (5 μmoles/rat)	0.191±0.010(6)**	0.197±0.014(6)**	0.106±0.008(3)
NaF (50 μmoles/rat)	0.277±0.037(6)**	0.203±0.023(6)**	0.102±0.005(6)

** Different from saline-saline controls at $P<0.01$. Estradiol was given intravenously in 0.15M NaCl and all other compounds were given by the intrauterine route in 0.3M NaCl twelve hours before sacrifice of animals. Data from Barker (13) and Smith and Barker (14).

inducers, their mechanisms of action appear to involve de novo synthesis of enzyme protein. An experiment was conducted to determine whether the actions of the three inducers was additive or synergistic in nature when given in combinations to the same animal. The results given in Table 2 indicate that the actions of estradiol and NADP are additive in nature (observed increase approximated the expected increase) while all combinations involving NaF appear to result in a synergistic effect (observed increase exceeded the expected increase). These results suggest that all three inducers are acting at independent molecular levels and that the actions of estradiol, NADP and NaF occur in sequential order at various sites of the overall process of enzyme induction.

REGULATION OF SYNTHESIS OF UTERINE G6PD AT THE TRANSCRIPTIONAL AND TRANSLATIONAL LEVELS BY ESTRADIOL

The effect of estradiol on the relative rates of synthesis of the apoenzyme for uterine G6PD was determined by measuring the rate of incorporation of ^{14}C-amino acids into immunoprecipitable uterine G6PD as generally described by Smith and Barker (15). Highly

Table 2

Additive and Synergistic Nature of the Effects of Multiple Inducers of Uterine Glucose-6-Phosphate Dehydrogenase (G6PD)

Treatment	n	G6PD activity (unit/uterus)	Observed increase	Expected increase if additive
Control	6	0.095±0.009		
NaF (50 μmol)	5	0.189±0.015	0.094	
NADP (5 μmol)	5	0.129±0.005	0.034	
Estradiol (5 μg)	5	0.184±0.005	0.089	
NADP + NaF	5	0.277±0.035	0.182	0.128
Estradiol + NADP	5	0.237±0.016	0.137	0.123
Estradiol + NaF	5	0.345±0.007	0.250	0.183
Estradiol + NADP + NaF	6	0.447±0.016	0.382	0.217

Total uterine G6PD activity expressed as a mean ± S.E. was determined 12 hours after intrauterine administration of either NADP or NaF. Where employed estradiol was given intravenously 4 hours before the intrauterine treatments to compensate for the lag phase of the uterine response to estradiol relative to the other inducers. Expected increase is the sum of the G6PD activity of the control plus the net observed increase in enzyme activity which is seen when each component of the combined treatments is given individually. Data from Smith and Barker (14).

specific antisera to rat liver G6PD were prepared by purification of G6PD from livers of "nutritionally induced" rats to homogeniety followed by immunization of rabbits with the pure enzyme. Antisera prepared in this manner crossreact and have identical enzyme activity titration points with rat liver G6PD and uterine G6PD from control, estradiol, NADP and NaF induced ovariectomized mature rats. The antisera precipitate a single labeled protein from uterine cytosols which were labeled in vivo with ^{14}C-amino acids and this labeled protein migrates on SDS polyacrylamide gel electrophoresis at a point equal to the migration of pure rat liver G6PD subunits. The precipitation of ^{14}C-labeled G6PD from uterine cytosols by the antisera can be completely blocked by the addition of an excess of pure liver G6PD. Administration of radiolabeled amino acids directly into the uterine lumen by a simple non-surgical technique involving administration of material through each of the two cervical openings while the animals are under light ether anesthesia (13) allows synthesis of high specific activity preparations of uterine proteins. When corrected for specific radioactivity of the labeled precursor in the tissue, the incorporation of a labeled amino acid into a specific protein during a measured interval of time allows for direct comparison of the relative rates of synthesis of the proteins between a variety of animal treatment groups. Using this general technique, the effects of estradiol on the relative rates of synthesis of uterine G6PD have been measured (15). During the first four hours after estradiol injection both total uterine G6PD activity and G6PD synthesis rates remained at control levels. From 4 to 8 hours after hormone injection, which coincides with the end of the lag period preceding the increase in total uterine G6PD activity, the rate of G6PD synthesis increased 4-fold. From 12 to 16 hours after hormone treatment the enzyme synthesis rates were increased 18-times the control rate and then the synthesis rates were reduced to 10 to 12-times the control rate during the period from 20 to 48 hours after estradiol injection. Total uterine G6PD activity was maximal after 36 hours and then decreased even though G6PD synthesis rates remained elevated and nearly constant during this interval of time. Direct assessment of the effects of NADP and NaF on the *de novo* rate of G6PD synthesis was similarly assessed, and the synthesis rates were found to be increased 2 to 8-fold and 9-fold, respectively (14, 15 and unpublished observations).

Effect of Estradiol on the Rate of Translation of the G6PD mRNA

A modification of the above general method for measurement of G6PD synthesis was employed to evaluate the effect of estradiol on the time required to translate uterine G6PD under *in vivo* conditions. The average transit time, which is the length of time required for a ribosome, after becoming attached to the G6PD mRNA, to complete and release immunoreactive G6PD into the cytosol was measured. The assay technique was first described by Fan and Penman (16) for use in estimating the rate of translation of total cytosol proteins in cultures of Chinese hamster ovarian cells. The Fan and Penman technique involves determination of the difference in the initial time required to observe a linear rate of incorporation of a labeled amino acid into *total* protein (nascent and released protein chains) and the initial time required to observe a linear rate of incorporation of the amino acid into released proteins found in the cytosol fraction of the cell or tissue. The initial time required to begin the linear rate of incorporation of a labeled amino acid into nascent plus released protein chains defines the time required to equilibrate and charge tRNA with the labeled amino acid in preparation for its use in protein synthesis. The additional time required to establish the initial linear rate of labeling of a specific protein in the released protein fraction represents one-half of the time required for "average ribosomes" to transit the specific mRNA. This is because only after 50% of the nascent chains for the specific protein are completed in the presence of the labeled amino acid will *all* of the positions occupied by the labeled amino acid in the nascent chains (including the last chain to be initiated and the next to be terminated) of the specific protein be labeled at the same uniform rate from the pool of labeled amino acyl tRNA.

We applied this technique *in vivo* to estimate the effect of estradiol on the ribosome transit time for uterine G6PD (17). Groups of animals were given either ^{3}H-leucine or ^{3}H-glutamate by the intrauterine route for various intervals of time from 2 to 16 minutes followed by quick freezing of the tissues and preparation of post-mitochondrial fractions (15,000 X g supernatants which contain nascent plus released protein chains) and cytosol fractions (105,000 X g supernatants which contain only released protein chains). G6PD was precipitated from the cytosol fractions using the immunoprecipitation technique previously described and the incorporation of label into each fraction as a function of pulse interval was plotted. Half-transit times of 2.1 and 2.8 minutes were obtained in the two independent experiments for G6PD synthesis in control animals while estimates of 0.7 and 1.3 minutes and of 1.6 and 1.8 minutes were obtained in rats given estradiol for 12 and 24 hours, respectively. These results indicated that the average total times required to translate the uterine G6PD mRNA were 4.9, 2.0 and 3.4 minutes in control, 12-hour estradiol and 24-hour estradiol treated rats, respectively. These results suggest that 12 and 24 hours after estradiol treatment, there is a 2.5-and 1.5-fold increase, respectively, in the rate of G6PD mRNA translation into the apoenzyme. Similar activation of the translation rate of protein synthesis in the chick oviduct by estrogens have been observed by Palmiter (18). The mechanisms of activation of the translation process are uncertain, but it is possible that in the uterine G6PD system, the estrogen effect could be manifest indirectly through an increased amount of NADP which could facilitate the final stages of translation by binding the nascent G6PD chain to remove steric hinderances caused by the open configuration of the growing and very large peptide chain. Alternatively, a mechanism similar to that proposed by Sharma and Borek (19, 20) could exist in which the estrogen-dependent formation of specific minor species of tRNA present in rate limiting amounts could facilitate the synthesis of proteins from messengers which contain unique triplet codons requiring these tRNA molecules for completion of the protein. Some preliminary evidence we have obtained also suggests that direct estrogen-receptor interaction with uterine ribosomes may activate the rate of peptide elongation during early estrogen action.

Effect of Estradiol on the Level of Uterine G6PD mRNA

An assay for uterine G6PD mRNA has been developed in our laboratory based on the translation of rat uterine mRNA into immunoprecipitable G6PD by a messenger-dependent rabbit reticulocyte cell-free protein synthesis system (21). Uterine RNA was isolated by a modification of the guanidine hydrochloride method of Strohman _et al_. (22). The RNA was assayed directly for its ability to code for G6PD synthesis in the nuclease-treated rabbit reticulocyte lysate system described by Pelham and Jackson (23). With this general system, we observed a linear increase in the incorporation of ^{35}S-methionine into protein as increasing amounts of uterine RNA was added to a maximum of 0.007 A_{260} units of RNA in a 25µl translation assay. The amount of mRNA activity for G6PD was measured by immunoprecipitating the translation products with anti-rat liver G6PD, followed by SDS-polyacrylamide gel electrophoresis of the labeled immunoprecipitate. The total radioactivity in three gel regions coinciding with uterine G6PD, uterine pre-G6PD and a predominent nascent chain of uterine G6PD which accumulates both during the reticulocyte cell-free

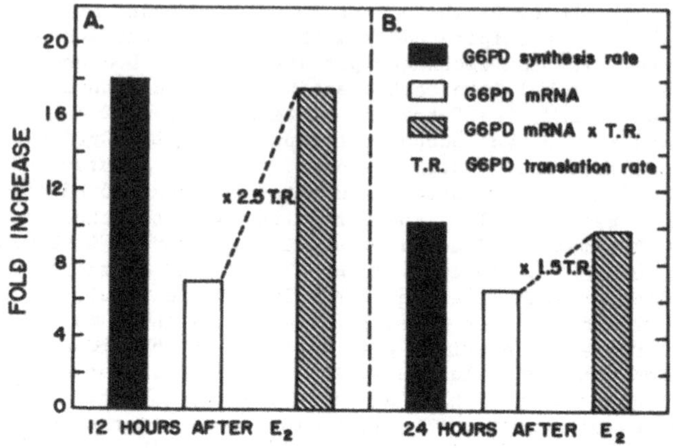

Fig. 6. Effect of estradiol on the fold-increase in the in vivo rate of synthesis of uterine glucose-6-phosphate dehydrogenase, the fold-increase in the amount of G6PD mRNA in the uterus and the fold-increase in the in vivo rate of translation of uterine G6PD mRNA. Data taken from Smith and Barker (15), Adams and Barker (21) and Donohue et al. (17), respectively.

synthesis and the in vivo uterine synthesis of G6PD were taken as total uterine G6PD mRNA activity in the uterine RNA extract. The total amount of G6PD mRNA present in the rat uterus increases 7-fold and 6.5-fold at 12 and 24 hours after estradiol treatment, respectively.

A summary of the effect of estradiol on the fold-increase in the rates of uterine G6PD synthesis, the fold-increase in the uterine pool of G6PD mRNA and the G6PD translation rates are given in Fig. 6. Twelve hours after estradiol treatment, the rate of G6PD synthesis is increased 18-fold relative to control rates and this increase in rate of enzyme synthesis can be accounted for by the translation of a 7-fold greater pool of G6PD mRNA at a rate that is 2.5-times greater than that seen in control animals. The decrease rate of G6PD in synthesis at 24 hours relative to that seen at 12 hours appears to be due to a decrease in the rate of translation of the mRNA to a rate that is only 1.5-fold that seen in control animals. Preliminary studies we have made suggest that elevated NADP levels may participate in regulation of the rate of translation of the uterine G6PD mRNA.

REGULATION OF THE RATE OF PROCESSING OF UTERINE PRE-G6PD BY ESTRADIOL

The amino-terminus of rat liver and uterine G6PD is pryoglutamate. Since methionine is thought to be the initiating amino acid for all eukaryote proteins, it is apparent that G6PD must exist at some time, either as a nascent protein chain or a complete and released precursor molecule with an excess of one or more amino acids on its amino-terminus. As part of the study to estimate the transit time for uterine G6PD, we injected ^{3}H-glutamate as the labeled precursor and estimated the amount of time required to detect ^{3}H-labeled pyroglutamate at the amino-terminus of the G6PD immunoprecipitate. The earliest time that ^{3}H-pyroglutamate was found at the amino-terminus of uterine G6PD was 16, 4 and 8 minutes for control, 12-hour estradiol and 24-hour estradiol treated animals, respectively. This difference in labeling time can partially be accounted for by the difference in time required to initiate the incorporation of ^{3}H-glutamate into total uterine protein. However, if one subtracts the time required to establish the initial incorporation of label into the nascent protein chains from the time required to detect labeled pyroglutamate at the amino-terminus of the enzyme, it is obvious that a significant reduction in the time required to process the amino-terminus of newly synthesized uterine G6PD occurs in response to estradiol treatment (Fig. 7). Since labeled G6PD is released and present in the cytosol which does not contain pyroglutamate as its amino-terminus, these results further suggest that G6PD exists in the cytosol as a released pre-G6PD molecule which is processed by some event or process which itself is regulated by estradiol.

REGULATION OF TURNOVER OF UTERINE CYTOSOL PROTEINS INCLUDING G6PD BY ESTRADIOL

The most popular model proteins used for studies of the mechanism of regulation of protein levels and/or protein synthesis in estrogen target organs are proteins which are secreted by the target cells. These include the popular chick oviduct ovalbumin, the amphibian or avian hepatic vitellogenin and the rabbit uterine uteroglobin systems. All such studies strongly suggest that steroids act on their target organs primarily if not exclusively at a transcriptional level. Berlin and Schimke (24) first suggested that the regulation of enzyme levels in a tissue was due to a balance between the rate of enzyme synthesis and the rate of enzyme degradation. Studies of the effects of estrogen on the rate of intracellular enzyme degradation are not appropriate to the above systems due to their elimination from their cells of origin by secretion rather than degradation mechanisms. We developed a method to measure the effect of estradiol on the rate of degradation of uterine cytosol proteins including G6PD (25). Total uterine proteins were pulse-labeled by intrauterine administration of (1-^{14}C) glutamate 12 to 16 hours into the uterine

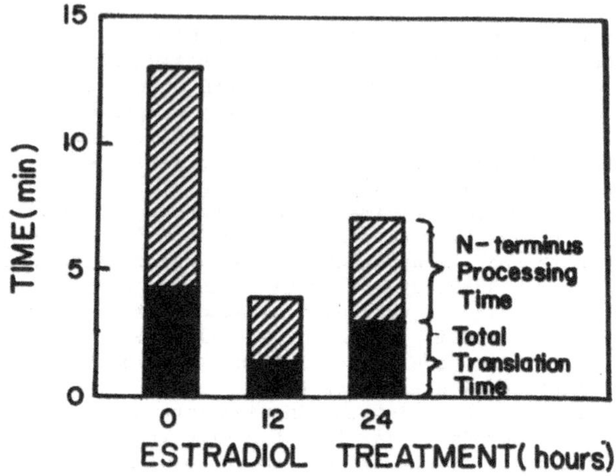

Fig. 7. Estimates of the effect of estradiol on the total transit time of ribosomes on the mRNA for G6PD and the time required to process the newly synthesized G6PD to a form which contains pyroglutamate at its amino-terminus in the uterus of the ovariectomized mature rat. Data taken from Donohue et al. (21).

response to estradiol. After 48 hours the protein biosynthetic stimulus caused by the initial estradiol treatment was nil and the amount of the precursor remaining in the tissue was reduced to less than 0.005% of that present during the protein pulse labeling interval. The effect of a second injection of estradiol on the rate of loss of ^{14}C-glutamate labeled proteins in the uterine cytosol is given in Table 3. The loss of radioactivity from the uterine cytosol proteins over a 24 hour period is decreased from 58% in saline-treated controls to 20% in estradiol-treated rats. The loss of radioactivity from immunoprecipitable uterine G6PD is decreased from about 65% to 0% by the actions of estradiol. These results clearly indicate that estradiol inhibits the rate of loss of uterine cytosol proteins and that there must be some difference in the rate of loss of different proteins since the actions of estradiol are more complete for G6PD than for other proteins. The mechanism of degradation of uterine cytosol proteins is uncertain; however, lysosomes are considered to be prime candidates for the intracellular degradation of proteins in other tissues (26-28). It is of interest and likely relevant to the present observed inhibition of uterine glucose-6-phosphate dehydrogenase degradation (and total cytosol protein degradation) that during estrogen action in its various target organs there is a migration of lysosomes from the cytosol to the nucleus (29). While the exact mechanism and function of the nuclear migration of lysosomes may be unclear, depletion of lysosomes from the cytoplasm could account for the inhibition of the degradation of proteins which reside in the cytoplasm of uterine tissue.

Table 3

Effect of estradiol on retention of radioactivity derived from (1-^{14}C) glutamate in total uterine glucose-6-phosphate dehydrogenase, (G6PD) perchloric acid-insoluble material (protein), and free uterine pool of (1-^{14}C) glutamate

Treatment at 48th hour	Time after treatment	G6PD		PCA-insoluble radioactivity	(1-^{14}C)Glutamate pool
		Activity	Radioactivity		
	hour	units/uterus	dpm/uterus	dpm/uterus	dpm/uterus
None	0	0.25	68	58,000	1,745
Saline	6	0.24	65	51,700	1,940
	12	0.22	49	30,000	950
	24	0.18	24	24,300	457
Estradiol	6	0.32	68	62,600	145
	12	0.35	74	55,900	99
	24	0.56	70	46,600	-

Estradiol-treated ovariectomized mature rats were given 2.0 μCi of (1-^{14}C) glutamate at 12, 13, 14 and 15 hours (8 μCi/rat) after intravenous injection of 5 μg of estradiol. Forty-eight hours after the initial estradiol treatment, seven groups of 20 identically treated rats were given either estradiol or saline. At the indicated times after treatment, identically treated animals were killed and the total uterine G6PD activity and the total radioactivity contained in immunoprecipitable uterine G6PD uterine perchloric acid (PCA)-insoluble material, and uterine (1-^{14}C) glutamate pool were determined. Data from Smith and Barker (25).

SUMMARY

Observations described above indicate that regulation of a specific enzyme in the uterus by estradiol involves both direct and indirect control signals. Estradiol probably initiates the general synthesis of uterine RNA, among which is found the G6PD mRNA and it may exert a direct action on the translational capacity of uterine ribosomes. The activity of the HMP pathway is accelerated and NADP levels are increased in response to estradiol treatment, prior to an increase in G6PD level, and these indirect factors appear to exert control of uterine G6PD synthesis at the translational level. The increased utilization of the HMP pathway prior to the increase in G6PD levels raises the important question of whether an increase in other estrogen-induced enzymes cause a response or metabolic event to operate at a greater rate or whether the utilization of an existing enzyme at a greater rate causes "adaptive-type" changes in enzyme levels. With the HMP pathway system, it appears that estrogen-induced lipid synthesis occurring in direct response to hormone-receptor interactions or indirectly in response to increased glucose or nutrient uptake by the tissue is responsible for events leading to both the increased utilization of the HMP pathway and the synthesis of the NADP coenzyme in the uterus and these in turn play an important role in regulation of G6PD synthesis.

The amount of uterine G6PD present in the uterus is controlled by the direct and indirect estrogen induced signals at a minimum of four different molecular levels. First, it appears that at the time of maximum rate of enzyme synthesis, 12 hours after estradiol injection, there is a 7-fold increase in G6PD mRNA levels. Second, there is a 1.5 to 2.5-fold increase in the rate of translation of the G6PD mRNA into completed and released G6PD apoenzyme. Third, estradiol appears to induce the activity of some process or enzyme which is rate limiting in the processing of a pre-G6PD molecule into the predominant pyroglutamate-containing form of the enzyme which is present in the uterine cytosol. Fourth, estradiol appears to inhibit the turnover or degradation of uterine cytosol proteins including G6PD. These observations suggest that estradiol and possibly the estradiol-receptor complex may exert control, of tissue enzyme levels directly or indirectly, at multiple points in the synthesis of RNA and protein and at various protein processing events in estrogen target organs such as the uterus.

ACKNOWLEDGEMENTS

This work was supported by a research grant HD-02851 from the National Institute of Child Health and Human Development.

REFERENCES

1. Bonsignore A and DeFlora A (1972) Regulatory properties of glucose-6-phosphate dehydrogenase. In: Current Topics in Cellular Regulation, Vol. 6, BL Horecker and ER Stradtman, eds, Academic Press, New York, p 21-62.

2. Levy HR (1979) Glucose-6-phosphate dehydrogenases. Adv Enzym 48:97-192.

3. Holten D (1972) Relationships among the multiple molecular forms of rat liver glucose-6-phosphate dehydrogenase. Biochim Biophys Acta 268:4-12.

4. Yoshida A (1972) Micro method for determination of blocked NH_2-terminal amino acids of protein: Application to identification of acetylserine of phosphoglycerate kinase and pyroglutamine acid of glucose-6-phosphate dehydrogenase. Anal Biochem 49:320-325.

5. Singh D and Squire PG (1975) Bovine adrenal glucose-6-phosphate dehydrogenase. Int'l J Peptide & Protein Res 7:179-184.

6. Donohue TM Jr, Mahowald TA and Barker KL (1977) Identification and labeling of the NH_2-terminal residue of uterine glucose-6-phosphate dehydrogenase. Fed Proc 33:799 (abstract).

7. Baquer NZ and McLean P (1972) Evidence for the existence and functional activity of the pentose phosphate pathway in the large particle fraction isolated from rat tissues. Biochim Biophys Res Commun. 46:167-174.

8. Barker KL and Warren JC (1966) Estrogen control of carbohydrate metabolism in the rat uterus: Pathways of glucose metabolism. Endocrinology 78:1205-1212.

9. Moulton BC and Barker KL (1971) Synthesis and degradation of glucose-6-phosphate dehydrogenase in the rat uterus. Endocrinology 89:1131-1136.

10. O'Dorisio MS and Barker KL (1970) Effects of estradiol on the levels of pyridine nucleotide coenzymes in the rat uterus. Endocrinology 86:1118-1126.

11. O'Dorisio MS and Baker KL (1976) Effects of estradiol on the biosynthesis of pyridine nucleotide coenzymes in the rat uterus. Biol Reprod 15:504-510.

12. Aizawa Y and Mueller GC (1961) The effects in vivo and in vitro of estrogens on lipid synthesis in the rat uterus. J Biol Chem 236:381-386.

13. Barker KL (1967) Cofactor induced synthesis of D-glucose-6-phosphate: NADP oxidoreductase in the uterus. Endocrinology 81:791-797.

14. Smith ER and Barker KL (1976) Effects of sodium fluoride on glucose-6-phosphate dehydrogenase activity in the rat uterus. Biochim Biophys Acta 451:223-237.

15. Smith ER and Barker KL (1974) Effects of estradiol and nicotinamide adenine dinucleotide phosphate on the rate of synthesis of uterine glucose-6-phosphate dehydrogenase. J Biol Chem 249: 6541-6547.

16. Fan H and Pen S (1970) Regulation of protein synthesis in mammalian cells. II. Inhibition of protein synthesis at the level of initiation during mitosis. J Mol Biol 50:655-670.

17. Donohue TM Jr, Mahowald TA and Barker KL (1979) Posttranscriptional control of glucose-6-phosphate dehydrogenase synthesis in the uterus by estradiol. Fed Proc 38:329 (abstract).

18. Palmiter R (1972) Regulation of protein synthesis in chick oviduct. II. Modulation of polypeptide elongation and initiation rates by estrogen and progesterone. J Biol Chem 247:6770-6780.

19. Sharma OK and Mays LL (1973) Enhancement of the synthesis of a hormone induced protein by transfer ribonucleic acids. J Biol Chem 248:7622-7624.

20. Sharma OK and Borek E (1976) A mechanism of estrogen action on gene expression at the level of translation. Cancer Res 36: 4320-4329.

21. Adams DJ and Barker KL (1979) Regulation of glucose-6-phosphate dehydrogenase mRNA levels in the uterus by estradiol. Fed Proc 38:399 (abstract).

22. Strohman RC, Moss PS, Micou-Eastwood J, Spector D, Przybyla A, and Paterson B (1977) Messenger RNA for myocin polypeptides: Isolation from single myogenic cell cultures. Cell 10:265-273.

23. Pelham HRB and Jackson RJ (1976) An efficient mRNA-dependent translation system from reticulocyte lysates. Eur J Biochem 67: 247-256.

24. Berlin CM and Schmike RT (1965) Influence of turnover rates on the responses of enzymes to cortisone. Mol Pharmacol 1:149-156.

25. Smith ER and Barker KL (1977) Effect of estradiol and nicotinamide adenine dinucleotide phosphate on rate of degradation of uterine glucose-6-phosphate dehydrogenase. J Biol Chem 252: 3709-3714.

26. Segal HL and Dunaway GA Jr (1975) In: Intracellular Protein Turnover (Schmike RT and Katunuma N, eds). Academic Press, New York, p 223.

27. Natori Y (1975) In: Intracellular Protein Turnover (Schmike RT and Katunuma N, eds). Academic Press, New York, p 237.

28. Schmike RT (1975) In: Intracellular Protein Turnover (Schmike RT and Katunuma N, eds). Academic Press, New York, p 173.

29. Szego CM (1975) In: Lysosomes in Biology and Pathology (Dingle JT and Dean RT, eds). American Elsevier Publishing Co., New York, p 385.

DISCUSSION

KATZENELLENBOGEN: Ken, I believe you've shown that progesterone diminishes the estradiol stimulated glucose-6-phosphate dehydrogenase activity. With your more specific probes now, where do you think progesterone is acting?

BARKER: We have just completed some studies with Dr. Lloyd Swanson who is doing a sabbatical in our lab and is studying this issue. Progesterone appears to have no effect on synthesis of this enzyme in response to estrogen during the first 36 hours. After 36 hours, progesterone becomes active, probably due to the induction of receptor proteins for progesterone. The specific response that we have observed so far is that progesterone blocks the ability of estradiol to continue the induction of G6PD synthesis. In other words, progesterone becomes a direct antagonist to estrogen action on enzyme synthesis. I suspect, that the estrogen effect on degradation of G6PD and cytosol, and proteins in general, may continue in the presence of progesterone. However, we have not established this yet. If my suspicion is correct, during proestrus an abundance of estradiol and no progesterone might be present, to induce estrogen dependent protein synthesis. After formation of the active corpus luteum, when both progesterone and estrogen are produced simultaneously, progesterone may selectively inhibit the synthesis of estrogen-induced proteins, and estrogen could continue to block turnover of those proteins so they persist and can be used in this tissue for an extended period.

KATZENELLENBOGEN: Does progesterone affect the messenger for this protein?

BARKER: We have not yet measured the messenger pool in the presence of progesterone.

SHAPIRO: I wonder if you have or are contemplating fractionating the ribosomal system to look at the possibility of a cytosolic protein being added to the 40S or 60S ribosome to account for the increase in transit time.

BARKER: We have thought of several alternatives to explain the post-transcriptional control for this enzyme. Some preliminary experiments we have done suggest that NADP may be involved. We think the growing G6PD peptide wraps around the NADP to form the NADP binding site on the enzyme. This may facilitate pulling the protein off the ribosome so it could be translated faster. Another very intriguing possibility, related to the observation by Baglionni, is that the levels of glucose-6-phosphate in a tissue may directly affect the rate of initiation of protein synthesis by ribosomes. I think perhaps this may be the mechanism of the action of the fluoride effect which blocks glycolysis and probably causes an increase in G6P levels in this tissue. I would add one additional possibility. If one homogenizes uteri in something other than tris-EDTA an abundance of what we previously have been calling cytosol estradiol receptor appears to be present on microsomes or ribosomes. We can find a very close correlation between the amount of tightly bound estrogen receptor attached to isolated ribosomes and their ability to synthesize proteins, in general. I think that the estrogen receptor is likely to play a direct role in controlling the function of uterine ribosomes.

LOBL: Do you have an explanation for the immediate activation of certain things such as lipid biosynthesis?

BARKER: I don't really have an explanation. I'm inclined to think that the estrogen receptor may regulate several different molecular events, including the activation of fatty acid synthetase. Also, the early increase in permeability and glucose uptake may allow more glucose to be metabolized to produce precursors for lipid synthesis.

GERSCHENSON: The story on lipid synthesis reminds one of some of the classic experiments by Tata (1970), showing that each time you have a major increase in protein synthesis, first you have an increase in lipid synthesis. His hypothesis was there was a need for more membrane synthesis for rough endoplasmic plasma reticulum.

BARKER: I think it all fits.

GLASSER: I don't think it's appropriate for me to give somebody else's data, but I would alert people to the work of Lawrence Chan in our department. In short summary, Chan has indicated a direct transcriptive effect of estrogen on synthesis of VLDL, which goes back to the original Meuller finding that Dr. Barker mentioned.

Reference:

Tata, JR (1970). Regulation of protein synthesis by growth and developmental hormones. In: Biological Actions of Hormones, Vol 1, G Litwack, ed p 89-133.

The Endometrium

13

Steroid Regulation of Endometrial Peroxidase

Eugene R. DeSombre
C. Richard Lyttle

INTRODUCTION

Research over the last two decades has significantly increased our knowledge about how steroid hormones act on their target tissues. Numerous experimental approaches have contributed to the expanding knowledge of the mechanism of steroid hormone action. The early studies during the 1950's emphasized the effect of steroid hormones on metabolic processes in various target tissues. The direction of research in this field changed drastically, however, following reports of the preparation of tritiated estrogens of sufficiently high specific activity to allow investigation of the tissue localization of the hormone using physiologic amounts of estrogen. The now classic studies by Jensen and Jacobson (1), showing that target tissues for estrogens contained unique components, subsequently called receptors, which effected specific uptake and prolonged retention of estrogens, caused a period of intense investigation during the 1960's to understand the nature of the interaction of a steroid hormone with its target cell, particularly as mediated by its specific receptor protein. Figure 1 illustrates current knowledge about the estrogen-receptor interaction with its target cell (2-5). After entering the cell, probably by a passive diffusion process, the estrogen (E) associates with the extranuclear estrogen receptor protein. This cytosol receptor is present in excess amounts over the minute amounts of steroid entering the target cell and shows the well-documented high affinity and steroid specificity for estrogens. The association of estrogen with its receptor protein endows the complex with a new capability, that is, the ability to undergo a steroid-dependent, energy-requiring activation process. Although a steroid-dependent activation of a cytoplasmic receptor is a common feature of steroid-dependent cells (6,7), with estrogen the change effected by this activation can be identified by a characteristic change in sedimentation coefficient of the complex, from the 4S sedimentation form of the native complex to a 5S form. As indicated in Figure 1, data presented by Notides (8) and also by Jungblut (9) suggest that the steroid-dependent activation results in a dimerization to the 5S complex. Most important, activation results in the steroid-receptor complex with increased affinity for nuclei and chromatin or, as studied in vitro, DNA cellulose columns (5). It is this property which results in the binding of the activated complex to various chromatin sites, an association which apparently leads to the gene tran-

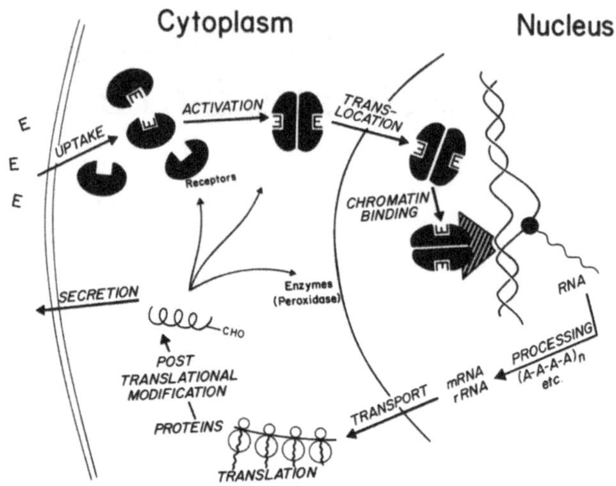

Fig. 1. Schematic representation of the interaction of estrogen with a target cell, showing the sequential interaction pathway of estrogen with the cytoplasmic receptor as a prelude to subsequent RNA and protein synthetic responses in the hormone-stimulated cell.

scriptional events recognized to result from exposure of the target cells to estrogen.

Coupled with the emerging knowledge of the steroid interaction pathway and receptor modulation by steroids has been recent advance in the purification, analysis, synthesis and amplification of specific gene products and their m-RNA under control of various hormones. Examples of such hormone-regulated specific proteins are ovalbumin (10-12), tryptophan oxygenase (13), growth hormone (14), mouse mammary tumor virus (15), uteroglobin (16) and prolactin (17).

While major effects on transcription and translation in the uterus after administration of estrogen to the immature animal have been characterized, the complex phenomena associated with estrogen-induced growth of the atrophic uterus makes the study of this biologic endpoint extremely complicated as a means to elucidate the details of the receptor-chromatin interaction related to gene transcription. As has been evident from the recent studies of the steroid regulation of ovalbumin synthesis in the oviduct, there is considerable utility to the study of a specific protein whose concentration is closely regulated by a steroid hormone. Several specific uterine proteins, synthesized in response to estrogen, have been studied. Best known is the so-called "induced protein", IP, first reported by Notides and Gorski (18) and studied by the laboratories of Kaye and Lindner, Katzenellenbogen and Gorski as well as others (16,19,20). From the viewpoint of steroid hormone action, a particularly interesting uterine marker protein is the progesterone receptor. Although it has been known for some time that the uterine concentration of progesterone receptor is regulated by estrogen (21-23), recent investigations have begun to unravel the details of the hormonal modulation of this marker (24-26). While obviously important to understanding the hormonal modulation of function of the uterus, the progesterone receptor is present in such minute quantities that its use to elucidate estrogen-dependent regulation of gene transcription, as indicated by hormone-dependent increases in progesterone receptor m-RNA, will be technically very difficult. Thus, there is some attraction to studying marker enzymes which are present in substantially larger amounts in the mammalian uterus and endometrium. Indeed, a number of enzymes involved in carbohydrate synthesis have been found to increase in the uterus after estrogen treatment, but in general the extent of such increases due to estrogen have been rather small (27). Nonetheless, studies in Barker's laboratory (28, this volume) have indicated that the de novo rate of synthesis of uterine glucose 6-phosphate-dehydrogenase increases as much as 18-fold by 12 to 16 hours after estradiol administration to the rat.

Increases in uterine peroxidase (donor: hydrogen-peroxide oxidoreductase, E.C. 1.11.1.7) content after estrogen administration were reported over 20 years ago by Stotz and co-workers (29) but subsequently attributed to an influx of eosinophils into the tissue (30). More recent evidence, both biochemical (31,32) and histochemical (33-35), clearly indicates that the enzyme is endogenous to the uterus and is located in the endometrial epithelium. Although the capability of uterine peroxidase and hydrogen peroxide to participate in the metabolism of ^{14}C-estradiol has been the basis for one of the frequently used assays of uterine peroxidase (36), it has not been established that the enzyme actually participates in uterine metabolism of estradiol in vivo. In fact, a recent report from Jellinck's laboratory (37) indicates that it is unlikely that uterine peroxidase functions in vivo to limit the duration of estrogen action. Histochemical studies done at the University of Chicago suggests that the estrogen-induced peroxidase accumulation occurs only in those tissues, such as the epithelium of the uterus, vagina, and carcinogen-induced mammary tumor, whose growth is affected by estrogen (35,38). Electron micrographic studies of localization of the oxidation product of diaminobenzidine, indicate that the enzyme resides in the endoplasmic reticulum and nuclear membrane, but not plasma membrane, of the epithelial cells. Hence while a general competition of peroxidase and receptor for estradiol within the target cell is unlikely, it is nonetheless possible that at certain locations, such as the nuclear membrane, the enzyme could be available for the metabolism of estrogens. Independent of such possible biologic activity related to estrogen metabolism, the magnitude of the induction of endometrial peroxidase makes the enzyme a particularly interesting and useful marker to study estrogen action in this target organ.

This chapter will summarize our present knowledge on the induction and regulation of endometrial peroxidase as a specific protein marker and will outline the state of our knowledge of the relationship of the estrogen-receptor interaction to control of peroxidase synthesis.

MATERIALS AND METHODS

Animals

Sprague Dawley derived female rats were obtained from ARS/Sprague Dawley, Madison, WI or King Animal Laboratories, Oregon, WI. Female lactating rats, each fostering a litter of ten female pups, were obtained from King Animal Laboratories. The animals arrived in our laboratory at least two days prior to use and each mother and litter was housed in a separate cage. The animals were kept under 12 hour light/dark periods. Immature animals were received at 20 days of age and studied at 21 to 23 days of age. Bilateral ovariectomy was performed using ether anesthesia at least one week prior to use of the animal. For the experinent comparing the uterine responses to estradiol administered to ovariectomized and hypophysectomized rats, 30 day-old Holtzman rats were hypophysectomized (Hormone Assay Laboratories, Chicago) or ovariectomized in our laboratory, both at one week prior to initiation of the experiment.

Chemicals

Estradiol, estrone, estriol, diethylstilbesterol, norethindrone (19-nor-17α-ethynyl-4-androsten-17β-ol-3-one), cycloheximide (3 [2(3,5-dimethyl-2-oxo-cyclohexyl)2-hydroxyethyl]glutarimide), emetine hydrochloride and actinomycin D were obtained from Sigma Chemical Company; progesterone from Schwarz Mann; R5020 (17,21-dimethyl-19-norpregna-4,9,-diene-3,20-dione) and R2858 (moxestrol, 11β-methoxy-19-nor-1,3,5(10)-pregnatrien-20-yne-3,17-diol) were obtained by courtesy of Dr. J.P. Raynaud, UCLAF. Medrogestone (6,17-dimethyl-6-dehydroprogesterone) and clogestone (3β,17α-diacetoxy-6-chloropregna-4,6-diene-20-one) were kindly supplied by M. Givner, Ayerst Laboratories, Montreal. Parke Davis, CI628, 1-[2-(p [α(p-methoxyphenyl)-β-nitrostyryl] phenoxy)ethyl] pyrolidine monocitrate, was kindly supplied by Dr. Jerry Reel, Parke Davis Company. These substances were dissolved in ethanol followed by dilution in saline to the appropriate concentration for administration. Injection of steroids and hormones was subcutaneous and control animals received vehicle alone. Actinomycin D, cycloheximide and emetine were administered by intraperitoneal injection.

Experimental Procedures

For experiments with neonatal rats the pups in each litter were kept with the foster mother but marked as two groups, providing five animals for the estrogen treated and control groups at each age. After injection, the pups were returned to the foster mother until sacrificed by decapitation, 20 hours later. The older animals also were sacrificed by decapitation, four to eight animals per group. The entire uterus from oviduct to cervix was quickly removed, dissected free of fat and connective tissue, nicked, blotted on hard filter paper to excise luminal fluid, and weighed. Each uterus was minced with a scissors into a 12 ml polycarbonate tube with the exception of the uteri of 4 day old animals where groups of 5 uteri were combined and for the sedimentation analysis studies for estrogen receptor where five to 20 uteri were pooled prior to homogenization. Uteri were homogenized in 10 mM Tris-HCl, pH 7.2 buffer (25 mg of tissue/ml except for sedimentation analysis where 100 mg/ml was used) for 10 second intervals with ice cooling, using a Polytron PT 10 ST homogenizer at setting 6. After removal of aliquots for DNA analysis (39), the homogenates were centrifuged at 2 C for 45 min at 39,000 x g, or at 250,000 x g in those experiments where cytosols were to be assayed for estrogen receptor content by sedimentation analysis. The hypotonic supernatant fraction contains little peroxidase activity by guaiacol assay. The peroxidase activity was solubilized by rehomogenizing the sediment with 10 mM Tris-HCl, pH 7.2 buffer containing 0.5 M $CaCl_2$ as previously reported (40) and the extract collected by centrifugation for 45 min at 39,000 x g, 2 C.

For the purification of rat uterine peroxidase, 100 adult female rats were given two daily injections of 5 μg of estradiol. 20 hr after the last injection the animals were sacrificed. The uteri were removed, pooled, minced and homogenized at a concentration of 50 mg/ml in 10 mM Tris-HCl, pH 7.2 buffer at 2 C. The homogenate was centrifuged for 45 min at 39,000 x g. After decanting the supernatant fluid, the pellet was resuspended in the original volume of 0.5 M $CaCl_2$ in 10 mM Tris, pH 7.2 buffer and the extract collected following centrifugation for 45 min at 39,000 x g, 4 C. The extract was further purified by affinity chromatography on Con-A Sepharose, from which the peroxidase was eluted with the specific eluent α-methylmannoside, and by hydrophobic interaction chromatography on Phenyl Sepharose, elution effected with the addition of 50% (V/V) ethylene glycol to the extraction buffer, similar to the previous report from our laboratory for the purification of rat mammary tumor peroxidase (41). Final purification was effected by gel filtration on Sephadex G200, also conducted in the enzyme extraction buffer.

Peroxidase assays were performed as previously reported (40), measuring the rate of oxidation of guaiacol at 25 C. The assay mixture contained 13 mM guaiacol and 0.3 mM hydrogen peroxide in the extraction buffer. The reaction was started by addition of enzyme and the linear initial rates, measured on a Gilford Model 3401 automated enzyme analyzer, were converted to enzyme units, defined as the amount of enzyme which produced an increase of 1 adsorbance unit per min at 470 nm at 25 C.

For sedimentation analysis of cytosol receptor, the hypotonic uterine cytosol was incubated at 2 C for 30 min with 10 mM Tris, pH 7.2 buffer containing 500 nM diethylstilbesterol or with buffer alone. Following this, tritiated estradiol, final concentration 5 nM, was added to each aliquot and after an additional 60 min at 2 C, 200 μl samples were layered on cold, preformed, 5-20% sucrose gradients in 10 mM Tris, pH 7.2 buffer. After centrifugation at 250,000 x g for 16 hours, the tubes were punctured at the bottom and successive 100 μl fractions were collected by displacement with paraffin oil. Following addition of a toluene-Triton X-100 scintillation fluid, the samples were counted for tritium content in a Packard Model 3330 scintillation counter at approximately 30% efficiency.

RESULTS AND DISCUSSION

The endometrium of the uterus of the immature or castrate rat has insignificant amounts of peroxidase activity. Previous studies in our laboratory (40,42-45) have shown that estrogens effect a dose-dependent increase in the amount of peroxidase in the immature rat uterus. After a single dose of estradiol the uterine peroxidase content, detectable as enzymatic activity by four to six hours, increases for the first twenty hours and then diminishes, Figure 2. Because of the sensitivity of the enzymatic assay for peroxidase we are able to measure the enzyme content in individual rat uteri. Thus, unlike other responses studied, such as IP where pools of uteri are required for assay, the individual animal variation of the peroxidase response can be deter-

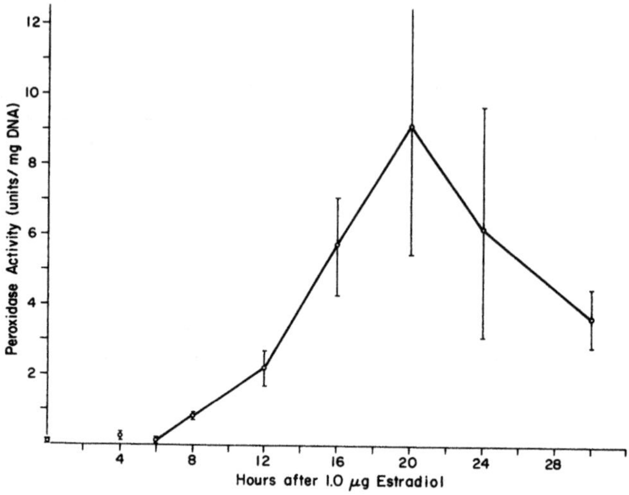

Fig. 2. Time course for the estrogen induction of rat uterine peroxidase. Twenty-one day old female rats were given 1.0 g estradiol and, at the times indicated, groups of 5 animals were sacrificed. The individual uteri were assayed for peroxidase as detailed in the Materials and Methods section. Results presented as mean values ± S.D. From DeSombre and Lyttle (45).

mined. It can be seen in Figure 2 that significant animal variation is observed especially near the peak time of induction, 20 hours. Whether these large animal variations represent differences in the sensitivity of individual animals for the estrogen induction of endometrial peroxidase, or whether they represent differences in the timing of peroxidase response cannot be answered at the present time. Morphologic evidence, however, suggests that within the endometrium of a single uterus, there are significant cell to cell differences in peroxidase induction after estrogen. It is not uncommon to observe a cell strongly positive for peroxidase staining by histochemical methods, between two cells completely negative for the enzyme (35). Such, possibly cell cycle dependent, differences in the sensitivity of individual endometrial cells to exogenous estrogen are believed to explain at least in part the large standard errors seen in the time of induction study, Figure 2.

Even though the uterine response of peroxidase activity following a single physiologic dose of estrogen is so dramatic, multiple doses of estradiol cause further major increases in uterine peroxidase activity, Figure 3. Upon two and three days of sequential administration of estradiol one continues to observe further major stimulation of endometrial peroxidase activity. These increases in endometrial peroxidase clearly parallel the increases in uterine weight and uterine RNA content in the same estradiol treated animals. As is also seen with the parameters of uterine growth, the uterine content of peroxidase reaches

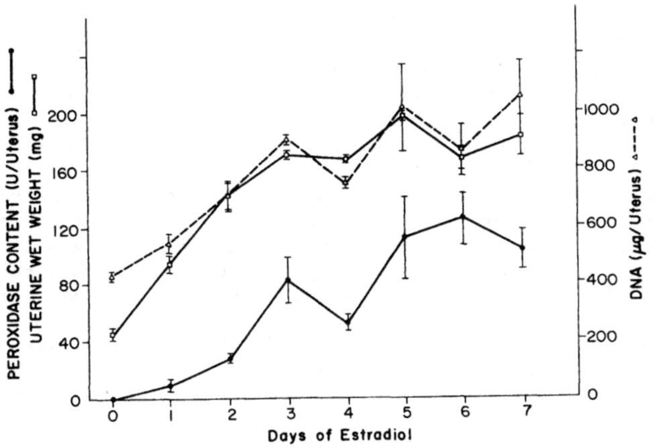

Fig. 3. Effect of estradiol treatment on rat uterine wet weight, DNA and peroxidase content. Ovariectomized rats received 1.0 µg estradiol per day and were sacrificed in groups of 5 animals, 20 hrs after the last injection of estradiol. Results presented as mean values ± S.E.M. From DeSombre and Lyttle (43).

a plateau in rats given 1 µg of estradiol per day for 5 to 7 days. This plateau level in uterine peroxidase is similar to the level of the enzyme seen in the mature animal (43). As is evident from Figure 3, the uterine increase in peroxidase content, even though consisting entirely of the endometrial response, closely parallels the increases in weight and DNA content suggesting that peroxidase is a reasonable marker for the more complicated, but commonly studied, growth effects of estrogen on the uterus. As we have reported elsewhere (43) the uterine peroxidase content varies during the estrous cycle. The concentration is highest during proestrus and estrus and is significantly lower at metestrus reaching a minimum during diestrus. Administration of estradiol to the rat in metestrus or diestrus causes a significant increase in the uterine peroxidase content 20 hours later, reaching a level essentially the same as that seen during estrus. However, administration of estradiol to the estrous or proestrous animal does not effect a significant increase in the already elevated uterine concentration of the enzyme.

The response in peroxidase seen in the rat uterus appears to relate closely to the estrogenic activity of various estrogens. As we have shown earlier (40), estrogenic steroids such as estrone and estriol, which have approximately one order of magnitude lower affinity for the estrogen receptor than does estradiol, similarly require approximately a ten-fold increase in dose to be able to effect a similar induction of peroxidase. Each of these steroids also shows a dose-dependent induction of the endometrial enzyme, nonetheless. Jellinck and Newcombe have recently also reported a good correlation between the uterotrophic activity of a variety of estrogens and the ability of these steroids to effect increases in uterine peroxidase (46). The response in uterine peroxidase following estrogen administration is not unique to the laboratory rat. We have reported (42) on comparing four common laboratory animals, the hamster, guinea pig, rat and mouse that the extent of uterine peroxidase stimulation in each of these species appears to correlate with the extent of the uterine weight increase on estradiol treatment. Although each of these laboratory animals showed a significant response to administered estradiol, the extent of the response varied dramatically, from about a 2-fold peroxidase stimulation (1.4-fold increase in uterine weight) in the hamster uterus to an almost 300-fold increase in peroxidase concentration (4.5-fold increase in uterine weight) in the mouse uterus on two days of estrogen treatment. In view of the clear evidence from morphologic studies that peroxidase expression is limited to endometrial and epithelial tissue whereas the biochemical assays, as represented in Figures 2 and 3, are based upon the peroxidase activity per unit uterine weight, it is apparent that the extent of the estrogen-dependent peroxidase induction in the endometrium is very dramatic indeed, even more so than is represented by the increases seen in Figures 2 and 3. Although peroxidase is a secretory product and is found in the luminal fluid (35), the tissue content is so dramatically greater than the concentration in the luminal fluid that it is probable that this major cellular product has a major physiologic role. The intracellular function of the enzyme, however, still remains to be elucidated.

RNA and Protein Synthesis Requirement for the Peroxidase Response

Until the reagents necessary for quantitation of the specific messenger RNA for peroxidase are available and one can demonstrate that following administration of estrogen there is an increase in the messenger RNA for this specific marker, the description of the increase in peroxidase elicited by estrogen as induction must be used with reservation. Especially when assessing enzymatic activity one must be concerned with the possible activation of a pre-existing protein as an alternative possibility for the apparent stimulation. Although peroxidase can effect binding and subsequent metabolism of estrogen, there is no evidence that the hormone is able to directly increase uterine content of peroxidase. Moreover, the dramatic estrogen-dependent increases in uterine peroxidase require prior macromolecular synthesis, consistent with de novo synthesis of new protein. As shown in Table 1 actinomycin D, an inhibitor of RNA synthesis, as well as cyclohexamide and emetine, inhibitors of protein synthesis, are effective inhibitors of the estrogen-dependent increases in uterine peroxidase when these inhibitors are administered along with estrogen. In addition, the temporal relationship of the actinomycin D and emetine inhibition of estrogen-dependent uterine peroxidase expression are consistent with a process involving gene regulation. As reported elsewhere (45) from time course studies of actinomycin D and emetine inhibition of estrogen-dependent increases in uterine peroxidase, the requirement for RNA synthesis for the peroxidase induction precedes by about two hours the requirement for protein synthesis for the 20 hour enzyme response.

Peroxidase Induction in Hypophysectomized or Ovariectomized Rats

Estradiol induction of endometrial peroxidase can be observed in the ovariectomized and hypophysectomized, as well as in the immature, rat.

TABLE 1. INHIBITION OF ESTRADIOL-DEPENDENT INCREASES IN UTERINE PEROXIDASE BY INHIBITORS OF RNA AND PROTEIN SYNTHESIS

Treatment	Peroxidase Activity[a] Units/g	% of E2
Saline	0.05 ± 0.03	0.6
E2 (1 μg)	8.47 ± 3.36	100.0
E2 (1 μg) + Actinomycin D (150 μg)	0.76 ± 0.67	8.9
E2 (1 μg) + Cycloheximide (250 μg)	0.43 ± 0.17	5.0
E2 (1 μg) + Emetine (1.5 mg)	0.51 ± 0.14	6.0

[a]Peroxidase activity by guaiacol assay of $CaCl_2$ extracts of uteri of rats 20 hours after treatment as shown, ± S.D.

However, as shown in Table 2, the response to a single dose of estradiol

TABLE 2. ESTRADIOL INDUCTION OF PEROXIDASE IN OVARIECTOMIZED AND HYPOPHYSECTOMIZED RATS

	HYPOPHYSECTOMIZED[a]		OVARIECTOMIZED[a]	
	Uterine Weight (mg)	Peroxidase (Units/g)	Uterine Weight (mg)	Peroxidase (Units/g)
Control	23.2 ± 1.2	0.0	28.4 ± 0.9	0.0
1 day E2 (5 μg)	38.8 ± 1.7	0.6 ± 0.2	58.0 ± 1.6	48.0 ± 13.6
2 days E2 (5 μg)	54.5 ± 3.0	40.0 ± 13.2	103.0 ± 5.8	77.6 ± 14.8

Results given as mean values ± S.E.M.

is much less dramatic in the hypophysectomized animal than the ovariectomized animal. This decreased responsiveness of the hypophysectomized animal is observed both in uterine weight and peroxidase. Following two days of administration of estrogen to the hypophysectomized animal the increases in both weight and peroxidase content of the uterus are more dramatic. Nonetheless, neither the weight nor the peroxidase concentration of the uterus of the estrogen-treated hypophysectomized rat reach the comparable level of these parameters in the estrogen treated castrate animal after 2 days of treatment. In fact, it appears that after 2 days of estrogen treatment the uterus of the hypophysectomized animal resembles that of the castrate given only one day of estrogen treatment. It is possible that the decreased biosynthetic capability of the uterus of the hypophysectomized animal, as represented by decreased polysome content among other things, may be largely responsible for the initial lack of responsiveness to estrogen. It is also possible, as has been suggested by Sonnenshein (47), that the pituitary is directly responsible for some of the estrogen-induced response of the uterus. Nonetheless, the clear evidence that estrogen can effect increase in peroxidase in the uterus of the hypophysectomized animal argues for the direct action of estrogen upon the uterus, at least one not requiring a pituitary factor for the actual induction.

Antiestrogens and Peroxidase Induction

It has been known for some time that certain triphenylethylene derivatives exhibit antiuterotrophic activity with regard to estrogens. These compounds, similar in structure to the prototype MER-25 (48), are able to reduce the uterine uptake of tritiated estradiol in vivo and in vitro (49). Although the antiestrogens are competitive inhibitors of estrogen binding to its cytoplasmic receptor and early investigations ascribed the antagonist property to this capability, more recent evidence (44,50-52) suggest that a prolonged nuclear occupancy of the estrogen receptor protein and a concomitant, prolonged depression of the cytoplasmic receptor capacity following administration of antiestrogen are probably of greater biologic significance. Studies of the effect of the antiestrogen, Parke-Davis CI628, on the estrogen stimulation of uterine peroxidase support this latter view. Figure 4 shows

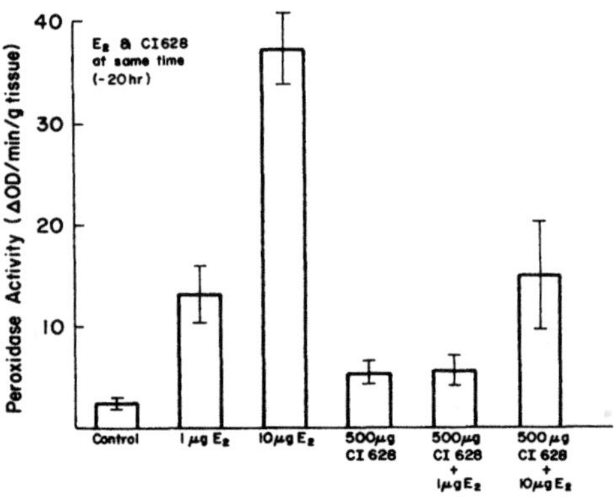

Fig. 4. Effect of the antiestrogen, CI628, on induction of estrogen-dependent rat uterine peroxidase. Immature female rats, five per group, were treated with estradiol, CI628 or combinations of the two compounds and after 20 hrs the animals were sacrificed and uteri assayed for peroxidase. Results given as mean values ± S.E.M. From DeSombre and Lyttle (43).

the results of an experiment in which CI628 and estradiol were administered alone and in combination to determine their ability to affect uterine peroxidase levels in immature rats. Although in this experiment even the control animals had a low level of endogenous peroxidase, significant increases in peroxidase were seen with 1 μg of estrogen and even more dramatic increases were observed with 10 μg of the hormone. Twenty hours after a very large, 500 μg dose of CI628 there was a small, but significant, increase in uterine peroxidase, indicative of the partial agonist activity of this antiestrogen. Administration of this high dose of antiestrogen with 1 μg of estradiol suppressed the peroxidase induction to that seen with the antiestrogen alone. With the higher dose of estrogen, 10 μg of estradiol, the antiestrogen administered concomitantly could only partially inhibit the dramatic increase due to estrogen. It is apparent from Figure 4 that the ratio of antiestrogen to estrogen is important since the high ratio of antiestrogen to estrogen could completely suppress the increase seen with estrogen while being only partially effective at a lower ratio. If the effect of antiestrogen is due to a depletion of cytoplasmic estrogen receptor, prior treatment with the antiestrogen should be more effective than simultaneous treatment. As shown in Figure 5 there is

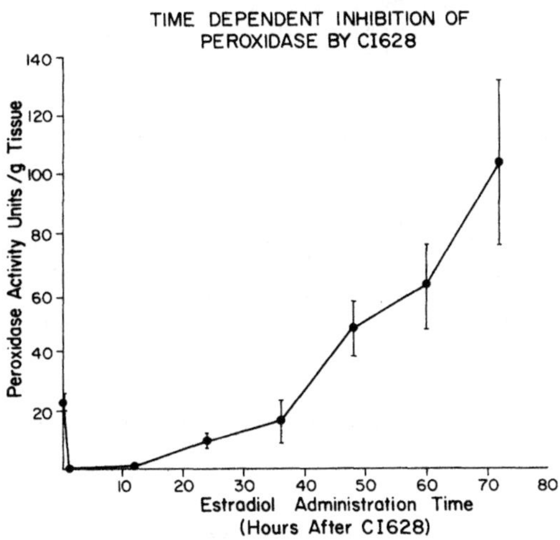

Fig. 5. Time-dependent inhibition of estradiol stimulated rat uterine peroxidase by the antiestrogen, CI628. Two-hundred μg of CI628 were administered to immature female rats. At various times thereafter, from 0 to 72 hours later, groups of five animals were given 5 μg of estradiol and 20 hrs after estrogen the rats were sacrificed and uteri assayed for peroxidase activity. Results presented as mean values ± S.E.M. From DeSombre and Lyttle (44).

clearly a time-dependent inhibition of estrogen induction of peroxidase when the antiestrogen is administered first. Because the ratio of CI628 to estradiol in this experiment was only 40, concomitant administration of CI628 did not effect a complete inhibition of the estrogen-induced peroxidase. However, when estradiol was given either one hour or 12 hours after CI628, times which for all practical purposes the cytosol estrogen receptor is absent, no peroxidase induction was seen.

At later times which allowed partial recovery of cytoplasmic receptor, one to two days after antiestrogen, there was a partial induction of peroxidase by estrogen. Finally, by three days when the cytoplasmic receptor is fully replenished, occasionally even to a level higher than found in the untreated uterus, the estrogen inducibility of peroxidase is maximal. These studies therefore show a remarkable correlation of the effect of CI628 on the depletion of cytosol estrogen receptor and the blocking of estrogen induction of the endometrial enzyme, peroxidase. Previous studies by McNabb, Jellinck (52) using the antiestrogen, nafoxidine or U11100A, had also shown that this antiestrogen was an effective inhibitor of the estrogen-induced peroxidase. However these investigators, using the water soluble product peroxidase assay, reported that pretreatment of animals with nafoxidine was less effective than administering both the estrogen and antiestrogen at the same time. Preliminary studies in our laboratory have indeed indicated that there are significant differences in the activities of various antiestrogens, differences seen in their agonist activities when used alone, and also in their ability to antagonize estrogen-induced increases of uterine weight or peroxidase activity. It will be important to relate these differences to the effects of antiestrogen upon estrogen receptor in the uterus.

Progesterone Antagonism of Peroxidase Induction

Progesterone has been recognized for some time to be an antagonist of estrogen action (53,54). An earlier report from our laboratory in collaboration with Anderson (55) demonstrated the progesterone antagonism of estrogen-dependent increases in uterine peroxidase in normal and pregnant adult female rats, using the histochemical assay for peroxidase. As shown in Table 3, progesterone is a potent inhibitor of

TABLE 3. INHIBITION OF ESTROGEN-INDUCED UTERINE PEROXIDASE BY VARIOUS PROGESTINS[a]

	Peroxidase Activity (% of E2 alone)		
	100 μg[b]	500 μg[b]	1000 μg[b]
Progesterone	48.4	26.7	19.0
R5020	31.9	9.4	9.6
Norethindrone	31.7	4.2	3.7
Medrogestone	72.8	36.1	40.1
Clogestone	72.2	73.0	71.1

[a]Immature rats received 1 μg estradiol (E2) on day one and either 1 μg E2 alone or simultaneously with the progestin 24 hours later. Twenty hours after the second injection the animals were sacrificed and the uteri assayed for peroxidase activity as described in the Materials and Methods section.

[b]Dose of progestin given with E2 on day 2.

estrogen-induced endometrial peroxidase, assayed biochemically in the immature rat. For the experiment described in Table 3, immature rats were first primed with estradiol for one day to effect an increase in the tissue level of progesterone receptor and then challenged with estradiol alone or in the presence of various progestins. As can be seen, progesterone shows a dose-dependent inhibition of estrogen-induced endometrial peroxidase which appears to level off at a dose of 500 μg. Increasing the amount of progesterone to 1000 μg does not substantially increase the inhibition even though approximately 20% of the peroxidase activity still remains. Other progestins are also found to be effective. Table 3 shows that two very potent progestins, R5020 and norethindrone, appear to be even more active antagonists of the estrogen-induced peroxidase response than is progesterone itself. These steroids have a significantly higher affinity than progesterone for the progestin receptor and also have been shown to possess greater biologic potency with regard to standard assays of positive action (maintenance of pregnancy, deciduoma formation) and antagonism of estrogen-induced uterine growth (56). As supported by more detailed dose response studies, the maximum activity of progesterone, R5020 and norethindrone are observed with doses in the 250 μg to 500 μg dose range, despite the fact that the extent of the maximum inhibition varies among these three progestins. Interestingly, the two less potent progestins in this assay, medrogestone and clogestone, did not show significantly increased potency at doses up to 2 mg per rat, despite the fact that neither of these steroids had equaled the potency of progesterone at the doses shown in Table 3. These results suggest that the weaker progestins not only may have a different dose response curve but may also show decreased maximum potency, at least as regards inhibition of estrogen stimulated uterine peroxidase. The least active steroid in the study, clogestone, while an active progestin in the rabbit, has been found to be practically inactive in rats (57).

The well documented effect of progestins to stimulate the amount of the estradiol metabolizing enzyme, 17β-hydroxysteroid dehydrogenase, of the mammalian uterus, as reported by Tseng and Gurpide (58,59), does not appear to be responsible for the observed effects of progesterone. This enzyme converts the more active estrogen, estradiol, to the less active estrone, Figure 6, and by increasing such conversion progestins could reduce the estrogenic potency of estradiol. However, as shown in Figure 7, progesterone is able to antagonize the estrogen induction of endometrial peroxidase when the estrogen is estrone or diethylstilbesterol as well as estradiol itself. Since neither estrone or diethylstilbesterol would be converted to less active estrogens by the dehydrogenase, it is unlikely that the progestin antagonism depends upon induction of this metabolizing enzyme. Furthermore, while progesterone has been clearly found to increase the 17β-hydroxysteroid dehydrogenase activity in the human uterus, a recent report suggests that in the rat the uterine activity of this enzyme is stimulated by estrogen and reduced by progesterone administration (60).

Although studies from a number of laboratories, including our own (55), have confirmed Clark's report (61) that progestin administration decreases the replenishment of the cytosol estrogen-receptor complex following administration of estradiol, recent studies in our laboratory suggest that this effect of progesterone is insufficient to explain the inhibitory effect of progesterone on estrogen-dependent endometrial peroxidase. Most important in this regard is that progesterone, even given following estradiol, is able to effect inhibition of the peroxidase response due to estrogen. As shown in Table 4, progesterone given

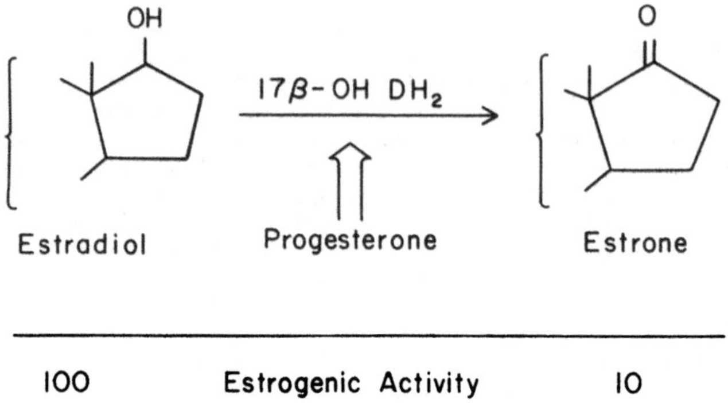

Fig. 6. Schematic description of progesterone antagonism of estradiol action as mediated by progesterone induction of the uterine enzyme 17β-hydroxysteroid dehydrogenase. This enzyme is capable of converting estradiol to estrone, a change corresponding to a 10-fold reduction in estrogenic activity of the steroid.

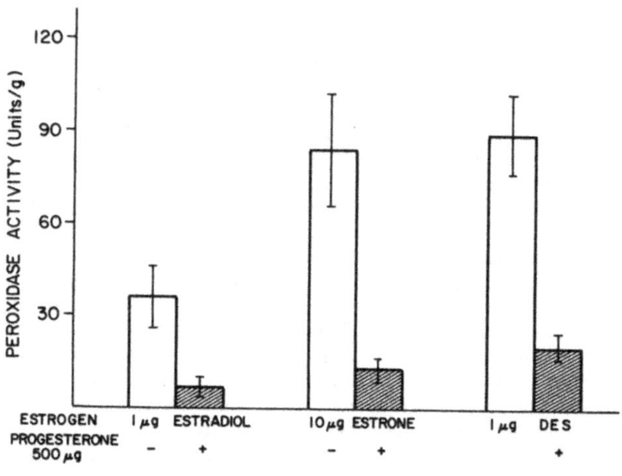

Fig. 7. Progesterone antagonism of uterine peroxidase induction by several estrogens. Groups of five immature rats were treated with the indicated dose of estradiol, estrone, or diethylstilbesterol (DES), alone or each along with 500 μg of progesterone. Twenty hours after treatment the animals were sacrificed and their uteri assayed for peroxidase activity. Results presented as mean values ± S.E.M., open bars representing animals given only estrogen, cross-hatched bars results from animals given estrogen and progesterone. From DeSombre and Lyttle (43).

TABLE 4. TIME COURSE OF PROGESTERONE-DEPENDENT INHIBITION OF ESTROGEN INDUCTION OF UTERINE PEROXIDASE

Treatment time[a] (hours after E2)	Peroxidase Activity[c] Units/g	% of E2 alone
Control[b]	11.95 ± 4.8	100.0
0	4.14 ± 1.6	34.6
1	2.02 ± 1.9	16.9
2	0.70 ± 0.4	5.9
4	1.03 ± 0.5	8.6
6	4.62 ± 2.3	38.7
11	11.57 ± 3.6	96.0

[a]Treatment time is the time, in hours, after 1 μg estradiol (E2) that 500 μg progesterone was administered. In each case all animals were sacrificed 20 hours after E2 for assay of uterine peroxidase.

[b]Control animals received no progesterone.

[c]Peroxidase activities given as mean values of 5 uteri per group ± S.E.M.

up to four hours after estradiol dramatically reduces the peroxidase present twenty hours after estrogen. By six hours after estrogen the progesterone inhibition is reduced and it is no longer seen by eleven hours. Clearly, by one or two hours after administration of estradiol in vivo the estrogen receptor complex has left the cytosol and is localized in the nucleus. These data therefore suggest that the progesterone effect, probably mediated through progesterone receptor, acts at a point subsequent to initial nuclear binding of the estrogen receptor complex. Our preliminary studies with progesterone are consistent with a block of the estrogen-dependent peroxidase induction occuring prior to RNA synthesis since the timing of the progesterone affect, Table 4 is similar to the timing of the inhbition of estrogen-dependent peroxidase induction seen after administration of actinomycin D (45). Obviously such a temporal relationship of progesterone antagonism is inconsistent with a process requiring new receptor synthesis, a process which is significantly delayed in time. In order to understand the molecular mode of action of this progesterone antagonism it will be important to determine whether the progesterone-receptor complex can effect release of estrogen-receptor complex from chromatin.

Ontogeny of the Peroxidase Response in the Developing Postnatal Rat

One very interesting model system for studying the factors important to the biologic response of the uterus to estrogen is that of the developing postnatal rat. Studies of the estrogen sensitivity of the postnatal rat uterus have consistently shown that the tissue is able to respond to hormone significantly before puberty. Most parameters of response which have been studied, however, show no significant estrogen stimulation in animals younger than 10 days old but generally show an estrogen response in animals older than 15 days of age. An exception to this is the response in induced protein, IP, which has been found by both Katzenellenbogen and Greger (62) and Walker et al. (63) to be stimulated by estrogen in the five day old rat. As shown in Figure 8

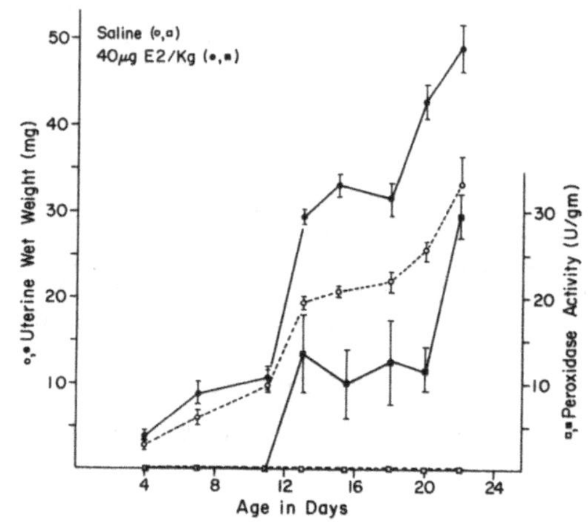

Fig. 8. Effect of estradiol on uterine weight and uterine peroxidase concentration in the postnatal female rat. Estradiol (40μg/Kg body weight, closed symbols and solid line) or saline (open symbols, dashed lines) was administered subcutaneously to five pups each from the same foster mother fed litter and the pups were sacrificed 20 hrs later for assay of uterine weight (circles) and uterine peroxidase (squares). Values given as means ± S.E.M. From Lyttle, Garay and DeSombre (64).

the uterus of the untreated rat, up to 21 days of age, does not contain any endogenous peroxidase. Treatment of rats, 11 days of age or less, with a significant dose of estradiol (40μg/Kg) is unable to induce any measureable peroxidase in the uteri of these rats and, furthermore, shows no significant stimulation of uterine weight. However the uterus of the 13 day old rat showed a significant sensitivity to estradiol as found both in the induction of significant amounts of uterine peroxidase and by the significant increases in uterine wet weight, 20 hours after administration of the hormone. In all rats 13 days of age or older a similarly dramatic stimulation of uterine weight and peroxidase content was seen after administration of a single dose of estradiol. Although, as shown by Raynaud (65), the early postnatal rat blood contains high concentrations of the estradiol binding protein, α-fetoprotein, it appears that the ability of α-fetoprotein to decrease the amount of circulating estrogen is not the reason for the delayed uterine sensitivity to estradiol. In particular, as shown in Figure 9, when similar studies were carried out with the synthetic estrogen R2858, an estrogen which does not show appreciable affinity for α-fetoprotein,

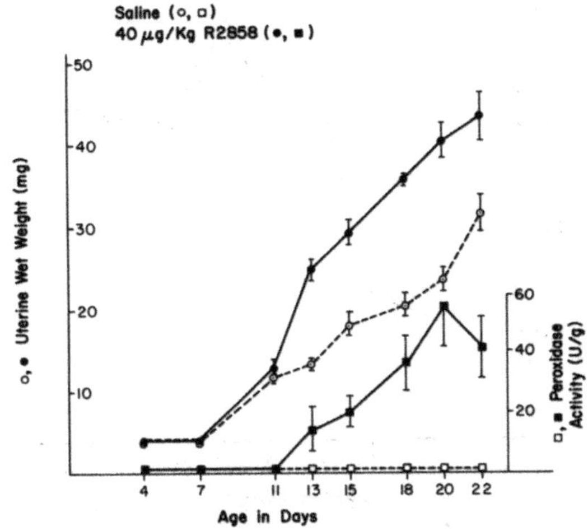

Fig. 9. Effect of the synthetic estrogen, R2858, on uterine wet weight and uterine peroxidase concentration in the postnatal female rat. Protocol, symbols and procedures as detailed in Figure 8 except that the same body weight dose of R2858 rather than estradiol was used.

the same pattern of estrogen sensitivity during development was seen. In animals 11 days of age and younger the estrogen again elicited no response in either uterine wet weight or peroxidase content. While the uterus grew significantly by seven and 11 days, estrogen could not effect further growth. The R2858 did stimulate increases in uterine weight and uterine peroxidase in animals 13 days of age or older. The nonsteroidal estrogen, diethylstilbesterol, also an estrogen with little affinity for α-fetoprotein, is similarly ineffective in the stimulation of uterine growth or peroxidase in animals younger than 11 days but, like estradiol and R2858, is an active estrogen in older pups as we have recently reported (64). These results suggest that the estrogen inducibility of uterine peroxidase in the postnatal rat correlates very well with the estrogen stimulation of uterine weight and that peroxidase appears to be a good marker for the sensitivity of the uterus to estrogen.

In an effort to relate the uterine sensitivity to estrogen to the estrogen receptor we are studying the ontogeny of the uterine receptor and the interaction of estrogen with its receptor in the developing uterus. As shown in Figure 10, the estrogen receptor content of the five and seven day old rat uterus is low but detectable. Between seven and nine days of age there appears to be a significant increase in the estrogen receptor content of the uterus. The concentration of cytoplasmic 8S receptor in the nine day old rat uterus is about the same as that seen in the 21 day old animal, even though the latter but not the former uterus is fully responsive to estrogen. Because, as noted by

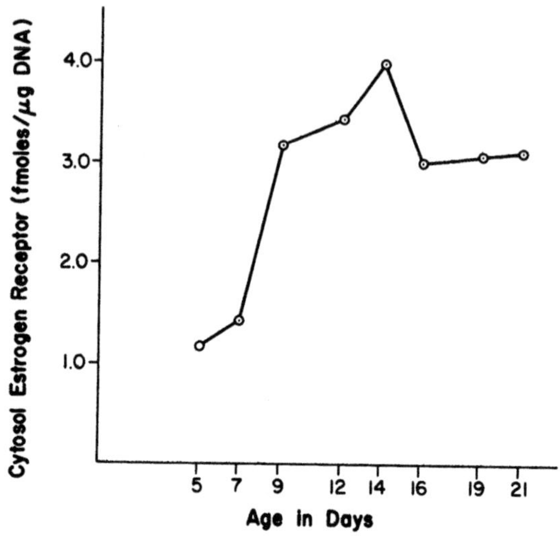

Fig. 10. Cytosol estrogen receptor content of postnatal female rat uteri. Hypotonic uterine cytosols were analyzed by sedimentation methods as described in Materials and Methods section. Diethylstilbesterol inhibitable binding of tritiated estradiol in 8S and aggregate regions of sucrose gradients were measured to obtain the amount of cytosol estrogen receptor in the uteri of the untreated rats at the various days after birth.

others (66), uterine cytosol of early postnatal rats often contains appreciable amounts of a nonreceptor 4S estradiol binding component, the data presented in Figure 10 corresponds only to 8S receptor complex from sedimentation analysis. The binding of tritiated estradiol to this 4S component is inhibited by preincubation with excess estradiol, but not diethylstilbesterol, so that it is most probable that the binding is due to α-fetoprotein. However quantitation of "receptor" under commonly employed conditions using inhibition by nonradioactive estradiol as commonly practiced in the field indeed gives erroneous results due to the presence of this protein. Our results shown in Figure 10 agree with those of Somjen, Kaye and Lindner (66) who also used sedimentation methods. Recent studies in our laboratory have indicated that when exposed to estrogen in vivo or in vitro the uterine cytosol receptor of the nine or ten day old animal is fully capable of nuclear transmigration and shows the same physical characteristics of estrogen receptor in 21 day old, fully responsive uterus. Therefore this model system provides the means by which one can compare responsive and nonresponsive uterine tissues which have similar amounts of physically comparable estrogen receptor. This provides an interesting model to study possible post receptor blocks to estrogen-dependent gene expression.

In order to be able to dissect the nature of estrogen effects on gene regulation in the endometrium using the enzyme peroxidase as marker it will be important to have available antibody to endometrial peroxidase to be able to quantitate levels of specific peroxidase m-RNA. Therefore recent efforts in our laboratory have been directed to the purification of uterine peroxidase for characterization and preparation of antibody. As shown in Table 5 a recent purification utili-

TABLE 5. PURIFICATION OF RAT UTERINE PEROXIDASE[a]

Fraction	Total Enzyme (Units)[b]	Total Protein (mg)	Specific Activity (U/mg)	Purification Factor
Homogenate	4678	4738	0.98	1
$CaCl_2$ extract	18650	1026	18.18	18.5
Con-A Sepharose	8040	11.6	691	704
Phenyl Sepharose	4233	2.02	2091	2134
Sephadex G200	2586	0.41	6223	6350

[a]From uteri of 100 mature, estradiol treated female rats.

[b]By guaiacol assay, see Materials and Methods section.

zing: $CaCl_2$ extraction of the enzyme from estrogen-treated rat uteri, affinity chromatography on Conconavalin A Sepharose, hydrophobic interaction chromatography on Phenyl Sepharose and finally gel exclusion chromatography on Sephadex G200, have resulted in an approximate 6000-fold purification of the enzyme from rat uterus. The final material has a specific activity of over 6000 units/mg protein, a specific activity higher than that recently reported (67) for thyroid peroxidase claimed to be the highest specific activity for a mammalian peroxidase. As is evident from Table 5, solubilization of the enzyme with $CaCl_2$ provides about a four-fold increase in enzyme activity even though all the peroxidase assays, including that of the homogenate, were carried out in the presence of $CaCl_2$. The Con-A affinity chromatography step clearly is a very effective means of purifying uterine peroxidase, and its elution by α-methylmannoside clearly indicates the uterine enzyme has carbohydrate side chains with a terminal mannose. Current efforts in our laboratory are directed to production of antibodies to this purified rat uterine peroxidase. With such antibodies we expect to have the tools necessary to readily detect hormone-dependent changes in marker protein content, independent of enzyme activity, and to relate the amount of marker protein to its messenger RNA under various hormone conditions. Although the biologic function of peroxidase in the endometrium is unknown, studies of the regulation of this porphyrin-containing, complex glycoprotein can provide important information to elucidate the macromolecular details of the estrogen receptor interaction and particularly its relation to gene transcription.

ACKNOWLEDGEMENTS

These investigations were supported by grants from the American Cancer Society, BC-279, and the National Cancer Institute DHEW, CA 21525. We are indebted to Richard Garay, Peter Chioros, Restituto Dizon, Jeffrey Wheat and Leighton Toney for valuable technical assistance.

REFERENCES

1. Jensen, E.V. and Jacobson, H.I. (1960). In: Biological Activities of Steroids in Relation to Cancer, G. Pincus and E.P. Vollmer, editors, Academic Press, New York, pp 161-174.
2. Jensen, E.V. and DeSombre, E.R. (1973). Science, 182, 126-134.
3. O'Malley, B.W. and Means, A.R. (1974). Science, 183, 610-620.
4. Gorski, J. and Gannon, F. (1976). Annu. Rev. Physiol., 38, 425-450.
5. Yamamoto, K.R. and Alberts, B.M. (1976). Annu. Rev. Biochem., 45, 721-746.
6. Jensen, E.V., Numata, M., Brecher, P.I. and DeSombre, E.R. (1971). In: The Biochemistry of Steroid Hormone Action, R.M.S. Smellie, editor, Academic Press, London, pp 133-159.
7. Liao, S. (1975). Int. Rev. Cytol., 41, 87-172.
8. Notides, A., Hamilton, D.E. and Auer, H.E. (1975). J. Biol. Chem., 250, 3945-3950.
9. Little, M., Szendro, P., Teran, C., Hughes, A. and Jungblut, P.W. (1975). J. Steroid Biochem., 6, 493-500.
10. Chan, L. and O'Malley, B.W. (1978). Ann. Internal Med., 89, 694-701.
11. Palmiter, R.D., Mulvihill, E.R., McKnight, G.S. and Senear, A.W. (1978). Cold Spring Harbor Symp. Quant. Biol., 42, 639-647.
12. Robins, D.M. and Schimke, R.T. (1978). J. Biol. Chem., 253, 8925-8934.
13. Schultz, G., Beato, M. and Feigelson, P. (1973). Proc. Natl. Acad. Sci. U.S.A., 70, 1218-1221.
14. Martial, J.A. Baxter, J.D., Goodman, H.M. and Seeburg, P.H. (1977). Proc. Natl. Acad. Sci. U.S.A., 74, 1816-1820.
15. Ringold, G.M., Yamamoto, K.R., Tomkins, G.M. Bishop, J.M. and Varmus, H.E. (1975). Cell, 6, 299-305.
16. Beato, M., editor (1980). Steroid Induced Uterine Proteins, Elsevier/North Holland Biomedical Press, Amsterdam, in press.
17. Shupnik, M.A., Baxter, L.A., French, L.R. and Gorski, J. (1979). Endocrinology, 104, 729-735.
18. Notides, A. and Gorski, J. (1966). Proc. Natl. Acad. Sci. U.S.A., 56, 230-235.
19. Somjen, D., Kaye, A.M. and Lindner, H.R. (1974). Molecular Cellular Endocrinol. 1, 77-88.
20. Katzenellenbogen, B.S. and Gorski, J. (1972). J. Biol. Chem., 247, 1299-1305.
21. Leavitt, W.W. and Blaha, G.C. (1972). Steroids, 19, 263-271.
22. Rao, B.R., Wiest, W.G. and Allen, W.M. (1973). Endocrinology, 92, 1229-1240.
23. Milgrom, E., Thi, L., Atger, M. and Baulieu, E.E. (1973). J. Biol. Chem., 248, 6366-6374.
24. McGuire, W.L., Raynaud, J.P. and Baulieu, E.E., editors (1977). Progesterone Receptors in Normal and Neoplastic Tissues, Raven Press, New York.
25. Leavitt, W.W., Chen, T.J. and Evans, R.W. (1978). In: Steroid Hormone Receptor Systems, W.W. Leavitt and J.H. Clark, editors, Plenum Press, New York, pp 197-222.
26. Saffran, J., Loeser, B.K. and Faber, L.E. (1978). In: Steroid Hormone Receptor Systems, W.W. Leavitt and J.H. Clark, editors, Plenum Press, New York, pp 223-239.
27. Baquer, N.Z. and McClean, P. (1972). Biochem. Biophys. Res. Commun., 48, 729-734.

28. Smith, E.R. and Barker, K.L. (1974). J. Biol. Chem., 249, 6541-6547.
29. Lucas, F.V., Neufeld, H.A., Utterback, J.G., Martin, A.P. and Stotz, E. (1955). J. Biol. Chem. 214, 775-780.
30. Klebanoff, S.J. (1965). Endocrinology, 76, 301-311.
31. Jellinck, P.H. and Lyttle, C.R. (1972). Adv. Enzyme Regul., 11, 17-33.
32. Jellinck, P.H., McNabb, T., Cleveland, S. and Lyttle, C.R. (1976). Adv. Enzyme Regul., 14, 447-465.
33. Brokelman, J., and Fawcett, D.W. (1969). Biol. Reprod. 1, 59-71.
34. Churg, A. and Anderson, W.A. (1974). J. Cell Biol., 62, 449-459.
35. Anderson, W.A., Kang, Y. and DeSombre, E.R. (1975). J. Cell Biol., 64, 668-681.
36. Lyttle, C.R. and Jellinck, P.H. (1972). Biochem. J., 127, 481-487.
37. Keeping, H.S. and Jellinck, P.H. (1978). J. Steroid Biochem., 9, 1049-1054.
38. DeSombre, E.R., Anderson, W.A. and Kang, Y. (1975). Cancer Res., 35, 172-179.
39. Burton, K. (1956). Biochem. J., 62, 315-323.
40. Lyttle, C.R. and DeSombre, E.R. (1977). Proc. Natl. Acad. Sci. U.S.A., 74, 3162-3166.
41. DeSombre, E.R. and Lyttle, C.R. (1978). Cancer Res., 38, 4086-4090.
42. Lyttle, C.R. and DeSombre, E.R. (1977). Nature, 268, 337-339.
43. DeSombre, E.R. and Lyttle, C.R. (1979). In: Steroid Hormone Receptor Systems, W.W. Leavitt and J.H. Clark, editors, Plenum Press, New York, pp 157-171.
44. DeSombre, E.R. and Lyttle, C.R. (1978). In: Hormones, Receptors, and Breast Cancer, W.L. McGuire, editor, Raven Press, N.Y., pp 181-197.
45. DeSombre, E.R. and Lyttle, C.R. (1980). In: Steroid Induced Uterine Proteins, M. Beato, editor, Elsevier/North Holland Biomedical Press, Amsterdam, in press.
46. Jellinck, P.H. and Newcombe, A. (1977). J. Steroid Biochem., 8, 1193-1195.
47. Sonnenschein, C. and Soto, A.M. (1978). J. Steroid Biochem., 9, 533-537.
48. Lerner, L.J., Holthause, F.J., Jr. and Thompson, C.R. (1958). Endocrinology, 63, 295-318.
49. Jensen, E.V. Jacobson, H.I., Smith, S., Jungblut, P.W., and DeSombre, E.R. (1972). Gynec. Invest., 3, 108-122.
50. Clark, J.H., Peck, E.J., Jr. and Anderson, J.N. (1974). Nature, 251, 446-448.
51. Katzenellenbogen, B.S. (1978). In: Hormones, Receptors and Breast Cancer, W.L. McGuire, editor, Raven Press, N.Y., pp 135-157.
52. McNabb, T. and Jellinck, P.H. (1976). Steroids, 27, 681-689.
53. Lerner, L.J. (1964). Recent Prog. Hormone Res., 20, 435-490.
54. Brenner, R.M. (1969). In: The Mammalian Oviduct, E.S.E. Hafez and R.J. Blandau, editors, University of Chicago Press, Chicago, pp 203-229.
55. Anderson, W.A., DeSombre, E.R. and Kang, Y. (1977). Biol. Reprod., 16, 409-419.
56. Raynaud, J.P. (1977). In: Progesterone Receptors in Normal and Neoplastic Tissues, W.L. McGuire, J. P. Raynaud and E.E. Baulieu, editors, Raven Press, New York, pp 9-21.

57. Revesz, C., Banik, U.K. and Herr, F. (1967). Steroids, 10, 291-305.
58. Tseng, L. and Gurpide, E. (1973). Endocrinology, 93, 245-248.
59. Tseng, L. and Gurpide, E. (1975). Endocrinology, 97, 825-833.
60. Wahawisan, R. and Gorell, T.A. (1979). Abstr. Endocrine Soc. Meeting, p 215.
61. Hseuh, A.J.W., Peck, E.J., Jr. and Clark, J.H. (1975). Nature, 254, 337-339.
62. Katzenellenbogen, B.S. and Greger, N.G. (1974). Molecular Cellular Endocrinol., 2, 31-42.
63. Walker, M.D., Gozes, I., Kaye, A.M., Reiss, N. and Littauer, U.Z. (1976). J. Steroid Biochem., 7, 1083-1085.
64. Lyttle, C.R. Garay, R.V. and DeSombre, E.R. (1979). J. Steroid Biochem., 10, 359-363.
65. Raynaud, J.P. (1973). Steroids, 21, 249-258.
66. Somjen, G.J., Kaye, A.M. and Lindner, H.R. (1974). Molecular Cellular Endocrinol., 1, 341-353.
67. Alexander, N.M. (1977). Endocrinology, 100, 1610-1620.

DISCUSSION

BARKER: Have you ever looked for the induction of the uterine peroxidase in a mature ovariectomized female rat?

DESOMBRE: Yes, we can induce it in a mature ovariectomized animal as well as in a hypophysectomized animal, although the extent of induction in the hypophysectomized animal to a single dose is less and requires several doses. I think this is again a question of building up a ribosomal network which will allow the synthesis.

BAULIEU: Did you study the kinetics of the inhibition by progesterone?

DESOMBRE: No. We are in the process of doing that, but we haven't done that yet.

14

Reevaluation of Histamine in Implantation

S.K. Dey
D.C. Johnson

The biochemical and physiological events during the preimplantation stages of pregnancy, as well as the implantation of the blastocyst, depend upon a precise hormonal balance which is regulated by ovarian progesterone and estrogen. Despite considerable research, it is still not clear how estrogen initiates decidualization or implantation in the progesterone primed uterus. A local pro-inflammatory reaction accompanied by an increase in uterine stromal capillary permeability at the site of blastocyst attachment has been considered to be one of the earliest discernible events and a prerequisite for implantation (Psychoyos, 1967; Finn & McLaren, 1967; McLaren, 1968). On the basis of this and several other findings, it was proposed that the release of histamine, a vasoactive amine, by estrogen is responsible for induction of implantation (reviewed by Nalbandov, 1971). However, Shelesnyak's theory of histamine induction of decidualization or implantation was challenged by many investigators and did not gain general acceptance (reviewed by DeFeo, 1967).

Renewed interest for histamine participation has been generated by the findings of two kinds of receptors, referred to as H_1 and H_2, for this amine (Ash & Schild, 1966; Black, Duncan, Durant, Ganellin & Parsons, 1972). Rabbit blastocyst and endometrial cell membranes have been shown to carry H_2 and H_1 receptors respectively (Dey, Villanueva & Abdou, 1979). Systemic administration of a combination of mepyramine, an H_1 receptor blocker and burimamide, an H_2 receptor blocker, was effective at interfering with implantation, whereas, replacement of burimamide with metiamide, another kind of H_2 receptor blocker, did not prevent implantation in the rat (Brandon & Wallis, 1977; Brandon & Raval, 1979). On the other hand, implantation induced by histamine in delayed implanting rats, under subthreshold doses of estrogen, can be blocked by the combined administration of mepyramine and metiamide (Brandon & Raval, 1979). Such findings are confusing and may contribute to misunderstanding of histamine actions. Quite obviously many more questions must be answered before we can unequivocally decide on a role for histamine in the implantation process. The questions addressed in this communication are: 1) what are the possible sources of histamine? 2) does inhibition of histamine formation interfere with embryo development and implantation? and 3) how could histamine be involved with implantation?

Sources of Histamine

The histamine forming capacity of tissues can be examined by determining their histidine decarboxylase (HDC) activity using the following reaction:

$$\text{L-histidine-}^{14}\text{COOH} \xrightarrow[\text{pyridoxal-5-phosphate}]{\text{histidine decarboxylase}} \text{HISTAMINE} + {}^{14}CO_2$$

The enzyme activity is expressed in terms of the amount of $^{14}CO_2$ evolved in an acid medium, trapped, and counted in a liquid scintillation spectrometer. Using this method, HDC activities of intact blastocysts recovered on day 6 of pregnancy, or homogenates (20,000g supernatant) of blastocysts recovered on days 5 or 6 have been determined. In addition, the enzyme activity of rabbit endometrial homogenates as well as day 6 blastocysts cultured for 24 hr, i.e. actually day 7 blastocysts, has been measured. The results are presented in Figure 1. The endometrial tissue did not show

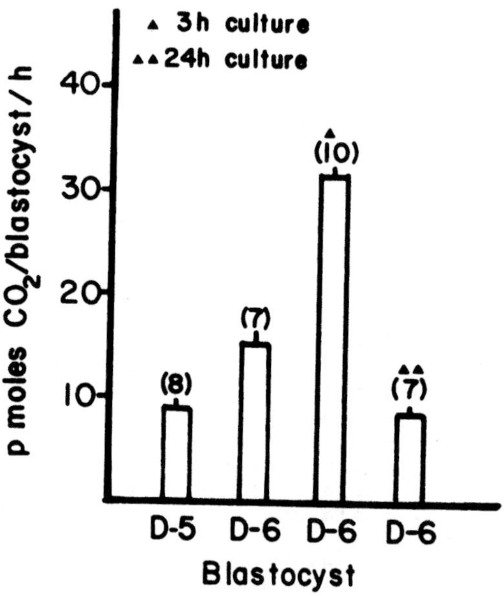

FIGURE 1. Histidine decarboxylase activity in rabbit blastocysts removed on day 5 or day 6 of pregnancy. Parentheses indicate number of determinations. Enzyme activity was measured in 20,000g homogenates except for day 6 intact embryos cultured for 3 hr.

any HDC activity in our assay. In contrast, blastocysts exhibited considerable enzyme activity; the day 6 blastocysts had about 40% more activity than did those of day 5, or those of day 6 cultured for 24 hr. The day 6 blastocysts cultured for 3 hours showed about 53% more HDC activity than did the homogenates of non-cultured blastocysts. Thus these results clearly indicate that the rabbit blastocyst could be a source of considerable histamine. While the endometrium did not appear to contain HDC activity, we must consider that histamine may be limited to mast cells and because of their limited numbers, our assay system would not detect their HDC activity. The details of the methods used as well as the results will be published in Biology of Reproduction (Dey, Johnson & Santos, 1980).

Effect of Inhibition of Histidine Decarboxylase Activity on Implantation

DL-α-methylhistidine dihydrochloride (DL-α-MH) is a specific competitive inhibitor of L-histidine in the HDC reaction (Taylor, Leinweber & Braun, 1973). Considering that rabbit blastocysts have histamine forming capacity, the effect of inhibiting this action upon the rate of implantation seemed appropriate.

On day 5 of pregnancy (day 1=24 hr post coitum), rabbits were anesthetized and their uteri exteriorized. In each animal, TC-199 media (0.2 ml) containing 6 mg of L-histidine was instilled into one uterine lumen and the same volume containing an equal amount of DL-α-MH was placed into the contralateral lumen. In separate experiments, 0.2 ml of media containing 4 mg of DL-α-MH was placed into one uterine lumen, while the contralateral lumen received an equal volume containing a combination of 4 mg of DL-α-MH and 6 mg of L-histidine. Right and left uterine horns were selected randomly for these treatments. On day 12 the does were killed, the uteri and ovaries examined for the presence and number of implantation sites, and the corpora lutea (ovulation points) counted.

As shown in Table 1, intrauterine instillation of DL-α-MH on the day preceding normal implantation caused a significant reduction in the rate of implantation when compared to normal rates in uteri treated with L-histidine; 23.8 vs 96.4%. The implantation rate was restored to almost normal level by combining L-histidine with DL-α-MH (25.5 vs 80.8%).

Effect of Inhibiting Histamine Formation Upon Embryo Development

The histamine forming capacity of the rat fetus is quite large, but this significantly drops about 24 hr prior to parturition (Kahlson, 1962). While a growth promoting function has been suggested for this amine during fetal development, no previous reports have discussed the necessity for histamine in preimplantation embryo development. Our results with rabbit blastocysts have indicated that a his-

TABLE 1. The effect of inhibiting histidine decarboxylase activity upon implantation in the rabbit.

Treatment (mg)		NO.of CL	NO.of IS	IS/CL (%)
L-H	DL-α-MH			
6	--	5.1±0.7*	4.9±0.5*	96.4±3.6*[a]
--	6	4.0±0.5	1.0±0.4	23.8±7.9[b]
--	4	5.4±0.6	1.6±0.6	25.5±9.4[c]
6	4	5.3±0.7	4.0±0.4	80.8±8.5[d]

Animals were treated on day 5 of pregnancy in groups of 7. CL=Corpora Lutea; IS=Implantation sites; L-H=L-histidine; DL-α-MH=DL-α-methylhistidine dihydrochloride. *Mean±S.E.M. a vs b: $p<.02$, c vs d: $p<.02$ (compared between observations in the same animal by Wilcoxon-matched-pairs signed-rank test). a vs c: $p<.01$, b vs c & a vs d: NS (comparing observations between different animals by Mann-Whitney test).

TABLE 2. The effect of inhibiting histidine decarboxylase activity of the mouse embryo upon its development in culture.

Treatment††	No. cultured*	% blastocysts	% morulae	% undeveloped
Media	63 (7)	77.0±4.8†[a]	9.2±5.6†	13.8±5.3†
L-H	100 (9)	83.1±4.1[a]	12.0±4.7	4.9±1.6
DL-α-MH	85 (9)	12.0±7.4[b]	34.5±9.9	53.5±11.9
L-H + DL-α-MH	58 (5)	84.5±6.8[a]	11.5±5.2	4.0±4.0

Numbers with the same superscripts are not significant from each other. L-H=L-histidine HCl; DL-α-MH=DL-α-methylhistidine dihydrochloride. *4-8 cell embryos, Numbers in parentheses indicate the number of experiments. †Mean±S.E.M., ††100 μg/ml. a's vs b: $p<.001$.

tamine forming capacity may be an essential part of normal growth and development of the embryo as well as implantation. We do not know, however, if such a need for histamine is shared with other mammalian species. An obvious difficulty in such studies is the paucity of embryonic tissue available for study. We have used embryo culture techniques to give us at least some circumstantial evidence that histamine formation is also required for the mouse.

Mouse embryos were cultured in Whitten's medium for 48 hr under an atmosphere of 90% N_2+5% O_2+5% CO_2(Whitten,1971). As shown in Table 2, about 77±4.8% of the 4-8 cell embryos developed to the blastocyst stage within 48 hr under the conditions used for culture. Addition of L-histidine hydrochloride to the culture medium did not interfere with embryonic development (83.1±4.1% developed into blastocysts), whereas, inclusion of DL-α-MH, to inhibit histamine formation, drastically retarded blastocyst development (12±7.4% blastocysts). A large number of embryos were arrested at the compacted morula stage. The culture of embryos in the presence of L-histidine hydrochloride and DL-α-MH completely prevented the inhibition of embryonic development that was seen with the inhibitor alone. These results suggest that the mouse preimplantation embryo has histamine forming capacity and furthermore, that it is necessary for normal blastocyst development.

Histamine Potentiation of Estrogen Induction of Implantation

Brandon and Raval (1979) observed that implantation could be induced in the delayed implanting rat, ovariectomized on the 3rd day of pregnancy and maintained with progesterone, by combining histamine with a subthreshold dose of estrogen. However, the mechanism by which histamine was acting is not clear. An attempt has been made to explore the possible mechanisms of histamine participation in implantation by adopting designs used in other studies.

Rats (Holtzman strain) weighing 250-280g were hypophysectomized, under ether anesthesia, on the 3rd day of pregnancy and thereafter maintained with progesterone (2mg/rat/day, subcutaneously). This method of obtaining delayed implantation has the advantage of not disturbing the ovary and oviduct. The animals were divided into 6 groups and subjected to various treatments. The experimental design is shown in Figure 2.

Groups I, II & III

The rats in these groups were divided into subgroups. While all the animals received an intravenous injection of estradiol, dissolved in saline, on day 8, some received an intraperitoneal injection of histamine dihydrochloride (300 μmole/kg body weight) immediately after administration of estradiol. One subgroup (Ic, Table 3) of animals received two more injections of histamine 4 hr apart on the same day as the estrogen treatment.

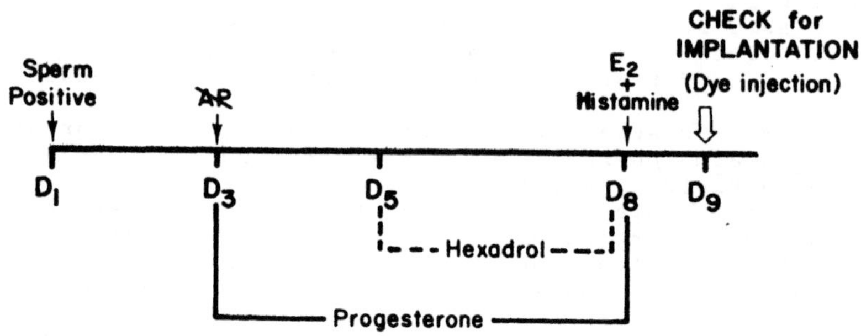

FIGURE 2. Experimental design explained in the text.

Groups IV, V & VI

All rats in these groups received an intravenous injection of estradiol (20 ng/rat in 0.2 ml of saline) on day 8 of pregnancy, but those of groups V and VI also received 0.1 mg (days 5 and 6) and 0.2 mg (days 7 and 8) of dexamethasone (Hexadrol, Organon Laboratories) subcutaneously. Group VI, in addition to estradiol and dexamethasone, received an injection of histamine (300 μmole/kg body weight, I.P.) immediately after estradiol injection and a second dose (150 μmole/kg body weight, I.P.) 4 hr later.

On day 9 (24 hr after estradiol injection), the animals of all groups were injected intravenously with 1 ml of 2% Chicago Blue B solution in saline 20 minutes before sacrifice to delineate implantation sites. The uteri were flushed with saline to recover blastocysts. Only the rats with either implantation sites or blastocysts were included in the experimental results.

As shown in Table 3, histamine was capable of increasing the number of implantation sites in the progesterone-treated delayed implanting rats under subthreshold amounts of estrogen (Groups I, II & III). Multiple injections of histamine were more effective than a single dose. The lowest dose of estrogen tested was completely ineffective at inducing implantation and a single dose of histamine did not signifi-

TABLE 3. Effect of histamine on implantation in delayed implanting rats

Group	E_2† (ng/kg)	Histamine (µmole/kg)	Hexadrol (µg/rat)	No. of IS/horn** (mean ± s.e.m.)	Blastocysts recovered (mean ± s.e.m.)
I a	20	--	--	0 (8)	7.75 ± 0.88
I b	20	300	--	2.88 ± 0.77(5)	7.00 ± 1.38
I c	20	300 x 3	--	0.3 ± 0.3(8)	4.25 ± 1.47
II a	30	--	--	0.14 ± 0.09(7)	6.14 ± 1.60
II b	30	300	--	2.22 ± 1.00(9)	5.30 ± 0.52
III a	40	--	--	2.90 ± 0.12(5)	7.80 ± 0.73
III b	40	300	--	5.44 ± 0.60(8)	5.73 ± 1.01
IV	20*	--	--	6.00 ± 0.32(5)	4.80 ± 1.56
V	20*	--	100x2 days 200x2 days	0.35 ± 0.24(10)	9.40 ± 0.82
VI	20*	300 + 150	" " "	4.14 ± 0.65(7)	7.43 ± 1.09

Numbers in parentheses indicate the number of rats. *20 ng E_2/rat ≅ 80 ng/kg. IS: Implantation sites. **Ic different from Ia & Ib at $p<.005$, IIb different from IIa at $p<.05$, IIIb different from IIIa at $p<.05$, V different from IV & VI at $p<.005$, IV different from VI at $p<.025$. †E_2: Estradiol-17β.

cantly improve the rate (Groups Ia & Ib). However, three doses did cause a profound rise in the implantation rate (Group Ic). Another important observation revealed from this study is that the glucocorticoid (Hexadrol) suppressed implantation inducible by estrogen in delayed implanting rats. This inhibition, however, was partially reversed by an injection of histamine immediately after estradiol administration followed by a second injection 4 hr later (Groups IV, V & VI).

Discussion

The highlights of our present investigation are: (i) rabbit blastocysts and endometrial cell membranes carry histamine receptors, (ii) rabbit, and possibly mouse, preimplantation embryos can generate histamine, (iii) histamine, generated by the preimplantation embryo, may participate in its development and implantation, (iv) histamine has an additive effect in inducing implantation in delayed implanting rats treated with subthreshold amounts of estrogen and (v) finally, dexamethasone suppressed implantation, inducible by estrogen in delayed implanting rats, and this inhibition was partially overcome by histamine.

Now the question arises as to how these findings can be combined with those of others to explain the relationship between histamine and implantation. The hypothetical model presented below may be worth consideration (Figure 3).

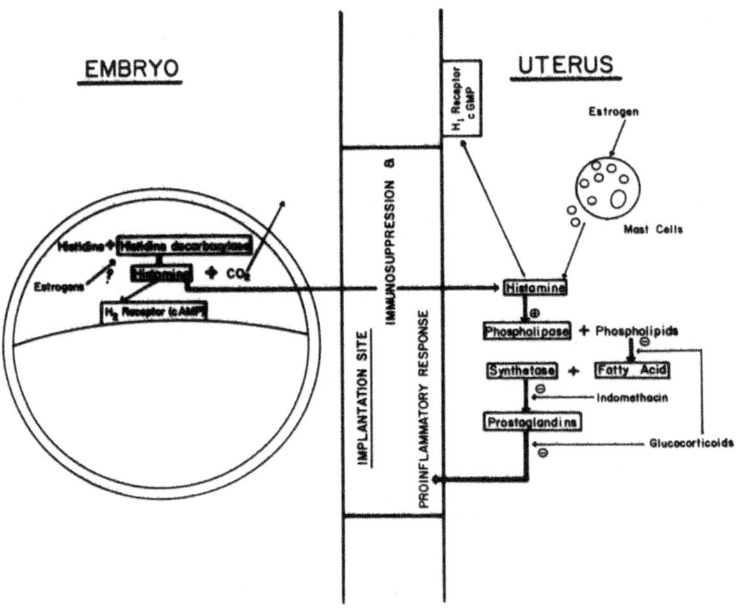

FIGURE 3. Hypothetical relationship of histamine in implantation.

The process of implantation is restricted to a specific area in the uterus and requires the presence of a blastocyst. Because this process is an interaction between the uterus and the blastocyst, and because the blastocyst could be a source of histamine, it seems likely that an action of histamine would be linked between a blastocyst and the uterus. The liberation of histamine and the subsequent edematous response are known to take place in the uterus within a few hours of estrogen stimulation (Szego, 1965). A similar temporal sequence of events would be expected in the uterus after a nidatory surge of estrogen. However, a pro-inflammatory type of reaction at the site of blastocyst attachment is observed about 20-24 hr after the estrogen surge. Furthermore, if uterine histamine mobilization is responsible for the implantation process, why is the response localized at the site of blastocyst attachment and how does the embryo implant in the pseudopregnant rat with low histamine content (Marcus & Shelesnyak, 1968)? These findings cast doubt upon the role of uterine histamine in implantation.

A local inflammatory reaction, observed at the site of blastocyst attachment, may be brought about by an alteration in cyclic-GMP as a result of histamine action through H_1 receptors in the endometrium. Secondly, histamine acting via H_2 receptors, on blastocyst cell membranes, may stimulate cyclic-AMP formation which in turn may be involved in modulating the uterine immunological responses toward the embryo (considered as an allograft) at the implantation site. Cyclic nucleotides have been shown to participate in implantation (references in Dey, Villanueva & Abdou, 1979). Alternatively, histamine participation may be mediated through generation of prostaglandins, which have been implicated in the process of implantation (Kennedy, 1977; Ottel, Koch, Kurischko & Schubert, 1979).

Liberation of the fatty acid precursor arachidonic acid from phospholipids, as a result of phospholipase A_2 activity, is considered the rate-limiting step in prostaglandin biosynthesis. In the lung and other tissues, histamine stimulates phospholipase A_2 activity, whereas, anti-inflammatory steroids inhibit this activity (Blackwell, Flower, Nijkamp & Vane, 1978; Flower & Blackwell, 1979). Could histamine derived from the embryo stimulate prostaglandin synthesis through phospholipase A_2 activity in the embryo (Shemesh, Milaguir, Ayalon & Hansel, 1979) or in the endometrium (Castracane & Jordan, 1975; Ham, Cirillo & Kuehl, 1975) at the site of implantation? If so, then we can postulate a mechanism for histamine in the process of implantation. Beneficial effects of a combination of histamine and $PGF_{2\alpha}$ in inducing implantation in delayed implanting mice have been reported recently (Saksena, Lau & Chang, 1976). Dexamethasone inhibition of implantation induced by estrogen in the delayed implanting rats and its partial reversal by histamine can be interpreted as indicative of a histamine-phospholipase A_2 process.

Histamine induced increase in the number of implantations in the delayed implanting rats under subthreshold amounts of estrogen cannot be easily explained on the basis of increased uptake and retention of estrogen as suggested by Brandon and Raval (1979). Our study shows that a single injection of histamine has a negligible effect on improving the implantation rate in delayed implanting rats treated with estrogen at a dose level of 20 ng/kg body weight (Group Ib, Table 3), whereas, three injections of histamine every 4 hr significantly increased the number of implantation sites (Group Ic, Table 3). At a dose level of 20 ng/kg, estradiol becomes undetectable in the serum within a few minutes (data not presented) and no detectable estrogen would be expected 4 hr later when the second injection of histamine was made.

Brandon and Raval (1979) reported interference with implantation by a combined treatment with burimamide, an H_2 receptor blocker, and mepyramine, an H_1 receptor antagonist. The failure to obtain such effects by the use of mepyramine and metiamide, another H_2 receptor blocker, in intact animals, as opposed to the reverse situation in the delayed implanting rats, seems conflicting and in need of explanation. Burimamide and metiamide share common properties as being H_2 receptor antagonists, although metiamide is the more potent in some actions. However, the degree and type of effect exercised by these compounds may vary between the different tissues, and even in the same tissue, under altered conditions. This is supported by the work of Fjalland (1979), who showed that cimetidine is 50 times more potent than burimamide in histamine stimulated atria preparation, but burimamide is 25 times more potent than cimetidine in the ilium preparation. The author suggested the existence of more than one kind of H_2 receptor; the same explanation may apply to the results obtained by Brandon and Raval.

Other important aspects of burimamide action should be mentioned; the compound is more potent than metiamide in terms of anti-inflammatory function (Brimblecombe, Duncan, Owen & Parsons, 1976), inhibition of histamine uptake (Cross, 1974), release of catecholamines (Brimblecombe, et al., 1976) and inhibition of 48/80-induced rat paw edema (Brimblecombe, et al., 1976). The initial phase of implantation is a pro-inflammatory type of reaction which results in increased capillary permeability at the site of blastocyst attachment. Thus, burimamide would seem to be the preferred compound, over metiamide, in interfering with this response in the intact rat; this is what was observed by Brandon and Wallis (1977) and Brandon and Raval (1979).

The inability of certain anti-histamines to interfere with implantation in intact animals may be due to several factors: (i) the process of implantation may not be dependent upon histamine, (ii) the anti-histamines may not reach the site of blastocyst attachment in sufficient concentrations during the critical time, (iii) the compounds may not reach the receptors of the blastocyst, (iv) anti-histamines may be completely ineffective because of a continuous source of histamine by the blastocyst, (v) anti-histamines may stimulate HDC activity in the blastocyst rather than block the activity (Håkanson, Larsson, Liedberg, Rehfeld & Sundler, 1977), and lastly, (vi) anti-histamines may alter the gonadotrophin or steroid hormone profiles by working via the pituitary or the ovary (Bohnet, Greiwe, Hanker, Aragona & Schneider, 1978; Knox, Lowry & Beck, 1979). All of these aspects are to be investigated carefully before we make any conclusion about the role of histamine in embryonic development and implantation. Inhibition of embryonic histamine may be a better approach to see whether the amine has any role in these processes. Our work with HDC inhibitors on implantation in the rabbit (Table 1) and mouse embryo development in culture (Table 2) seems encouraging in this respect.

Although changes in the metabolic pattern in the endometrium about the time of implantation have been considered to be attributed, at least partially, by the blastocyst-derived chemical messenger(s) (McLaren, 1969; Heald, O'Grady, O'Hare & Vass, 1975), the identity of the messenger(s) responsible for these changes has always been a speculation. Blastocysts in some rodents, for example, mice and rats, are not capable of initiating the implantation process in the uterus without a nidatory estrogen surge. On the other hand, implantation can occur in rabbits, hamsters, and guinea pigs in the absence of estrogen (Kwun & Emmens, 1974; Harper, Dowd & Elliott, 1969; Deanesly, 1960). Blastocyst dormancy during delayed implantation has been considered to be due to the appearance of a uterine inhibitor (Psychoyos, Bitton-Casimiri & Brun, 1975; Weitlauf, 1978). Perhaps a uterine inhibitor does not appear in those species where implantation can occur in the absence of estrogen and hence, delayed implantation does not exist in these species. It could be speculated that blastocyst-derived histamine may be sufficient in inducing implantation if the uterine environment is not under the influence of a uterine inhibitor. This idea is supported by the findings that dormant blastocysts become reactivated within a short time <u>in vitro</u> (Torbit & Weitlauf, 1975) and that blastocysts can implant ectopically even in the castrated animals (Kirby, 1967). The effect of histamine on increasing the number of implantation sites in the diapausing rats under subthreshold amounts of estrogen may be biphasic. Histamine may cause increased uptake and retention of estrogen in the uterus, which then removes the uterine inhibitor. Further, the histamine released from the reactivated blastocyst, superimposed on exogenous histamine, may trigger implantation either by itself or through stimulation of prostaglandin synthesis. The above analysis may also answer the question why administration of histamine alone cannot induce implantation in the delayed implanting rats in the absence of estrogen (data not presented).

Finally, we would like to emphasize that the control of early pregnancy is a complicated process and demands extensive research in the future.

ACKNOWLEDGEMENTS

We thank Miss Cheri Cox for typing the manuscript. This study was supported in part by NIH grant (HD-12304) and the Mid-America Cancer Center Program.

REFERENCES

Ash, A.S.F. and Schild, H.O. (1966). Receptor mediating some actions of histamine. Brit. J. Pharmac. Chemother. 27, 427-439.

Black, J.W., Duncan, W.A.M., Durant, C.J., Ganellin, C.R. and Parsons, E.M. (1972). Definition and antagonism of histamine H_2 receptors. Nature 236, 385-390.

Blackwell, G.J., Flower, R.J., Nijkamp, F.P. and Vane, J.R. (1978). Phospholipase A_2 activity of guinea pig isolated perfused lungs: stimulation and inhibition by anti-inflammatory steroids. Br. J. Pharmac. 62, 79-89.

Bohnet, H.G., Greiwe, M., Hanker, J.P., Aragona, C. and Schneider, H.P.G. (1978). Effects of cimetidine on prolactin, LH and sex steroid secretion in male and female volunteers. Acta Endocrinol. 88, 428-434.

Brandon, J.M. and Raval, P.J. (1979). Interaction of estrogen and histamine during ovum implantation in the rat. Eur. J. Pharmac. 57, 171-177.

Brandon, J.M. and Wallis, R.M. (1977). Effect of mepyramine, a histamine H_1 receptor antagonist, and burimamide, a histamine H_2 receptor antagonist on ovum implantation in the rat. J. Reprod. Fert. 50, 251-254.

Brimblecombe, R.W., Duncan, W.A.M., Owen, D.A.A. and Parsons, E.M. (1976). The pharmacology of burimamide and metiamide, two histamine H_2 receptor antagonists. Fed. Proc. 35, 1931-1934.

Castracane, V.D. and Jordan, V.C. (1975). The effect of estrogen and progesterone on uterine prostaglandin biosynthesis in the ovariectomized rat. Biol. Reprod. 13, 587-596.

Cross, S. (1974). Alteration of ^{14}C-histamine uptake in the presence of H_2 receptor antagonists. Proc. Aust. Physiol. Pharmacol. Soc. 5, 58.

Deanesly, R. (1960). Implantation and early pregnancy in ovariectomized guinea pigs. J. Reprod. Fert. 1, 242-248.

DeFeo, V.J. (1967). Decidualization. In: Cellular Biology of the Uterus (R.M. Wynn, Ed.), Appleton-Century-Crofts, New York, pp. 191-290.

Dey, S.K., Johnson, D.C. and Santos, J.G. (1979). Is histamine produced by the blastocyst required for implantation in the rabbit? Biol. Reprod. 21, 1169-1173.

Dey, S.K., Villanueva, C. and Abdou, N.I. (1979). Histamine receptors on rabbit blastocyst and endometrial cell membranes. Nature 278, 648-649.

Finn, C. and McLaren, A. (1967). A study of the early stages of implantation in mice. J. Reprod. Fert. 13, 259-267.

Fjalland, B. (1979). Evidence for the existence of another type of histamine H_2 receptor in guinea pig ileum. J. Pharm. Pharmacol. 31, 50-52.

Flower, R.J. and Blackwell, G.J. (1979). Anti-inflammatory steroids induce biosynthesis of a phospholipase A_2 inhibitor which prevents prostaglandin generation. Nature 278,456-459.

Håkanson, R., Larsson, L.I., Liedberg, G., Rehfeld, J.F. and Sundler, F. (1977). Suppression of rat stomach histidine decarboxylase activity by histamine: H_2 receptor-mediated feedback. J. Physiol. (Lond.). 269, 643-667.

Ham, E.A., Cirillo, V.J., Zanetti, M.E., and Kuehl, F.A. Jr. (1975). Estrogen directed synthesis of specific prostaglandins in uterus. Proc. Natl. Acad. Sci. U.S.A. 72, 1420-1424.

Harper, M.J.K., Dowd, D., and Elliott, A.S. (1969). Implantation and embryonic development in the ovariectomized-adrenalectomized hamster. Biol. Reprod. 1, 253-257.

Heald, P.J., O'Grady, J.E., O'Hara, A. and Vass, M. (1975). Nucleic acid metabolism of cells of the luminal epithelium and stroma of the rat uterus during early pregnancy. J. Reprod. Fert. 45, 129-138.

Kahlson, G. (1962). New approaches to the physiology of histamine. Perspectives in Biol. Med. 5, 179-197.

Kennedy, T.G. (1977). Evidence for a role for prostaglandins in the initiation of blastocyst implantation in the rat. Biol. Reprod. 16, 286-291.

Kirby, D.R.S. (1967). Ectopic autografts of blastocysts in mice maintained in delayed implantation. J. Reprod. Fert. 14, 515-517.

Knox, E., Lowry, S. and Beck, L. (1979). Prevention of ovulation in rabbits by anti-histamine. In: Ovarian Follicular Development and Function. (A.R. Midgley, Jr. and H.A. Sadler, Eds.), Raven Press, New York, pp. 159-163.

Kwun, J.K. and Emmens, C.W. (1974). Hormonal requirements for implantation and pregnancy in the ovariectomized rabbit. Aust. J. Biol. Sci. 27, 275-283.

Marcus, G.J. and Shelesnyak, M.C. (1968). Studies on the mechanism of nidation. XXXIII. Coital elevation of uterine histamine content. Acta Endocrinol. 57, 136-141.

McLaren, A. (1968). A study of blastocysts during delay and subsequent implantation in lactating mice. J. Endocrinol. 42, 453-463.

McLaren, A. (1969). Can a mouse blastocyst stimulate a uterine response before loosing the zona pellucida? J. Reprod. Fert. 19, 199-201.

Nalbandov, A.V. (1971). Endocrine control of implantation. In: The Biology of the Blastocyst. (R.G. Blandau, Ed.), University of Chicago Press, Chicago. pp. 383-392.

Ottel, M., Koch, M., Kurischko, A. and Schubert, K. (1979). A direct evidence for the involvement of prostaglandin $F_{2\alpha}$ in the first step of estrogen-induced blastocyst implantation in the spayed rat. Steroids 33, 1-7.

Psychoyos, A. (1967). The hormonal interplay controlling egg implantation in the rat. Adv. Reprod. Physiol. 2, 257-277.

Psychoyos, A., Bitton-Casimiri, V. and Brun, J.L. (1975). Repression and activation of the mammalian blastocyst. In: Regulation of Growth and Differentiated Function in Eukaryote Cells. (G.P. Talwar, Ed.), Raven Press, New York, pp. 509-514.

Saksena, S.K., Lau, I.F. and Chang, M.C. (1976). Relationship between oestrogen, prostaglandin $F_{2\alpha}$ and histamine in delayed implantation in the mouse. Acta Endocrinol. 81, 801-807.

Shemesh, M., Milaguir, F., Ayalon, N. and Hansel, W. (1979). Steroidogenesis and prostaglandin synthesis by cultured bovine blastocysts. J. Reprod. Fert. 56, 181-185.

Szego, C.M. (1965). Role of histamine in mediation of hormone action. Fed. Proc. 24, 1343-1352.

Taylor, R.J. Jr., Leinweber, F.J. and Braun, G.A. (1973). 4-imidazolyl-3-amino-2-butanone (MCN-A-1293), a new specific inhibitor of histidine decarboxylase. Biochem. Pharmac. 22, 2299-2310.

Torbit, C.A. and Weitlauf, H.M. (1975). Production of carbon dioxide _in vitro_ by blastocysts from intact and ovariectomized mice. J. Reprod. Fert. 42, 45-50.

Weitlauf, H.M. (1978). Factors in mouse uterine fluid that inhibit the incorporation of [^{3}H]uridine by blastocysts _in vitro_. J. Reprod. Fert. 52, 321-325.

Whitten, H.K. (1971). Nutrient requirements for the culture of preimplantation embryos _in vitro_. Adv. Bio. Sci. 6, 129-141.

DISCUSSION

BIGGERS: I have a question about the culture experiments. You start with four-cell embryos and your endpoint is the percent of expanded blastocysts. We studied the action of antiprostaglandins in a similar system and didn't find any effect of antiprostaglandins until blastocyst expansion, at the stage when the blastocyst is rapidly expanding from the force flow. From the two cell stage through the appearance of cavitation these antiprostaglandins had no effect. The antiprostaglandins were very specific for the fluid accumulation phase. What did you find? Can you be more precise about your results with antihistamines?

DEY: The inhibitor of histidine decarboxylase was added at the initiation of the cultures. We cultured the embryos 48 hours and looked for expanded blastocysts. It was observed that about 35% of the embryos stopped at the morula stage, 12% developed to the blastocyst stage, and the rest didn't develop at all. Next, I'm going to transfer those embryos to pseudopregnant animals to examine viability, i.e., whether treated embryos that develop to blastocysts in culture indeed form fetuses.

KENNEDY: I have a question about the inhibitor of histidine decarboxylase. You were overriding the effects of the inhibition not with histamine but with histidine, which presumably has to be converted to histamine to have an effect. How does this inhibitor work and why did histidine override the inhibition?

DEY: DL-α-methylhistidine is a competitive inhibitor of L-histidine for histidine decarboxylase. Exogenous L-histidine competes with DL-α-methylhistidine and overrides the inhibition of histamine formation.

PART IV
PROSTAGLANDINS AND THE UTERUS

The Endometrium

15

Endometrial Secretion of Prostaglandins During the Ovarian Cycle and Early Pregnancy

E.K. Inskeep
Laird Wilson, Jr.
W.R. Butler
D.J. Dierschke
G.R. Fritz
E. Knobil

That the prostaglandins are released in human menstrual fluid was first established in a series of studies by Pickles and coworkers during 1959 through 1967 (see Pickles, 1967 for references). Since that time, endometrial or uterine production of prostaglandins has been reported in a variety of mammals, including the ewe, cow, guinea pig, goat (see reviews by Flint and Hillier, 1975 and Horton and Poyser 1976), rat (Weems et al., 1975), mouse (Rankin et al., 1979), mare (Douglas and Ginther, 1976; Vernon et al., 1979a), monkey (Demers et al., 1974), hamster (Saksena et al., 1974) and rabbit (Scommegna et al., 1977; Harper et al., 1978) and in all segments of the oviduct in the hen (Hertelendy and Biellier, 1978). Still, relatively little has been learned about human endometrial secretion of the prostaglandins and the endocrine control of their secretion is not fully understood in any species.

Published with the approval of the Director of the West Virginia Agricultural and Forestry Experiment Station as Scientific Paper No. 1623 from the Division of Animal and Veterinary Sciences. Original work reported was supported by Hatch Project 224 (NE-72) and by NIH Contract 69-2215.

The interests of the senior author and his colleagues at West Virginia have centered around the role(s) of prostaglandins (PG) in either natural or induced luteolysis and in luteal maintenance during early pregnancy. Both of these phenomena have been shown to involve a local uteroovarian mechanism in the ewe (see Inskeep and Murdoch, 1980, for references). It is in this context that this group has examined uterine secretion of $PGF_2\alpha$ in ewes, rats, rhesus monkeys and pigs and of PGE_2 in ewes. The majority of this presentation will be limited to consideration of studies in the ewe and in primates. For the ewe, most of the work at West Virginia has been published and it will be summarized only. For the rhesus monkey, we will present data which have not been published elsewhere. The initial studies of tissues utilized the gerbil-colon bioassay (Wilson et al., 1972a) while the more recent studies of plasma and tissue have utilized specific radioimmunoassays for $PGF_2\alpha$ (Pexton et al., 1975c) and PGE_2 (Lewis et al., 1978). Bio-and radioimmuno-assays were preceded by thin layer and column chromatography, respectively, of extracted prostaglandins.

SECRETION OF $PGF_2\alpha$

The Ewe

Wilson et al. (1972a,b), Thorburn et al. (1973), Pexton et al. (1975a, b,c), Nett et al. (1976), Lewis et al. (1977, 1978) and Ottobre et al. (1978) have utilized samples of uterine tissue and venous plasma, the latter collected either acutely or by indwelling venous cannulae, to characterize the patterns of concentrations of $PGF_2\alpha$ during the estrous cycle and early pregnancy in the ewe. Three major points about uterine secretion of $PGF_2\alpha$ were revealed in these studies. First, concentrations in the endometrium and in uterine venous plasma were low early in the estrous cycle, but began to rise or exhibit peaks as soon as day 11 or 12 postestrus and increased especially on days 13 and 14. Second, a series of peaks, varying in frequency, magnitude and apparent duration were observed in plasma collected from the uterine vein or the utero-ovarian vein. Third, these peaks continued until estrus and concentrations of $PGF_2\alpha$ in endometrium and uterine venous plasma remained high at least through day 18 in pregnant ewes.

Variation in concentrations of $PGF_2\alpha$ in plasma was sometimes reduced in pregnant compared to nonpregnant ewes, endometrial levels of $PGF_2\alpha$ were somewhat higher in pregnant ewes and the number of peaks of $PGF_2\alpha$ observed by Nett et al. (1976) in uterine venous plasma was fewer in pregnant ewes. However, Inskeep and Murdoch (1980) have concluded in their review that pregnancy does not suppress endometrial secretion of $PGF_2\alpha$ into the uterine venous plasma. This conclusion is based upon concentrations of $PGF_2\alpha$ in the uterine venous plasma (Figure 1) and is reinforced by the finding that blood flow to the gravid uterine horn is increased during early pregnancy, especially on days 17 and 18 (Greiss and Anderson, 1970). It is at variance with the judgment by some authors (see review by Poyser and Maule Walker,1979), that pregnancy has its antiluteolytic effect by suppressing secretion of $PGF_2\alpha$. Workers who have made that judgment usually have accumulated data on very few ewes or depended upon assays of peripheral metabolites of $PGF_2\alpha$.

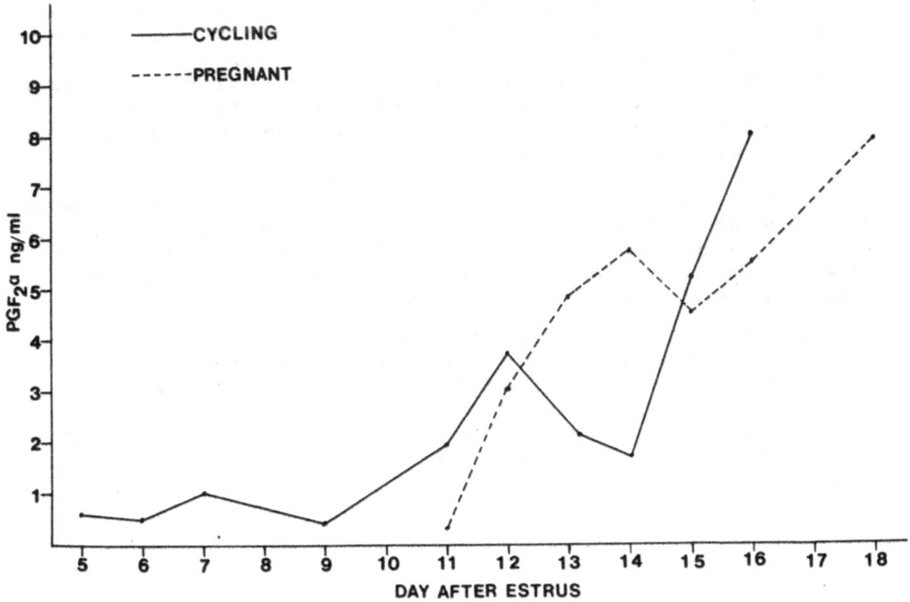

Figure 1. Composite patterns of concentrations of $PGF_{2}\alpha$ in uterine venous plasma of pregnant and non-pregnant ewes. Based upon pooled data of several studies at West Virginia.

The belief that pregnancy does not suppress endometrial production of $PGF_{2}\alpha$ is supported by the results of a thorough study by Ellinwood et al. (1979). These authors measured $PGF_{2}\alpha$ in endometrium, utero-ovarian venous serum, and flushings from the uterine lumen as well as synthesis of $PGF_{2}\alpha$ by endometrial slices in vitro. Five pregnant and five nonpregnant ewes were sampled on each of days 13, 15 and 17 postestrus. Concentrations of $PGF_{2}\alpha$ in pregnant ewes were higher than in non-pregnant ewes in the endometrium on day 15, the serum on day 13 and the uterine lumen on all three days. Secretion of $PGF_{2}\alpha$ in vitro by endometrial tissue from pregnant ewes was greater on day 15 than in samples from the nonpregnant ewes. In no case was $PGF_{2}\alpha$ significantly lower in pregnant than in nonpregnant ewes.

Other studies established that treatments known to shorten luteal life span in ewes, such as (1) intrauterine devices early in the estrous cycle (Wilson et al., 1972a; Pexton et al., 1975c), (2) intramuscular injections of high doses of estrogen on days 9 and 10 postestrus or on days 4 and 5 postestrus along with low doses of progesterone on days 1 to 5 (Ford et al., 1975), and (3) high doses of progesterone at estrus (Wilson et al., 1972a; Ottobre et al., 1978) all increased concentrations of $PGF_2\alpha$ in endometrium and uterine venous plasma at appropriate times prior to, and during, the induced luteal regression (Figure 2). In the case of treatment with progesterone at estrus (Ottobre et al., 1978), there were no effects on concentrations of LH immediately after estrus or peripheral concentrations of progesterone on days 4 to 7 postestrus. Thus, treatment with progesterone did not interfere with formation and development of corpora lutea. Rather, it caused an earlier onset of the series of peaks of secretion of $PGF_2\alpha$ which normally precede luteal regression. Luteolysis induced by any of these three treatments has been prevented by inhibiting synthesis of prostaglandins with indomethacin (see review by Inskeep and Murdoch, 1980). Thus, the effect of each of these luteolytic treatments appears to be mediated principally by increased secretion of $PGF_2\alpha$ by the uterus.

It is interesting that the intrauterine device is luteolytic in ewes and cows only if inserted when estrogen is dominant, while natural luteolysis and that induced by high doses of estrogen are initiated during periods of progesterone dominance. Warren and Hawk (1972) showed that exogenous progesterone inhibited luteolysis induced by intrauterine devices in ewes. Recently, Murdoch et al. (1978) have

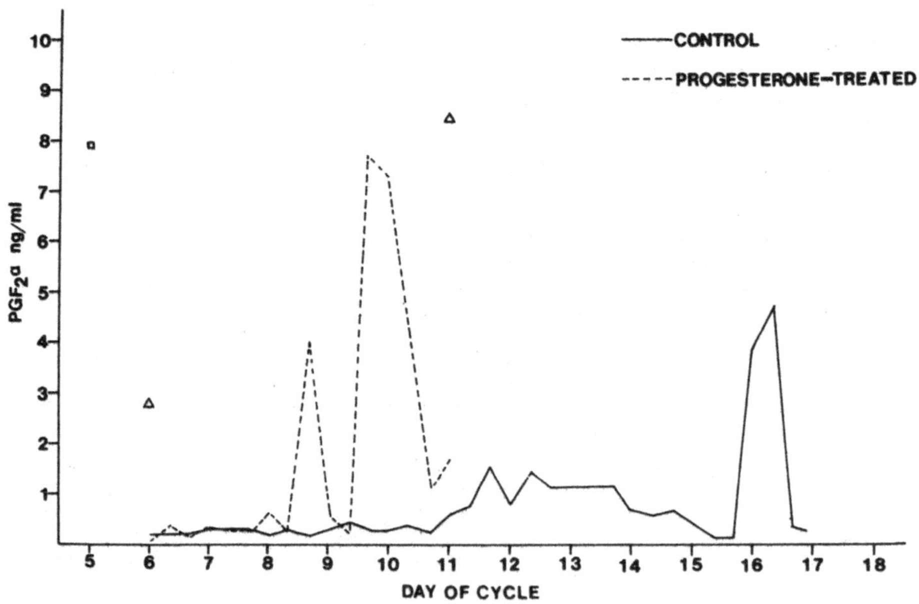

Figure 2. Effects of treatment with progesterone on days 0 and 1 (---, Ottobre, 1979), estrogen on days 4 and 5 or 9 and 10 (Δ, Ford et al., 1975) and intrauterine devices inserted on day 2 (□, Pexton et al., 1975c) on concentrations of $PGF_2\alpha$ in uterine venous plasma at selected sampling times.

shown that this inhibition can be accomplished locally by a progesterone-releasing intrauterine device. Use of this device was accompanied by a reduction in concentrations of $PGF_2\alpha$ in uterine venous plasma relative to those seen with an inert intrauterine device.

In the studies of effects of stage of cycle (Wilson et al., 1972a) and of intrauterine devices (Pexton et al., 1975c), there were no differences between uterine horns adjacent or opposite to corpora lutea in either endometrial or uterine venous plasma concentrations of $PGF_2\alpha$. Surprisingly, in a study described in more detail in a subsequent section, Alwachi et al. (1979) have reported that synthesis of $PGF_2\alpha$ by endometrium on two of the last six days of the cycle was lower if the ovary adjacent to the uterine horn being biopsied had been removed. Their method of collection of samples was unorthodox, however, and a total of only seven ewes was involved.

Primates; With Emphasis On The Rhesus Monkey

In contrast to the extensive work with ewes, only a few papers on uterine secretion of $PGF_2\alpha$ in primates have appeared in the literature. Most are case reports or involve only a few monkeys or women per stage studied. However, some valuable studies have been made. As early as 1966, van Dorp demonstrated synthesis of prostaglandins by homogenized human endometrial curettings in vitro. Downie et al. (1974) obtained endometrial curettings from 44 women undergoing sterilization and classified them into seven stages of the menstrual cycle by histological criteria. After pooling some small samples so as to have a minimum of .6g of tissue per extraction flask, they used a bioassay with rat fundal strips to estimate $PGF_2\alpha$ in two to five samples per stage at early, middle and late proliferative, early middle and late luteal and menstrual phases of the cycle. Levels of $PGF_2\alpha$ (ng/100 mg tissue) rose from 11 in early proliferative endometrium to 24 in mid-proliferative endometrium, then rose again to 67 in the mid-luteal phase and remained high through menstruation.

Wilks et al. (1973) examined concentrations of $PGF_2\alpha$ in peripheral plasma or serum of 16 healthy, nonpregnant women four times daily on days 1, 7 and 20 of 20 normal menstrual cycles (28 $\pm$ 2 days). They found no differences among days or times of day. Several studies (some recent ones include Lundstrom and Green, 1977 and Chan et al., 1979) have reported higher levels of $PGF_2\alpha$ in menstrual fluid and endometrium in women with dysmenorrhea. This difference was apparent in peripheral concentrations of metabolites of $PGF_2\alpha$ (Lundstrom and Green, 1977) but not for peripheral concentrations of $PGF_2\alpha$ itself (Wilks et al., 1973). Considerable relief of symptoms of dysmenorrhea has been achieved with prostaglandin synthetase inhibitors, even when these were administered after symptoms had begun (Larkin et al., 1979). These inhibitors reduced the concentration of bioassayable PG in menstrual fluid (Chan et al., 1979) and of metabolites of PGF in peripheral plasma (Lundstrom and Green, 1977). An intrauterine device which delivered 65 μg per day of progesterone reduced the total content of $PGF_2\alpha$ in menstrual fluid from women (Trobough et al., 1976).

In an unspecified number of rhesus monkeys, Demers et al. (1974) collected uterine luminal fluid continuously, removing samples from a special collection chamber daily. They presented data for 3 and 2/3 menstrual cycles in one monkey, which consistently had high concentrations of PGF in the uterine fluid at menses, low concentrations around day 5 and increasing levels from that point until mid-luteal phase. Concentrations were then stable or declined slightly until menses. In an ovariectomized monkey, PGF was low during six days of no treatment, rose during eight days of treatment with estrogen and declined slightly to a stable level during 10 days of estrogen plus progesterone, essentially duplicating the pattern seen in the cyclic monkey.

Experiment 1. Apparently, no thorough study of endometrial, myometrial or uterine venous plasma levels of $PGF_2\alpha$ in the monkey has been reported. Utilizing the facilities for primates at the University of Pittsburgh, concentrations of $PGF_2\alpha$ in uterine and ovarian venous plasma and contents and concentrations of $PGF_2\alpha$ in endometrium and myometrium were examined in rhesus monkeys. Six monkeys per stage were sampled on days 1-2, 6-8, 11-12, 16-17, and 22-26 in the first experiment. Each monkey was observed for three complete menstrual cycles before study. The cycle immediately prior to sampling averaged 27.2 ± 1.4 days in length.

Peripheral blood for assays of steriods and gonadotropins was collected from the femoral vein prior to laparotomy under sodium pentobarbital anesthesia. Each monkey also received 500 units of heparin before surgery. At laparotomy, the reproductive tract was exposed; insofar as possible the uterus was manipulated into position for blood collection by grasping the round ligament with forceps. The uterine branch of the ovarian vein (Ginther, 1976) on the side with a large follicle or a corpus luteum (active ovary) was clamped gently between the uterus and ovary. After venipuncture of the uterine vein, the sample was aspirated into a heparinized syringe through a 22 guage needle. This procedure was repeated for the inactive side. Ovarian venous samples were collected in the same order with the clamp placed so as to occlude flow from the uterine and tubal branches of the ovarian vein on each side. It was not always possible to obtain a collection from each of the four sites. A maximum of 12 ml was collected from each site and .1 ml of .1N HCl per ml of blood was added to each sample to retard any further synthesis of prostaglandin The samples were agitated and placed on ice. Plasma was harvested after centrifugation and stored frozen (-20C) until assay for $PGF_2\alpha$.

The animal was hysterectomized; the uterus was placed on ice and the endometrium dissected from the remainder (myometrium). These tissues were weighed, frozen on dry ice and stored at -20C until assay for $PGF_2\alpha$.

Some of the results of this experiment are presented in Figure 3. As expected, endometrial weights increased during the secretory phase of the cycle, while myometrial weights did not vary. Endometrial content of $PGF_2\alpha$ varied with stage of the cycle ($P < .01$) but endometrial concentration of $PGF_2\alpha$ (the use of which assumes a regression of content on weight of 1) did not vary significantly with stage. When endometrial content was adjusted by analysis of covariance for its actual pooled within stage regression on weight ($b = .632$; $P < .01$), there was no effect of stage on endometrial $PGF_2\alpha$ independent of its effect on endometrial weight. Myometrial $PGF_2\alpha$ varied only with myometrial weight ($b = .113$; $P < .05$).

Uterine venous concentrations of $PGF_2\alpha$ did not vary with stage of the cycle but were higher ($P < .05$) in the uterine vein adjacent to the inactive ovary (23.6 ng/ml) compared to the vein adjacent to the active

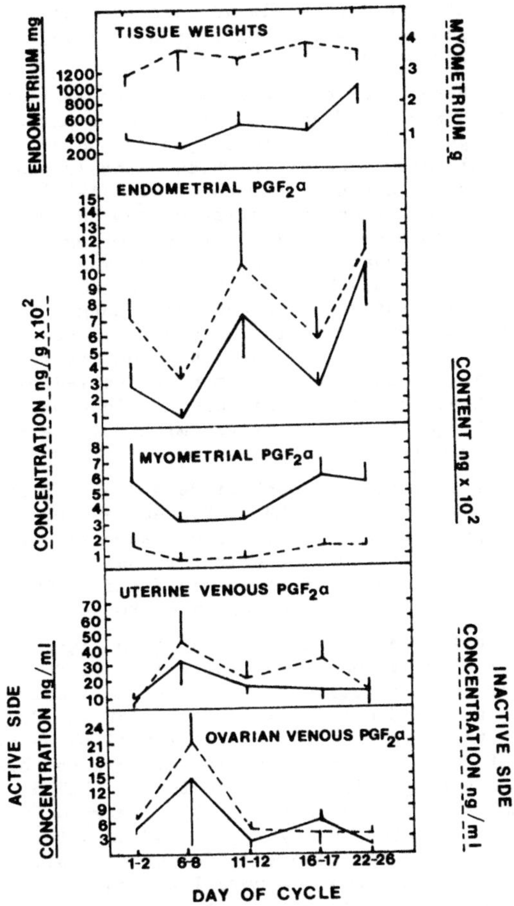

Figure 3. Characteristics of endometrium and myometrium and prostaglandin $F_2\alpha$ in these tissues and in uterine and ovarian venous plasma at five stages of the menstrual cycle in rhesus monkeys.

ovary (17.5 ng/ml). This difference probably reflects some increased release of $PGF_2\alpha$ due to handling the uterus (Roberts et al., 1975) since the inactive side was always collected after the active side. Uterine venous $PGF_2\alpha$ was not related to endometrial weight, endometrial $PGF_2\alpha$ or to estradiol, estrone, total estrogens or progesterone in peripheral plasma collected just prior to surgery. Although no stage differences were detected, when one inspects the data (Figure 3), the lowest concentrations of endometrial $PGF_2\alpha$ and the highest concentrations of $PGF_2\alpha$ in uterine venous plasma were seen at the same time (early follicular phase) as when Demers et al. (1974) found the lowest levels of PGF in uterine fluid.

Experiment 2. Because of our interest in luteal life span and function and the lack of evidence that the uterus plays any role in regulating the corpus luteum in primates, a second experiment was conducted in luteal phase monkeys in which emphasis was placed on the ovaries rather than the uterus. Karsch et al. (1973) had reported that increasing concentrations of estradiol caused luteal regression without changing serum concentrations of gonadotropins. Subsequently, Butler et al. (1975) demonstrated that estrone was higher in ovarian venous plasma from the ovary bearing the corpus luteum than from the opposite ovary in late luteal phase monkeys. Both estrone and estradiol were four times higher in corpora lutea collected on days 8-13 after the peak of LH compared to days 4-6. The report by Shaikh and Klaiber (1974) that a sequential treatment of estradiol and $PGF_2\alpha$ was luteolytic in monkeys whereas either hormone alone was not, led us to question whether $PGF_2\alpha$ of ovarian origin might play a role, with estradiol, in luteolysis.

Five monkeys were sampled on each of days 2-4, 7-9 and 11-12 of the luteal phase (days after peak of LH). Procedures were the same as in experiment 1 except that the ovarian venous samples were collected first and the monkeys were ovariectomized rather than hysterectomized. The corpus luteum was weighed, divided and frozen. One portion was used for steroid assays and one for assay of $PGF_2\alpha$.

There were no differences among stages of the luteal phase in either ovarian or uterine venous concentrations of $PGF_2\alpha$ (Table 1). There were significant increases in both estrone (early, 123; mid, 325; and late, 471 μg/gm;) and estradiol-17β (82, 188 and 231 μg/gm, respectively) in the corpora lutea as the luteal phase progressed. Concentrations of $PGF_2\alpha$ were measured in only six corpora lutea because nine were lost in a single laboratory accident. $PGF_2\alpha$ was nondetectable in two samples collected on day 2, but averaged 667 $\pm$ 300 ng/gm for corpora lutea collected on days 7, 11 and 12 after the surge of LH. This contrasts with the report by Swanston et al. (1977) that $PGF_2\alpha$ was higher in young human corpora lutea and was not correlated with steroid levels in the corpus luteum. Auletta et al. (1978) have shown recently that exogenous infusion of estradiol (1 ng/min) increased ovarian venous PGF in rhesus monkeys and that simultaneous infusion of indomethacin prevented this response. Thus, it is possible that the physiological mechanism for luteolysis in the primate includes an increase in estradiol followed by an increase in $PGF_2\alpha$, both occuring within the corpus luteum, in contrast to the increase in $PGF_2\alpha$ occuring in the uterus in the ewe. At present the only clearly defined function for uterine $PGF_2\alpha$ in primates is a negative one, the causing or enhancement of dysmenorrhea.

Other Species

The pattern of secretion of $PGF_2\alpha$ during the estrous cycle seems to be similar in the cow to that reported for sheep.

Table 1. Concentrations of $PGF_{2}\alpha$ in Ovarian, Uterine and Peripheral Plasma of Luteal Phase Monkeys.

Variable	Stage of luteal phase: Early (day 4)	Mid. (day 8)	Late (days 13-14)
Number of monkeys	5	5	5
Venous concentration of $PGF_{2}\alpha$ (ng/ml)			
Ovarian vein - side of corpus luteum	10.9 $\pm$ 7.2	4.1 $\pm$ 1.3	9.0 $\pm$ 4.8
Ovarian vein - side opposite corpus luteum	8.3 $\pm$ 4.6	4.9 $\pm$ 1.5	11.0 $\pm$ 3.5
Uterine vein - side adjacent to corpus luteum	10.0 $\pm$ 3.7	2.6 $\pm$ .8	11.5 $\pm$ 6.1
Uterine vein - side opposite to corpus luteum	10.1 $\pm$ 8.6	3.1 $\pm$ .9	5.7 $\pm$ 2.4[a]
Peripheral	3.4 $\pm$ 1.0	.6 $\pm$ .1	.7 $\pm$ .2[a]

[a]Mean of four animals. $PGF_{2}\alpha$ was non-detectable in the fifth monkey.

Increases of $PGF_{2}\alpha$ in endometrium began by days 15 to 17 and persisted through the onset of estrus (Shemesh and Hansel, 1975). In uterine venous plasma, increases of $PGF_{2}\alpha$ had begun by day 14, were maximal on days 15 to 17, and were declining but still high on day 20 and at estrus. In uterine fluids of the cow, the highest amounts of $PGF_{2}\alpha$ were observed just before estrus (Lamothe et al., 1977; Thatcher et al., 1979).

Oxytocin, a luteolytic agent in the cow known to require a uterine horn adjacent to the corpus luteum to be effective, has been tested for its effect on uterine venous concentrations of $PGF_{2}\alpha$ on days 4, 5 and 6 of the estrous cycle (Milvae et al., 1978). Increases were detected at 30, 60, 120 and 240 minutes after oxytocin. Newcomb et al. (1977) examined increases in PGF over pretreatment levels in posterior vena caval plasma of heifers treated with oxytocin on days 2 to 7 postestrus and found the greatest response on day 3. In sheep, oxytocin increased release of PGF in anestrous ewes treated with estradiol (Sharma and Fitzpatrick, 1974) and from endometrium in vitro (Roberts et al., 1976).

Concentrations of $PGF_{2}\alpha$ in uterine venous plasma on day 18 postestrus in pregnant Holstein heifers were approximately one-half of those in non-pregnant heifers but concentrations in the endometrium did not differ (Hansel et al., 1978). The decrease in concentration of PGF in uterine venous plasma must be considered in light of the report by Ford et al. (1979) that blood flow to the uterine horn containing the conceptus increased two- to three-fold from day 14 to day 18 of pregnancy. So the actual secretion rate may not differ. However, the decreased concentration of $PGF_{2}\alpha$ in plasma corresponds to the finding of higher amounts of PGF in flushings of the uterine lumen in pregnant than in nonpregnant heifers on days 16 and 19 postestrus (Thatcher et al., 1979). In that case, the cow may be like the pig, in which pregnancy has been reported (Bazer and Thatcher, 1977) to alter the pattern of secretion of $PGF_{2}\alpha$, so that more of it moves toward the uterine lumen and less into the uterine venous plasma. Estradiol, a known luteotropic agent in the pig, produced an effect similar to pregnancy in that species (Frank et al., 1978). Whether a change in the direction of secretion of $PGF_{2}\alpha$ by the uterus is crucial to luteal maintenance by the embryo in any species, or alternatively, plays a role in attachment of the embryo as proposed for the rat (Kennedy, 1977; Kennedy and Zamecnik, 1978) and rabbit (Hoffman, 1978) is not clear. The same is true for production and metabolism of prostaglandins by the conceptus (Maule Walker et al., 1977; Shemesh et al., 1978).

Other than the sheep, the species which has been studied most extensively is the guinea pig. The group at Edinburgh (see reviews by Horton and Poyser, 1976 and Poyser and Maule Walker, 1979) has shown in a series of studies that the guinea pig endometrium secretes $PGF_{2}\alpha$ and that it is a uterine luteolytic hormone in that species. Intrauterine devices and luteolytic doses of estrogen caused premature release of $PGF_{2}\alpha$. Pregnancy, even in one uterine horn, reduced concentrations of $PGF_{2}\alpha$ in uterovarian venous plasma from both horns on day 15 and reduced the amounts of $PGF_{2}\alpha$ formed during incubation of homogenized day-15 uteri.

The effect of pregnancy on PGF in uterine venous plasma in the pony mare was examined by Douglas and Ginther (1976). They collected samples from 3 to 4 mares per stage at laparotomy under anesthesia. They found that concentrations of PGF (ng/ml) increased from low levels during estrus and on days 2 and 6 of diestrus (1.4 to 2.9) to 8.2 ± .8 on day 10 and further to 14.9 ± .5 on day 14 of diestrus, then declined to 6.4 ± 1.3 on day 18. Pregnant mares had significantly lower concentrations of PGF than diestrus mares on days 10 and 14 (4.3 and 9.3, respectively) but did not differ on day 18. Vernon et al. (1979a) obtained different results when they incubated endometrial strips from mares. Production of $PGF_{2}\alpha$ by the tissue from pregnant mares was maximal on days 18 and 20 post-ovulation and was as high or higher from days 8 through 20 as in diestrous mares. Further study revealed that the endometrium of the gravid horn produced more $PGF_{2}\alpha$ than the nongravid horn on day 18, whereas, there was no difference between horns in nonpregnant mares.

While more work will be necessary to resolve some the conflicting findings, it appears at this point that there are indeed species differences in the effect of pregnancy on endometrial secretion of $PGF_{2}\alpha$.

SECRETION OF PGE_2

The secretion of PGE_2 has received relatively little study, but is of particular interest in sheep because the antiluteolytic effect of pregnancy, like luteolysis, is mediated locally and because PGE_2 has been shown to have antiluteolytic activity (for a detailed review, see Inskeep and Murdoch, 1980). Wilson et al. (1972a) found PGE_2 in the endometrium of nonpregnant sheep and Larkin et al. (1979) have reported its synthesis by human endometrium in vitro. Castracane and Shaikh (1976) found that the presence of decidual tissue increased concentrations of PGE on day 10 of pseudopregnancy in rats.

Recently, four groups have investigated some aspects of uterine secretion of PGE_2 in sheep. First, Clark et al. (1977) found higher concentrations of PGE in uterine venous plasma in ewes pregnant 80 days or more compared to nonpregnant ewes. The second study was by Lewis et al. (1978), who determined concentrations of PGE_2 in uterine venous plasma collected from indwelling cannulae in pregnant and nonpregnant ewes on days 15 and 16 postestrus and in endometrium, uterine venous tissue and ovarian arterial tissue on day 16. They found no differences in concentrations of PGE_2 in endometrium or in uterine venous tissue. Concentrations of PGE_2 in uterine venous plasma at 15 sampling times averaged .7 ± .1 μg/ml in pregnant ewes and 1.2 ± 2 μg/ml in nonpregnant ewes and did not differ with pregnancy status. They did find that PGE_2 tended to be higher in the ovarian arterial tissue in pregnant ewes (210 ± 84 pg/mg) than in nonpregnant ewes (33 ± 8 pg/mg; $p < .1$).

In the third study, Ellinwood et al. (1979) collected single samples of utero-ovarian venous blood, under anesthesia, on days 13, 15 and 17 of the estrous cycle and pregnancy (5 ewes per subgroup) and assayed PGE_2 in serum. They also collected uterine luminal flushings and endometrial tissue from each ewe and examined the secretion of PGE_2 by a portion of the endometrial tissue in vitro. Concentrations of PGE_2 were higher in utero-ovarian serum and endometrial tissue and its secretion was higher by incubated endometrium of the pregnant ewes on days 15 and 17 than for the nonpregnant ewes. In uterine flushings, PGE_2 was higher in the pregnant ewes on all three days studied. Values did not vary with day in nonpregnant ewes, but in each case PGE_2 increased from day 13 to day 15 in pregnant ewes.

The fourth report, by Alwachi et al. (1979) included two experiments. In the first, PGE_2 was measured in caruncular and noncaruncular endometrium and myometrium collected from seven ewes on day 3, 5 (two ewes), 12, 15 (two ewes) or 16 of the estrous cycle. Increased PGE_2 was reported in both types of endometrium later in the cycle. The second experiment utilized seven nonpregnant ewes, in which "the left uterine horn was fistulated to the exterior", one ovary was removed from six of the ewes and endometrial biopsies were taken daily during the six days prior to estrus. There was no effect of day or of whether the uterine horn sampled was adjacent to an ovary on endometrial content or synthesis in vitro of PGE_2.

OTHER PROSTAGLANDINS

Prostaglandins other than E_2 and $F_2\alpha$ have received almost no attention, but certainly other products are formed in the uterus and may be important in reproductive functions. For example, decidual microsomes produced predominantly PGE_2, while myometrial microsomes produced predominantly 6-keto-$PGF_1\alpha$, the stable metabolite of prostacyclin, in the pregnant rat (Downing and Williams, 1977). In homogenized uteri of sheep and pseudopregnant rats, Jones et al. (1977) found that 6-keto-$PGF_1\alpha$ was produced in greater quantities than $PGF_2\alpha$; the reverse was true for diestrous guinea pig uteri. These results mean very little until the separate tissues are compared in different physiological states within the same species. However, further assessments of changes in 6-keto-$PGF_1\alpha$ as an index of production of prostacyclin, are indicated.

Normally, 13, 14-dihydro-15-keto-$PGF_2\alpha$ is considered to be a metabolite of $PGF_2\alpha$ formed mainly in the liver. But Lundstrom and Green (1977) reported detectable concentrations of it in some human endometrial samples. Lewis et al. (1977) found that 13, 14-dihydro-15-keto-$PGF_2\alpha$ was higher in uterine venous than in jugular plasma. Mean concentrations in uterine venous plasma for this metabolite were 2.15 ng/ml in nonpregnant ewes on days 11 through 16 and 2.18 ng/ml in pregnant ewes on days 11 through 16 and 18 and did not differ significantly with day. These values were correlated with those for $PGF_2\alpha$ ($r= .53$) and 15-keto-$PGF_2\alpha$ ($r= .74$) in uterine venous plasma. But, 13, 14-dihydro-15-keto-$PGF_2\alpha$ was below detectable concentrations (.6 ng/ml) in peripheral plasma, so it may be a secretory product of the uterus.

SOURCE OF UTERINE PROSTAGLANDINS AND REGULATION OF THEIR SECRETION

The endometrium is probably the major tissue source of uterine prostaglandins. Concentrations in myometrium in ewes in several of the studies discussed earlier sometimes varied with stage of the estrous cycle, but not with luteolytic treatments. Roberts et al. (1976) found that oxytocin increased release of $PGF_2\alpha$ from endometrium but not from myometrium in vitro. Intrauterine devices, which are effective only when estrogen is dominant, increased concentrations of $PGF_2\alpha$ in both caruncular and intercaruncular endometrium in ewes (Pexton et al., 1975c). Progesterone alone for 10 days increased $PGF_2\alpha$ in caruncles but not in the remainder of the uterus (Robinson et al., 1976) while 15 μg estradiol daily for 10 days was ineffective on either tissue, but estradiol on days 8-10 in addition to progesterone priming increased $PGF_2\alpha$ in both tissues. In recent studies by Huslig et al. (1979) activity of the prostaglandin-forming cyclo-oxygenase, although present in nearly all uterine cells, was increased at day 14 of the estrous cycle specifically in the caruncular endometrium. They speculated that stromal cells of the caruncles were responsible for the luteolytic surges of $PGF_2\alpha$ near the end of the estrous cycle.

The roles of progesterone and estrogen in regulating the physiologic secretion of $PGF_2\alpha$ remain unclear. That estrogen stimulated the secretion of PGF from a progesterone-primed uterus was proposed by Caldwell et al. (1972). In ovariectomized ewes, exogenous progesterone for 7 to 14 days increased the release of PGF from the uterus (Scaramuzzi et al., 1977). Estrogen given after pretreatment with progesterone was more effective than treatment for several days with either hormone alone. However, 25 μg estradiol-17β, in two doses 12 hours apart, increased $PGF_2\alpha$ in uterine venous plasma 12 hours after the second dose to as great a degree as the same treatment after 5 days of progesterone (Ford et al., 1975), while continued treatment with estradiol twice daily for 5 days (or 9 days in the study by Louis et al., 1977) did not sustain this level of secretion. Similarly, $PGF_2\alpha$ was increased in the superior vena cava 24 hours after either 50 μg or 1 mg of estradiol-17β in anestrous ewes (Sharma and Fitzpatrick, 1974). In studies of the control of uterine contractions in sheep, Rexroad (1978) treated ovariectomized ewes with a single injection of 45 μg estradiol-17β, 250 μg cycloheximide (in 4 doses at 2-hour intervals), or both, and measured $PGF_2\alpha$ and PGE_2 in anterior and posterior segments of myometrium and endometrium 24 hours later. He found no main effects of estradiol, but an increase in endometrial concentrations of $PGF_2\alpha$ after estradiol clearly contributed to an observed estradiol x cycloheximide x tissue interaction.

Destruction of follicles by electrocautery led to heavier corpora lutea on day 17 in ewes (Ginther, 1971) and destruction of follicles by x-irradiation delayed the regression of corpora lutea in ewes (Karsch et al., 1970) and dairy cows (Cowley et al., 1979). On the other hand, antisera to estradiol did not prevent or delay luteal regression in ewes (Fairclough et al., 1976) or beef heifers (Martin et al., 1978). Having observed no association between concentrations of estrogen and of $PGF_2\alpha$ at 8-hour intervals during the period when peaks of $PGF_2\alpha$ are first observed, but a close temporal association of increases in these two hormones during the final stages of luteolysis, Ottobre (1979) has proposed that estrogen may be involved in stimulating only the final surges of $PGF_2\alpha$. If this is correct, the antisera to estradiol must not have prevented estradiol from affecting the endometrium after progesterone alone had preset the initiation of greater release of $PGF_2\alpha$. More frequent sampling in intact ewes and further studies in ovariectomized ewes will be necessary to clarify these points.

Effects of estradiol-17β with and without pretreatment with progesterone on PGE and PGF in uterine tissue and venous plasma of rats were studied by Castracane and Jordan (1975). Estradiol alone (10 μg) increased uterine weight but had no effect on uterine contents of PGE and PGF over the next 24 hours. Estradiol did increase concentrations of both PGE and PGF in uterine venous plasma over at least the next four hours. Following progesterone pretreatment, estradiol resulted in increased concentrations of PGE and PGF in uterine venous plasma which persisted for as long as 12 hours.

Vernon et al. (1979b) treated ovariectomized pony mares with estradiol valerate or progesterone daily for 3 weeks or with estradiol valerate for 7 days followed by progesterone for 14 days, then incubated endometrial strips with progesterone or varying doses of estradiol. In vivo treatments did not alter endometrial content of PGF, but each stimulated production of PGF in vitro. Estradiol in vitro increased production of PGF in a dose-dependent manner, with tissue from progesterone-treated mares giving the greatest response. Progesterone in vitro had no effect, a result in contrast to that of Cane and Villee (1975) who found that progesterone inhibited synthesis of PGF by human endometrial cultures, whereas estrogen tended to increase such synthesis.

CONCLUSIONS

Considerable progress has been made in defining the patterns of secretion of $PGF_{2}\alpha$ by mammalian endometrium. Factors regulating this secretion are not fully understood and more work in this area will be needed in order to account for the variety of species differences in patterns of secretion described to date.

REFERENCES

Alwachi, S.N., Bland, K.P. and Poyser, N.L. (1979). Uterine prostaglandin F_2 alpha and E_2 production and content during the second half of the oestrus cycle of the sheep-possible local control of the uterus by the ovary. Prostaglandins Med. 3:23-32.

Auletta, F.J., Agins, H. and Scommegna, A. (1978). Prostaglandin F mediation of the inhibitory effect of estrogen on the corpus luteum of the rhesus monkey. Endocrinology 103,1183-1189.

Bazer, F.W. and Thatcher, W.W. (1977). Theory of maternal recognition of pregnancy in swine based on estrogen controlled endocrine versus exocrine secretion of prostaglandin F by the uterine endometrium. Prostaglandins 14,397-401.

Butler, W.R., Hotchkiss, J. and Knobil, E. (1975). Functional luteolysis in the rhesus monkey: ovarian estrogen and progesterone during the luteal phase of the menstrual cycle. Endocrinology 96, 1509-1512.

Caldwell, B.V., Tillson, S.A., Brock, W.A. and Speroff, L. (1972). The effects of exogenous progesterone and estradiol on prostaglandin F levels in ovariectomized ewes. Prostaglandins 1, 217-228.

Cane, E.M. and Villee, C.A. (1975). The synthesis of prostaglandin F by human endometrium in organ culture. Prostaglandins 9, 281-288.

Castracane, V.D., and Jordan, V.C. (1975). The effect of estrogen and progesterone on uterine prostaglandin biosynthesis in the ovariectomized rat. Biol. Reprod. 13, 587-596.

Castracane, V.D. and Shaikh, A.A. (1976). Effect of decidual tissue on the uterine production of prostaglandins in pseudopregnant rats. J.Reprod.Fert. 46,101-104.

Chan, W.Y., Dawood, M.Y., and Fuchs, F. (1979). Relief of dysmenorrhea with the prostaglandin synthetase inhibitor ibuprofen: Effect on prostaglandin levels in menstrual fluid. Am.J.Obstet. Gynecol. 135, 102-108.

Clark, K.E., Meldrum, D., Brinkman, C.R., III and Assali, N. (1977). Prostaglandin E levels in nonpregnant and pregnant sheep. Gyn. Invest. 8,89

Cowley, J.L., Ireland, J.J., Wortman, J.A.and Fogwell, R.L. (1979). Luteal function in cows following destruction of ovarian follicles at midcycle. J.Animal Sci. 49,Supp.1, 289.

Demers, L.M., Yoshinaga, K. and Greep, R.O. (1974). Prostaglandin F in monkey uterine fluid during the menstrual cycle and following steroid treatment. Prostaglandins 5, 513-519.

Douglas, R.H. and Ginther, O.J. (1976). Concentration of prostaglandins F in uterine venous plasma of anesthetized mares during the estrous cycle and early pregnancy. Prostaglandins 11, 251-260.

Downie, J., Poyser, N.L. and Wunderlich, M. (1974). Levels of prostaglandins in human endometrium during the normal menstrual cycle. J.Physiol. 236, 465-472.

Downing, I. and Williams, K.I. (1977). Differential prostaglandin production by microsomal fractions of rat pregnant uterus. Br. J. Pharmac. 51, 158P

Ellinwood, W.E., Nett, T.M. and Niswender, G.D. (1979). Maintenance of the corpus luteum of early pregnancy in the ewe. II. Prostaglandin secretion by the endometrium _in vivo_ and _in vitro_. Biol. Reprod. 21, 845-856.

Fairclough, R.J., Smith, J.F., Peterson, A.J. and McGowan, L. (1976). Effect of oestradiol-17β, progesterone and prostaglandin $F_2\alpha$ antiplasma on luteal function in the ewe. J.Reprod.Fert. 46, 523-524.

Flint, A.P.F. and Hillier, K. (1975). Prostaglandins and reproductive processes in female sheep and goat. In Prostaglandins and Reproduction, p. 271 (S.M.M. Karim, Editor) Lancaster, MTP Press.

Ford, S.P., Chenault, J.R. and Echternkamp, S.E. (1979). Uterine blood flow of cows during the oestrus cycle and early pregnancy: effect of the conceptus on the uterine blood supply. J.Reprod.Fert. 56, 53-62.

Ford, S.P., Weems, C.W., Pitts, R.E., Butcher, R.L. and Inskeep, E.K. (1975). Effects of estradiol-17β and progesterone on prostaglandins F in sheep uteri and uterine venous plasma. J. Anim. Sci. 41, 1407-1413.

Frank, M., Bazer, F.W., Thatcher, W.W. and Wilcox, C.J. (1978). A study of prostaglandin $F_2\alpha$ as the luteolysin in swine: IV. An explanation for the luteotrophic effect of estradiol. Prostaglandins 15, 151-160.

Ginther, O.J. (1971). Response of corpora lutea to cauterization of follicles in sheep. Amer.J.Vet. Res. 32,59-62.

Ginther, O.J. (1976). Comparative anatomy of uterovarian vasculature. Veterinary Scope 20 (1), 2-17.

Greiss, F.C., Jr. and Anderson, S.G. (1970). Uterine blood flow during early ovine pregnancy. Amer.J. Obstet. and Gynecol. 106, 30-38.

Hansel, W., Lukaszewska, J. and Beal, W. (1978). Maintenance of the bovine corpus luteum of early pregnancy. Proc. 11th Ann. Meeting, Soc. Study Reprod., Carbondale, Illinois, page 27A.

Harper, M.J.K., Valenzuela, G., and Hodgson, B.J.(1978). Accelerated ovum transport in rabbits induced by endotoxin. I. Changes in prostaglandin levels and reversal of endotoxin effect. Prostaglandins 15, 43-63.

Hertelendy, F. and Biellier, H.V.(1978). Prostaglandin levels in avian blood and reproductive organs. Biol. Reprod. 18, 204-211.

Hoffman, L.H. (1978). Antifertility effects of indomethacin during early pregnancy in the rabbit. Biol. Reprod. 18,148-153.

Horton, E.W. and Poyser, N.L. (1976). Uterine luteolytic hormone: A physiological role for prostaglandin $F_{2}\alpha$. Physiol. Reviews 56, 595-651.

Huslig, R.L., Fogwell, R.L. and Smith, W.L. (1979). The prostaglandin-forming cyclooxygenase of ovine uterus: relationship to luteal function. Biol. Reprod. (Submitted).

Inskeep, E.K. and Murdoch, W.J. (1980). Relation of ovarian functions to uterine and ovarian secretion of prostaglandins during the estrous cycle and early pregnancy in the ewe and the cow. In: Reproductive Physiology III (R.O.Greep, Editor) Baltimore, University Park Press, In press.

Jones, R.L., Poyser, N.L. and Wilson, N.H. (1977). Production of 6-oxo-prostaglandin $F_{1}\alpha$ by rat, guinea-pig and sheep uteri, in vitro. Br.J. Pharmac. 59, 436P-437P.

Karsch, F.J., Noveroske, J.W., Roche, J.F., Norton, H.W. and Nalbandov, A.V. (1970). Maintenance of ovine corpora lutea in the absence of ovarian follicles. Endocrinology 87, 1228-1236.

Karsch, F.J., Krey, L.C., Weick, R.F., Dierschke, D.J. and Knobil,E. (1973). Functional luteolysis in the rhesus monkey: the role of estrogen. Endocrinology 92, 1148-1152.

Kennedy, T.G. (1977). Evidence for a role of prostaglandins in the initiation of blastocyst implantation in the rat. Biol. Reprod. 16, 286-291.

Kennedy, T.G. and Zamecnik, J. (1978). The concentration of 6-keto-prostaglandin $F_{1}\alpha$ is markedly elevated at the site of blastocyst implantation in the rat. Prostaglandins 16, 599-605.

Lamothe, P., Bosquet, D. and Guay, P. (1977). Cyclic variation of F prostaglandins in the uterine fluids of the cow. J. Reprod. Fert. 50, 381-382.

Larkin, R.M., Van Orden, D.E., Poulson, A.M. and Scott, J.R. (1979). Dysmenorrhea: treatment with an antiprostaglandin. Obstetrics and Gynecology 54, 456-460.

Lewis, G.S., Jenkins, P.E., Fogwell, R.L. and Inskeep, E.K. (1978). Concentrations of prostaglandins E_2 and $F_{2\alpha}$ and their relationship to luteal function in early pregnant ewes. J. Anim. Sci. 47, 1314-1323.

Lewis, G.S., Wilson, Laird, Jr., Wilks, J.W., Pexton, J.E., Fogwell, R.L., Ford, S.P., Butcher, R.L., Thayne, W.V. and Inskeep, E.K. (1977). $PGF_{2\alpha}$ and its metabolites in uterine and peripheral venous plasma and endometrium of ewes during early pregnancy. J.Anim. Sci. 45, 320-327.

Louis, T.M., Parry, D.M., Robinson, J.S., Thorburn, G.D. and Challis, J.R.G. (1977). Effects of exogenous progesterone and oestradiol on prostaglandin F and 13, 14-dihydro-15-oxo prostaglandin $F_{2\alpha}$ concentrations in uteri and plasma of ovariectomized ewes. J. Endocr. 73, 427.

Lundstrom, V. and Green, K. (1978). Endogenous levels of prostaglandin $F_{2\alpha}$ and its main metabolites in plasma and endometrium of normal and dysmenorrhreic women. Am. J. Obstet. Gynecol. 130, 640-646.

Martin, T.E., Rawlings, N.C., Hill, J.R., Jr. and Henricks, D.M. (1978). Active immunization of the cow against oestradiol-17β. J. Reprod. Fert. 53, 173-178.

Maule Walker, F.M., Patek, C.E., Leaf, C.F. and Watson, J. (1977). The metabolism of prostaglandins $F_{2\alpha}$ and E_2 by non-pregnant porcine endometrial and luteal tissue and early pregnant porcine endometrial tissue, luteal tissue and conceptuses in vitro. Prostaglandins 14,557-562.

Milvae, R.A. and Hansel, W. (1978). $PGF_{2\alpha}$ concentrations during oxytocin-induced luteal inhibition in heifers. J.Anim.Sci. 47, Suppl. 1, 378.

Murdoch, W.J., Lewis, G.S., Inskeep, E.K. and Tillson, S.A. (1978). The effect of a progesterone-releasing intrauterine contraceptive device on uterine secretion of prostaglandin $F_{2\alpha}$and lifespan of corpora lutea in the ewe. Am. J. Ob. Gyn. 132, 81-86.

Nett, T.M., Staigmiller, R.B., Akbar, A.M., Diekman, M.A., Ellinwood, W.E. and Niswender, G.D. (1976). Secretion of prostaglandin $F_{2\alpha}$ in cycling and pregnant ewes. J. Anim. Sci. 42, 876-880.

Newcomb, R., Booth,W.D. and Rowson, L.E.A. (1977). The effect of oxytocin treatment on the levels of prostaglandin F in the blood of heifers. J. Reprod. Fert. 49, 17-24.

Ottobre, J.S. (1979). Regulation of the life span of corpora lutea in ewes. M.S. Thesis, West Virginia University.

Ottobre, J.S., Lewis, G.S. and Inskeep, E.K. (1978). The effect of treatment with progesterone at estrus on the time of uterine release of $PGF_2\alpha$ in ewes. J.Anim. Sci. 47, Suppl. 1, 381.

Pickles, V.R. (1967). The prostaglandins. Biol. Rev. 42,614-652.

Pexton, J.E., Weems, C.W. and Inskeep, E.K.(1975a). Prostaglandins F in uterine venous plasma, ovarian arterial and venous plasma and in ovarian and luteal tissue of pregnant and nonpregnant ewes. J.Anim.Sci. 41, 154-159.

Pexton, J.E., Weems, C.W. and Inskeep, E.K. (1975b). Prostaglandins F in uterine and ovarian venous plasma from nonpregnant and pregnant ewes collected by cannulation. Prostaglandins 9, 501-509.

Pexton, J.E., Ford, S.P., Wilson, L., Jr., Butcher, R.L. and Inskeep, E.K. (1975c). Prostaglandins F in uterine tissue and venous plasma of ewes with intrauterine devices. J.Anim.Sci. 41, 144-153.

Poyser, N.L. and Maule Walker, F.M. (1979). Antiluteolytic effect of the embryo. In: Maternal Recognition of Pregnancy, Ciba Foundation Symposium 64, pp. 261-281, Excerpta Medica. Amsterdam.

Rankin, J.C., Ledford, B.E., Jonnson, H.T.,Jr.and Baggett, B. (1979). Prostaglandins, indomethacin and the decidual cell reaction in the mouse uterus. Biol. Reprod. 20, 399-404.

Rexroad, C.E.,Jr. (1978). Cyclohexamide blockage of estradiol-17β induced contractions in ovariectomized ewes. Biol.Reprod. 19, 648-652.

Roberts, J.S., Barcikowski, B., Wilson, L.,Jr., Skarnes, R.C. and McCracken, J.A. (1975). Hormonal and related factors affecting release of $PGF_2\alpha$ from the uterus. J.Steroid Biochem. 6, 1091-1097.

Roberts, J.S., McCracken, J.A., Gavagan, J.E. and Soloff, M.S. (1976). Oxytocin stimulated release of prostaglandin $F_2\alpha$ from ovine endometrium in vitro: correlation with estrous cycle and oxytocin-receptor binding. Endocrinology 99, 1107-1114.

Robinson, J.S., Challis, J.R.G., Furr, B.J.A., Louis, T.M. and Thorburn, G.D. (1976). Is the sheep corpus luteum subject to tonic inhibition during the luteal phase of the estrous cycle? Europ. J. Obstet. Gynec. Reprod. Biol. 6,191-

Saksena, S.K., Lau, I.F. and Castracane, V.D. (1974). Prostaglandin mediated action of IUD's.II. F prostaglandins (PGF) in the uterine horn of pregnant rats and hamsters with intra-uterine devices. Prostaglandins 5, 97-106.

Scaramuzzi, R.J., Baird, D.T., Boyle, H.P., Land, R.B. and Wheeler, A.J. (1977). The secretion of prostaglandin F from the autotransplanted uterus of the ewe. J.Reprod. Fert. 49, 157-160.

Scommegna, A., Ilekis, J., Sotrel, G., and Auletta, F.J. (1977). The effect of intrauterine progesterone treatment on the endometrial prostaglandin F content in the rabbit. Fertil. Steril. 28: 581-586.

Shaikh, A. and Klaiber, E.L. (1974). Effects of sequential treatment with estradiol and $PGF_2\alpha$ on the length of the primate menstrual cycle. Prostaglandins 6, 253-262.

Sharma, S.C. and Fitzpatrick, R.J. (1974). Effect of oestradiol-17β and oxytocin treatment on prostaglandin F alpha release in the anoestrous ewe. Prostaglandins 6, 97-105.

Shemesh, M. and Hansel, W. (1975). Levels of prostaglandin F(PGF) in bovine endometrium, uterine venous, ovarian arterial and jugular plasma during the estrous cycle. Proc. Soc.Expt.Biol. Med. 148, 123-126.

Shemesh, M., Ailenberg, M., Milaguir, F., Ayalon, N. and Hansel, W. (1978). Hormone secretion by culture bovine pre- and postimplantation gonads. Biol. Reprod. 19, 761-767.

Swanston, I.A., McNatty, K.P. and Baird, D.T. (1977). Concentration of prostaglandin $F_2\alpha$ and steroids in the human corpus luteum. J.Endocr. 73, 115-122.

Thatcher, W.W., Wilcox, C.J., Bazer, F.W., Collier, R.J., Eley, R.M., Stover, D.G. and Bartol, F.F. (1979). Bovine conceptus effects prepartum and potential carryover effects postpartum. Beltsville Symposium III: Reproduction (H.W. Hawk, Editor) Montclair, New Jersey, Allanheld, Osmun and Co. pp. 259-276.

Thorburn, G.D., Cox, R.I., Currie, W.B., Restall, B.J. and Schneider, W. (1973). Prostaglandin F and progesterone concentrations in the utero-ovarian venous plasma of the ewe during the oestrous cycle and early pregnancy. J. Reprod. Fert. Suppl. 18, 151-158.

Trobough, G., Guiderian, J., Erickson, R., Tillson, S., and Pharriss, B. (1976). Dysmenorrhea and the action of intra-uterine progesterone on menstrual blood loss and prosta-glandin content of menstrual blood. Eight World Congress of Gynecology and Obstetrics, Excerpta Medica Foundation, p. 193.

Van Dorp, D.A. (1966). Biosynthesis of prostaglandins. Mem.Soc. Endocrinol. 14: 39-46.

Vernon, M.W., Zavy, M.T., Seamans, K., Asquith, R.L. and Shays, D.C. (1979a). Endometrial PGF production in the nonpregnant and pregnant mare. J.Anim. Sci. 49 (Suppl.1), 344.

Vernon, M.W., Zavy, M.T., Thatcher, W.W., Wilcox, C.J. and Sharp, D.C. (1979b). Steroid modulation of equine endometrial PGF production. Proceedings 12thAnn.Meeting, Soc. Study of Reprod. Quebec. p. 95A.

Warren, J.E., Jr. and Hawk, H.E. (1972). Inhibition by progesterone of IUD-induced luteal regression in the ewe. J.Anim.Sci. 35, 1001-1004.

Weems, C.W., Pexton, J.E., Butcher, R.L., and Inskeep, E.K. (1975). Prostaglandins F in uterine tissue and venous plasma of pseudopregnant rats: effect of deciduomata. Biol. Reprod. 13, 282-288.

Wilks, J.W., Wentz, A.C. and Jones, G.S. (1973). Prostaglandin $F_2\alpha$ concentrations in the blood of women during normal menstrual cycles and dysmenorrhea. J. Clin. Endocrinol. Metab. 37, 469-471.

Wilson, Laird, Jr., Cenedella, R.J., Butcher, R.L. and Inskeep, E.K. (1972a). Levels of prostaglandins in the uterine endometrium during the ovine estrous cycle. J.Anim. Sci. 34, 93-99.

Wilson, Laird, Jr., Butcher, R.L. and Inskeep, E.K. (1972b). Prostaglandin $F_2\alpha$ in the uterus of ewes during early pregnancy. Prostaglandins 1, 479-482.

DISCUSSION

GREENBLATT: Can you explain what happens when ovulatory inhibiting doses of an estrogen are given from Day 5 to 25 to patients for the alleviation of severe dysmenorrhea? It appears that the progesterone in the normal cycle is responsible for the dysmenorrhea since anovulatory cycles are usually free of pain. On the other hand, oral contraceptives also yield good results in about 90% of patients despite 21 days of both estrogen and progestogen. Can you correlate these observations with prostaglandin secretion for me? One other point: hCG given every second day in doses of 5,000 to 10,000 units to the normal woman from Day 21, will maintain the corpus luteum to the 35th day, but not beyond it.

INSKEEP: Progesterone given via an intrauterine device in the sheep suppressed uterine fluid $PGF_2\alpha$ levels, and a progesterone-delivering intrauterine device has been reported to suppress $PGF_2\alpha$ levels in the menstrual fluid in humans. That would account for effects of progesterone in the pill. Estrogen, on the other hand, seemed to increase PGF in uterine fluid collected from ovariectomized monkeys when given alone, but when progesterone was added to the estrogen therapy PGF levels were reduced somewhat (Demers et al, 1974). In a number of recent studies, prostaglandin synthetase inhibitors have been administered to humans and have relieved symptoms of dysmenorrhea and reduced the levels of prostaglandins in human menstrual fluid.

We didn't see anything to indicate an association of uterine production of $PGF_2\alpha$ during the menstrual cycle with luteolysis. I think exogenous hCG is maintaining the corpus luteum just as endogenous hCG would in pregnancy, Dr. Greenblatt. I think it does so by some mechanism that does not involve uterine levels of $PGF_2\alpha$. Dr. Abel has studied this in humans and she'll talk later today.

BAZER: The pig, sheep, cow and horse all tend to have an equal or greater endometrial production of $PGF_2\alpha$ in the pregnant state as compared to the nonpregnant state. We propose (some people think naively) that prostaglandins are sequestered in the pregnant pig uterus. This is a simple explanation. In the pig the facts that are available to support this notion apply not only to PGF but other aspects of histotroph secretion as well. For example, the purple protein begins to move into the stroma at the end of the estrous cycle in the nonpregnant animal, but doesn't in pregnancy. PGF is higher in uterine venous drainage in the nonpregnant state but not in the pregnant state, and this is also true of 13,14-dihydro-15-keto-$PGF_{2}\alpha$ (Shille et al, 1979 and Terqui and Thatcher). Therefore, the evidence indicates that a much simpler mechanism is operating in pigs than may be working in the sheep; that is, sequestering PGF to protect the corpus luteum. Bito et al (1976) at Columbia University have data that show that prostaglandins cannot move freely through cell membranes. Instead, they have to be actively transported in a number of tissues and reproductive tissues happen to fall into that category. There are tissues that will allow them to move freely, some that actively block their transport into the cell and others that actively transport them. I think that Bito's work is worth thinking about in some of these mechanisms.

INSKEEP: What has disturbed me relative to the possibility of uterine sequestering of prostaglandins is that although the uterine venous concentrations may decrease in some of these situations, there is an increase in uterine venous blood flow. There are data in both the cow (Ford et al, 1979) and the pig (Ford and Christenson, 1979) that show there are specific times when venous blood flow increases. We have to correlate those data on blood flow with the data on prostaglandin levels to begin to sort this out better. There's no question there are higher levels of both $PGF_{2}\alpha$ and PGE_{2} in the uterine lumen in Ellinwood's (1979) studies in the sheep, Thatcher's studies in the cow, and your studies in the pig, Dr. Bazer, and so this is a possibility that has to be investigated.

BAZER: I think this is why the metabolite studies by Shille et al (1979) and Terqui and Thatcher add to this concept in the pig. They found that the metabolite levels remain basal at 100-200 pg/ml in pregnancy, whereas there were definite increases to over 1 ng/ml in the nonpregnant animal. They have sampled from a static fluid pool in the peripheral plasma, i.e., not affected by changes in uterine blood flow.

ABEL: In Edinburgh, we have found that although there's no difference in concentration of $PGF_{2}\alpha$ in endometrium or in uterine venous plasma in pregnancy relative to the nonpregnant sheep, we do find a significant increase in PGE concentrations. Mapletoft et al (1975) showed that if you took either the uterine venous or the ovarian arterial blood from a unilaterally pregnant sheep, you could maintain the contralateral corpus luteum by transferring the blood flow. This suggests that there was a local mechanism coming from the pregnant side. Henderson et al (1977) showed that simultaneous infusion of PGE_{2} with $PGF_{2}\alpha$ could overcome the luteolytic effect of exogenous $PGF_{2}\alpha$. In preliminary studies using sheep we have shown that Day 15 embryonic tissue cultured alone or together with nonpregnant endometrium produces quite large amounts of PGE. Thus, the developing embryo may be the source of PGE and/or may stimulate PGE production in the endometrium in early pregnancy. I wonder whether it might be profitable to study both the blastocysts and the endometrium in the pregnant animal?

INSKEEP: Very definitely. The possibility that PGE is a local anti-luteolytic substance is an exciting prospect. We've seen in studies all these years opposite or opposing effects of substances, such as estrogen and progesterone, which are very much alike but differ slightly in structure. To me, an opposing effect of PGE_2 and $PGF_{2}\alpha$ in this situation is quite a nice concept to contemplate. The problem has been to demonstrate clearly that PGE_2 is anti-luteolytic. Different ones of us have studied this in different ways and have had more or less degrees of success. The studies of Henderson, et al which you've mentioned, are particularly exciting because they have been able to infuse PGE_2 for a period of time and maintain high progesterone levels in spite of having given $PGF_{2}\alpha$. The problem is that when they stopped the infusions progesterone levels declined and the corpora lutea regressed. Bolt at Beltsville has obtained similar results with infusion of epinepherine after $PGF_{2}\alpha$. Perhaps PGE_2 has to be continued for some period of time beyond when $PGF_{2}\alpha$ was given. There's a lot more that we have to learn about the potential role of PGE_2 in maintenance of the corpus luteum, but it is an attractive hypothesis. Shemesh et al (1978) has shown that cattle blastocysts produce both PGE_2 and $PGF_{2}\alpha$. This needs to be looked at further. The prostaglandin-containing extracts of endometrium and conceptus that Bruce Pratt prepared in our laboratory, which overcame the effect of a challenge with $PGF_{2}\alpha$ in nonpregnant ewes, were very high in PGE_2. We don't know what else is in these extracts because we haven't completely assayed all of the components.

References:

Bito, LZ, Wallenstein, M and Baroody, R (1976). The role of transport processes in the distribution and disposition of prostaglandins. Advances in Prostaglandins and Thromboxane Research. Vol. 1, p 297.

Demers, LM, Yoshinaga, K and Greep, RO (1974). Prostaglandin F in monkey uterine fluid during the menstrual cycle and following steroid treatment. Prostaglandins 5:513-519.

Ellinwood, WE, Nett, TM and Niswender, GD (1979). Maintenance of the corpus luteum of early pregnancy in the ewe. II. Prostaglandin secretion by the endometrium in vitro and in vivo. Biol Reprod 21: 845-856.

Ford, SP, Chenault, JR and Echternkamp, SE (1979). Uterine blood flow of cows during the oestrous cycle and early pregnancy: effect of the conceptus on the uterine blood supply. J Reprod Fert 56:53-62.

Ford, SP and Christenson, RK (1979). Blood flow to uteri of sows during the estrous cycle and early pregnancy: local effect of the conceptus on the uterine blood supply. Biol Reprod 21:617-624.

Henderson, KM, Scaramuzzi, R and Baird, DT (1977). Simultaneous infusion of prostaglandin E_2 antagonizes the luteolytic action of prostaglandin $F_{2}\alpha$ in vivo. J Endocrinology 72:379-383.

Mapletoft, RJ, DelCampo, MR and Ginther, OJ (1975). Unilateral luteotropic effect of uterine venous effluent of a gravid uterine horn in sheep. Proc Soc Exp Biol Med 150:129-133.

Shemesh, M, Ailenberg, M, Milaguir, F, Ayalon, N and Hansel, W (1978). Hormone secretion by cultured bovine pre- and postimplantation gonads. Biol Reprod 19:761-767.

Shille, VM, Karlbom, I, Einarsson, S, Larsson, K, Kindahl, H, and Edqvist, L-E (1979). Concentrations of progesterone and 15-keto-13, 14-prostaglandin $F_{2\alpha}$ in peripheral plasma during the estrous cycle and early pregnancy in gilts. Zbl Vet Med A 26:169-181.

The Endometrium

16

The Influence of the Embryo on Uterine Prostaglandin Production in the Human

Margaret H. Abel

Progesterone is required for the maintenance of pregnancy in all mammals. In most species the duration of pregnancy exceeds the length of the oestrus cycle and therefore persistence of the corpus luteum must occur if progesterone secretion is to continue. In species such as the mouse, rat and rabbit, the corpus luteum is required throughout gestation whereas in others, such as the sheep, cow and primates, progesterone secretion is taken over by the placenta after the first third of pregnancy although the corpus luteum persists until term.

If fertilization fails to occur luteal activity is prematurely terminated in the majority of species by a luteolytic substance of uterine origin. This luteolysin has now been identified as prostaglandin $F_2\alpha$ ($PGF_2\alpha$). (For a review see Horton and Poyser, 1976). Therefore if progesterone secretion is to continue after successful fertilization, it is necessary either to prevent the synthesis of $PGF_2\alpha$ by the uterus or to overcome its luteolytic action by production of a luteotrophic hormone. This definition of luteotrophic would include any substance which blocked the action of $PGF_2\alpha$ at the level of the corpus luteum.

It appears that different mechanisms operate in different species to maintain the corpus luteum in early pregnancy. Recent studies suggest that in the sheep the developing embryo secretes a luteotrophic factor which maintains progesterone output by a local action at the corpus luteum (Mapletoft et al, 1975). In contrast, inhibition of uterine $PGF_2\alpha$ production appears to be the mechanism by which luteal function is prolonged in the guinea pig. Decreased concentrations of $PGF_2\alpha$ in uterine venous blood from day 15 onwards in pregnant animals are parallelled by a decreased prostaglandin synthesizing capacity of uterine tissue in vitro (Poyser and Maule-Walker, 1979).

In the human there is no evidence for a luteolytic role of $PGF_2\alpha$ of uterine origin, since cyclic ovarian activity continues following hysterectomy (Beling et al, 1970), or in the congenital absence of Mullerian duct structures (Fraser et al, 1973). The stimulus for continued progesterone production following fertilization is thought to be chorionic gonadotrophin secreted by the early blastocyst (Kosasa et al, 1973). This hormone has been shown to prolong the life span of the corpus luteum in spontaneously cyclic women (Bradbury et al, 1950).

Despite its lack of involvement in luteolysis, the human uterus is capable of synthesizing prostaglandins and production of $PGF_2\alpha$ increases during the luteal phase of the menstrual cycle (Pickles et al, 1965; Downie et al, 1974; Levitt et al, 1975; Singh et al, 1975; Maathuis and Kelly, 1978). Under the influence of progesterone and oestradiol (Abel and Baird, 1980) secreted by the ovary, maximum $PGF_2\alpha$ concentrations are reached at the time of menstruation.

Following the discovery of "smooth muscle stimulants" in human menstrual fluid (Pickles, 1957), with the subsequent identification of $PGF_2\alpha$ and PGE_2 as the major components (Pickles and Hall, 1963; Eglinton et al, 1963), Pickles suggested that these compounds might be involved in the initiation of menstruation, or cyclic shedding of the outer endometrial layers; a process restricted to humans and other Old World primates. These prostaglandins have been shown to affect the contractility of uterine smooth muscle with $PGF_2\alpha$ acting to contract and PGE to relax the non-pregnant myometrium (Martin et al, 1978). It is possible therefore that increased production of $PGF_2\alpha$ within the endometrium towards the end of the cycle could be responsible for the marked constriction of the spiral arterioles which precedes the onset of menstrual bleeding as observed by Markee in his endometrial transplants in the rhesus monkey (Macaca mulatta) (Markee, 1940). Recent reports of abnormal concentrations of prostaglandins in the endometrium of women with various disorders of menstruation (Downie et al, 1974; Willman et al, 1976; Lundstrom and Green, 1978) support the idea that prostaglandins may be involved in the mechanism of menstruation. Since an intact endometrium is required if implantation of the fertilized ovum is to occur, it follows that menstruation must be prevented. It has recently been reported that the concentrations of $PGF_2\alpha$ and PGE_2 in endometrium from women in early pregnancy (Willman and Collins, 1976), in one instance as early as day 17 (Maathuis and Kelly, 1978), are significantly lower than levels measured during the menstrual cycle, suggesting that the presence of the conceptus may prevent the rise in concentrations of $PGF_2\alpha$ in the endometrium, which occurs during the luteal phase of the nonpregnant cycle. However, the mechanism of this reduction in endometrial prostaglandin concentrations is not known. The process of decidualization of the endometrium may be accompanied by biochemical changes such that the decidual cell has a reduced capacity to synthesize prostaglandins and/or is unable to respond to the stimulus which elicits prostaglandin synthesis in the non-decidualized cell.

Decidualization in the human describes the changes which occur in the endometrial stromal tissue under the influence of progesterone. Stromal cells enlarge and the cytoplasm becomes more conspicuous and stains with acidic dyes such as eosin. Predecidual changes are apparent by the late secretory phase of the cycle and if pregnancy ensues and progesterone secretion continues these changes are intensified such that the endometrium of pregnancy is often referred to as decidua. This contrasts with the situation in rats and rabbits where decidualization of the uterus cannot be hormonally induced but is a response to the presence of blastocyst within the uterus or alternatively can be induced by traumatization of the uterus (Krebhiel, 1937).

However the observation that both concentration of $PGF_{2\alpha}$ in the endometrium and the synthesizing capacity of this tissue are maximal in the mid to late secretory phase when predecidual changes are present in the stroma, does not support this idea. In addition there is no evidence at the present time to suggest that prostaglandin production is restricted to the stromal tissue. Abundant glandular epithelium is present in the endometrium in both the late secretory phase and in early pregnancy. It therefore appears likely that the conceptus itself may influence either the metabolism of prostaglandins or their synthesis within the endometrium.

We have recently had the opportunity to investigate the concentrations of prostaglandins in the endometrium of women with an ectopic pregnancy, where the embryo had implanted outside the uterus but in the Fallopian tube. Tubal pregnancies appear to be peculiar to the primate since, unlike other mammals such as the mouse or guinea pig, implantation in primates does not appear to be restricted to a limited period when the uterine environment is nonhostile to the invading blastocyst (RJ Aitken personal communication.) Therefore, if embryo transport along the Fallopian tube is either delayed or prevented due to occlusion of the tube, the blastocyst will implant in the epithelium lining the tube.

Endometrium was obtained from sixteen women, by curettage of the uterus after laparotomy for removal of a tubal pregnancy, ranging from five to fourteen weeks gestation. The group was subdivided according to whether or not there was a history of vaginal bleeding since the last menstrual period. These groups are referred to as bleeding and intact ectopics respectively. Occurrence of vaginal bleeding was taken as evidence of failure of the pregnancy due to lack of hormonal support from the embryo.

A comparison was made with concentrations of prostaglandins in endomentrium from eleven women undergoing therapeutic termination of a normal intra-uterine pregnancy, ranging from four to eleven weeks gestation. Endometrium was obtained by curettage prior to suction evacuation of the uterus. In addition, endometrium was obtained from twenty-one women with normal menstrual cycles undergoing laparoscopic sterilization. Tissue was homogenized in ice cold ethanol within two minutes of its removal and $PGF_{2}\alpha$ and PGE were measured by radioimmunoassay in reconstituted ethanol extracts as previously described (Abel et al, 1980). As shown in Figure 1, the concentrations of $PGF_{2}\alpha$ and PGE in endometrium from women with tubal pregnancies were comparable with those in endometrium from intra-uterine pregnancies, both being significantly lower ($p < 0.01$) than levels at any stage of the menstrual cycle. It appears therefore that contact between foetal and maternal tissues is not a prerequisite for the reduction in endometrial PG concentrations observed during early pregnancy and suggests instead that this effect is mediated humorally, by a substance secreted by the developing embryo. Such a factor is likely to act systemically although this study does not exclude the possibility that substances secreted by the embryo could reach the uterus via the Fallopian tube and exert their effect locally.

Concentrations of $PGF_{2}\alpha$ in endometrium from the bleeding ectopics remained significantly lower ($p < 0.05$) than concentrations in secretory endometrium, suggesting that if the embryo is acting to reduce prostaglandin concentrations in this tissue, this effect persists despite failure of the pregnancy. In addition, the degree of decidualization of the endometrium was variable in the nine women with an intact ectopic pregnancy, despite consistently low concentrations of prostaglandins, providing further evidence that the histological appearance of the endometrium does not appear to reflect its ability to synthesize prostaglandins.

There is little evidence to suggest that metabolism of prostaglandins within the endometrium is increased during pregnancy. Kierse et al, (1975) found that from seven weeks onwards tissues of trophoblastic origin, such as the chorion and placenta have much higher 15-prostaglandin dehydrogenase activity than other uterine tissues including myometrium and decidua. They show that in incubations of decidua with $^{3}HPGF_{2}\alpha$ approximately 85% of the radioactivity was recovered as $PGF_{2}\alpha$ after 30 minutes, whereas foetal membranes or placenta converted the primary prostaglandin to 15-keto-$PGF_{2}\alpha$ and 15-keto-13,14-dihydro-$PGF_{2}\alpha$ within a few minutes. This ability to metabolize prostaglandins be a mechanism which prevents the foetus being exposed to high levels of prostaglandins at the time of parturition. Therefore, the low concentrations of $PGF_{2}\alpha$ and PGE_{2} in the endometrium in early pregnancy are unlikely to result from increased metabolism by this tissue.

In order to determine whether decidual tissue could be stimulated to produce prostaglandin in vitro, we have used an organ culture system originally developed to investigate the endocrine control of prostaglandin synthesis by the endometrium throughout the menstrual cycle. Using this system we have shown that oestradiol-17β, at physiological concentrations, can stimulate a significant increase in $PGF_{2}\alpha$ production by luteal or secretory phase tissue, but is without effect on proliferative tissue. This suggests that exposure of the endometrium to progesterone in vivo during the luteal phase increases the prostaglandin synthesizing capacity of the tissue and enables it to respond to oestradiol in vitro. Since decidual tissue has been exposed to high levels of progesterone in vivo during the early weeks of pregnancy it might be expected to respond to oestradiol in vitro in a similar manner to secretory endometrium by an increased production of $PGF_{2}\alpha$.

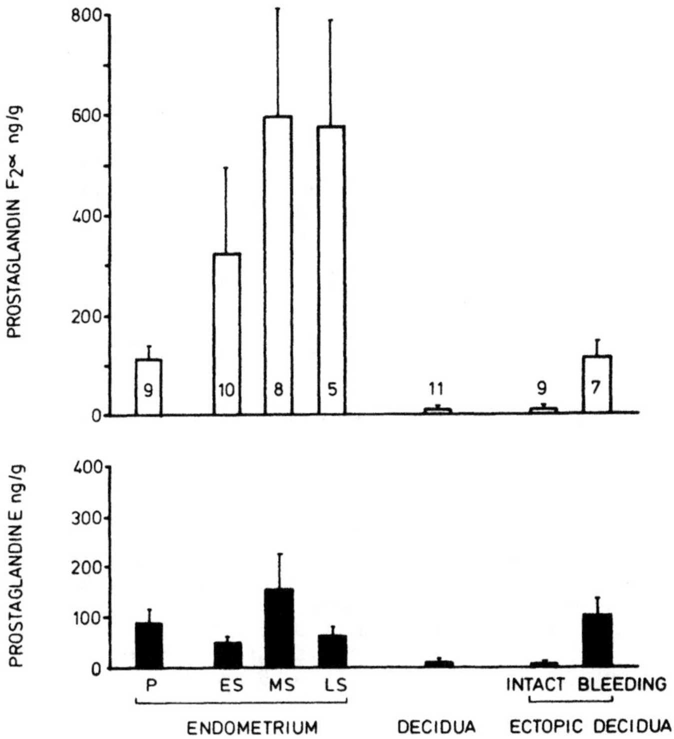

Figure 1. The concentrations of $PGF_{2}\alpha$ and PGE in endometrium throughout the normal menstrual cycle, (P, ES, MS and LS refer to proliferative, early, mid and late secretory endometrium, respectively); endometrium from intrauterine pregnancies, 6-11 weeks, (decidua) and endometrium from tubal pregnancies, 5-14 weeks, (ectopic decidua), intact and bleeding refer to the absence and presence respectively of vaginal bleeding since the last menstrual period.

Results are expressed in ng/g, wet weight of tissue, mean ± sem. The numbers in each category are shown in the upper half of the figure (from Abel et al, 1980).

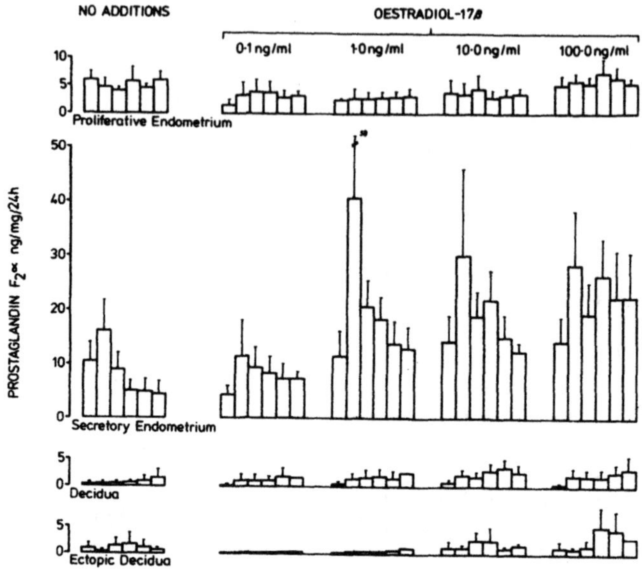

Figure 2. The production of $PGF_{2}\alpha$ by proliferative endometrium, 10-14 days; secretory endometrium, 20-26 days; endometrium from intrauterine pregnancies, 6-11 weeks (decidua); and endometrium from tubal pregnancies 5-14 weeks (ectopic decidua), maintained in organ culture alone and in the presence of 0.1, 1.0, 10.0 and 100.0 ng/ml oestradiol-17β for six days. Each histogram represents the mean ± sem output in ng/mg/24 hours (n = 5, 5, 5 and 4 respectively).

Decidual tissue from both intra-uterine gestations and ectopic pregnancies was maintained in Trowell's T_8 medium supplemented with 20% donor calf serum, antibiotics, fungicide and glutamine for periods of six days, in an atmosphere of air:carbon dioxide and oxygen:carbon dioxide at a pressure of 10 lb/sq in, using modified Kilner jars. The medium was replaced and the jar regassed every 24 hrs; $PGF_{2}\alpha$ and PGE were measured by radioimmunoassay of the medium without prior extraction. This method has been described in full elsewhere (Abel and Baird, 1980). The output of $PGF_{2}\alpha$ by proliferative endometrium, secretory endometrium and endometrium from intra-uterine and ectopic pregnancies incubated alone and with oestradiol-17β at concentrations ranging from 1.0 to 100.0 ng/ml as shown in Figure 2 and Figure 3. There was no stimulation of either $PGF_{2}\alpha$ or PGE in endometrium from intrauterine or ectopic pregnancies at any of

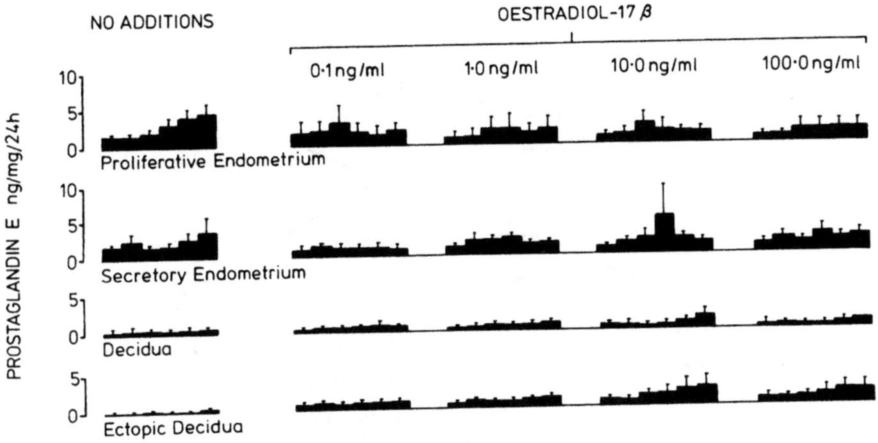

Figure 3. The production of PGE_2 by proliferative endometrium, 10-14 days; secretory endometrium, 20-26 days; endometrium from intrauterine pregnancies, 6-11 weeks (decidua); and endometrium from tubal pregnancies, 5-14 weeks (ectopic decidua) maintained in organ culture alone and in the presence of 0.1, 1.0, 10.0 and 100.0 ng/ml oestradial-17β for six days. Each histogram represents the mean ± sem output in ng/mg/24 hours (n = 5, 5, 5 and 4 respectively).

the concentrations of oestradiol-17β tested. It therefore appears that prostaglandin synthesis is actively inhibited in the endometrium during early pregnancy in the human. In addition, the inhibition appears to be prolonged since no response to oestradiol was seen during the six days of culture.

Since synthesis of both $PGF_{2}\alpha$ and PGE is prevented it is likely that inhibition occurs at a step in the synthetic pathway before the formation of the intermediate endoperoxides PGG_2 and PGH_2. These unstable products can breakdown nonenzymically to PGE_2 and $PGF_{2}\alpha$. Thus the conceptus may secrete a substance which inhibits synthesis of, or inactivates the cyclo-oxygenase enzyme. Alternatively it is possible that the inhibition could be exerted earlier in the synthetic pathway to prevent the mobilization of free arachidonic acid. The conversion of arachidonic acid to prostaglandins is outlined in Figure 4.

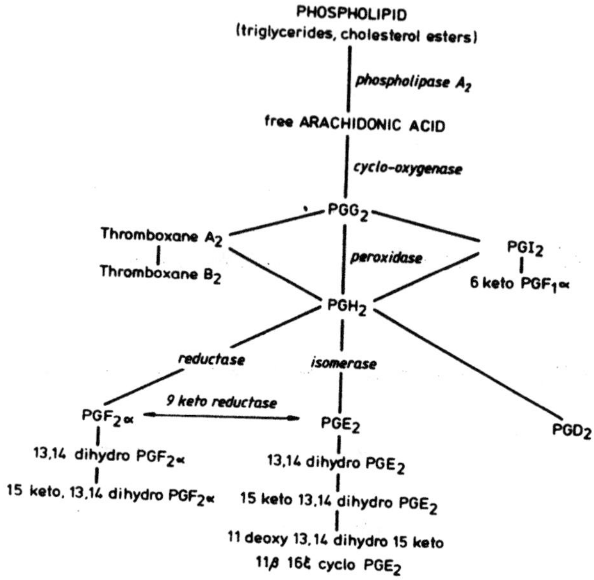

Figure 4. The arachidonic acid cascade.

Addition of arachidonic acid (2.5 μg/ml) to the culture medium did not stimulate prostaglandin production by endometrium from either intrauterine or ectopic pregnancies suggesting that the availability of this precursor was not rate limiting. However there is evidence that simply increasing the arachidonic acid content of the medium does not necessarily increase the concentration of free arachidonic acid within the cell, and therefore, to confirm that availability of arachidonic acid was not the rate limiting step, we investigated the ability of this tissue to metabolize ^{14}C-arachidonic acid to prostaglandins in vitro.

Tissue was homogenized in Tris/HCl buffer pH 7.4 and approximately 20 mg incubated with 0.5 μCi (2.76 μg) of ^{14}C-arachidonic acid in a final volume of 1.0 ml for 30 min at 37°C in a shaking water bath. After acidification, prostaglandins were extracted with 8 volumes of ether:ethyl acetate (3:1) and separated by a thin layer chromatography using the organic phase of a mixture of ethyl acetate:isooctane:acetic acid:water (11:5:2:10) (Sun et al, 1977). The products formed were visualised either by radioactive scanning of the plate or by autoradiography. Appropriate regions of the plate were then excised and the radioactivity counted in a scintillation counter. Using this technique we have shown that endometrium and myometrium differ in their ability to metabolize arachidonic acid to the intermediate endoperoxides and to convert these endoperoxides to the primary prostaglandins (Abel and Kelly, 1979). A homogenate of endometrium was found to metabolize arachidonic acid predominantly to a mixture of $PGF_{2}\alpha$ and PGE_2 and to a lesser extent PGD_2 whereas a similar preparation of myometrium showed relatively little activity, the major prostaglandin identified being 6-oxo-$PGF_{1}\alpha$, the metabolite of prostacyclin, PGI_2. Significant amounts of 6-oxo-$PGF_{1}\alpha$ were only seen when endometrial and myometrial homogenates were combined as shown in Figure 5. These observations may in part explain the recent reports that 6-oxo-$PGF_{1}\alpha$ is the major prostaglandin produced by the uterus in the rat, sheep and guinea pig (Fenwick et al, 1977; Jones et al, 1977).

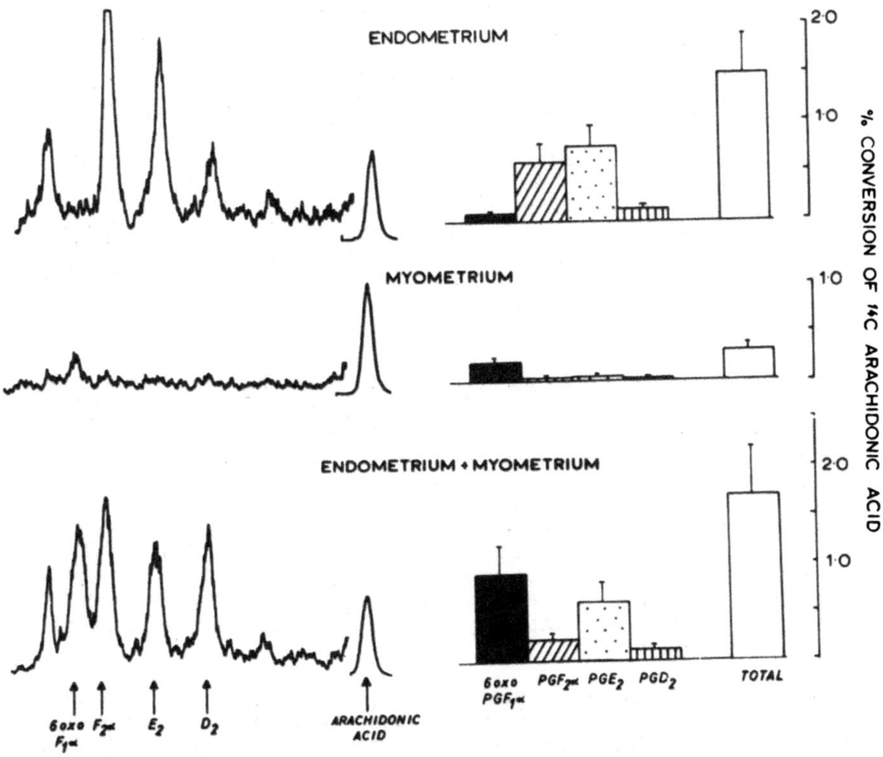

Figure 5. The conversion of arachidonic acid to prostaglandins by the human uterus. Left, a radio TLC scanning of the products isolated after incubation of ^{14}C-arachidonic acid with homogenates of endometrium, myometrium and a mixture of endometrium and myometrium. The positions of authentic prostaglandins run in the same system are indicated by the arrows, the arachidonic acid peak was scanned with a 30 fold reduction in sensitivity in each case. Right, the mean ± sem of eight separate incubations expressed as percentage conversion of the arachidonic acid added to 6-oxo-$PGF_{1}\alpha$, $PGF_{2}\alpha$, PGE_2 and PGD_2 (from Abel and Kelly, 1979).

Although oestradiol is known to stimulate prostaglandin production in vivo, and increased $PGF_{2}\alpha$ synthesis in the previously described organ culture, we have found that oestradiol has little effect on prostaglandin production in this broken cell preparation. In contrast a catechol metabolite of oestradiol, 2-hydroxy-oestradiol has been found to be a potent stimulator of both $PGF_{2}\alpha$ and PGE_2 production in this system (Kelly and Abel, 1980).

We have used this steroid to investigate the ability of endometrium from early pregnancy to metabolize ^{14}C-arachidonic acid to prostaglandins. The percentage conversions of arachidonic acid to 6-oxo-$PGF_{1}\alpha$, $PGF_{2}\alpha$, PGE_2 and PGD_2 by proliferative and secretory endometria are shown in Figure 6. Although oestradiol has little effect on prostaglandin production, 2-hydroxy-oestradiol stimulates both $PGF_{2}\alpha$ and PGE_2 production in proliferative endometrium and the conversion is significantly greater in secretory endometrium. However, in three samples of endometrium from early pregnancy there was virtually no conversion of arachidonic acid to prostaglandins and no response to stimulation with either oestradiol or 2-hydroxy-oestradiol. Since pregnant endometrium is unable to metabolise exogenous arachidonic acid to prostaglandins we conclude that the block to PG synthesis must be at the level of the cyclo-oxygenase enzyme. It is possible that 2-hydroxy-oestradiol may stimulate prostaglandin production by enhancing the conversion of PGG_2 to PGH_2 (RW Kelly, personal communication) and therefore failure of this steroid to stimulate production in the pregnant tissue may reflect absence of the endoperoxide intermediates.

Although it is not known how prostaglandin synthesis is prevented in early pregnancy, an obvious contender for the role of inhibitor is progesterone since this hormone has been shown to prevent oestradiol stimulated prostaglandin synthesis by the uterus in vivo in species such as the rat (Ham et al, 1975), and sheep (Baird, 1977). We have recently found that progesterone can inhibit output of $PGF_{2}\alpha$ and PGE_2 by both proliferative and secretory endometrium in vitro. In addition, progesterone can prevent the oestradiol induced stimulation of $PGF_{2}\alpha$ in secretory endometrium (Abel and Baird, 1980). Therefore the embryo may indirectly inhibit prostaglandin production in the endometrium by maintaining progesterone output by the corpus luteum through production of a luteotrophin.

However several factors argue against such a hypothesis. The concentration of $PGF_{2}\alpha$ and the synthetic capacity of the endometrium is high in the mid to late secretory phase when plasma concentrations of progesterone are comparable with those of early pregnancy (Tulchinsky and Hobel, 1973). In women with intact ectopic pregnancy concentrations of both $PGF_{2}\alpha$ and PGE_2 in the endometrium were consistently low despite variable plasma progesterone concentrations. In addition, the prolonged inhibition of prostaglandin synthesis in tissue from pregnant patients is inconsistent with the priming action of progesterone. If progesterone were acting to inhibit synthesis in vivo one would still expect to see a response to oestradiol in vitro.

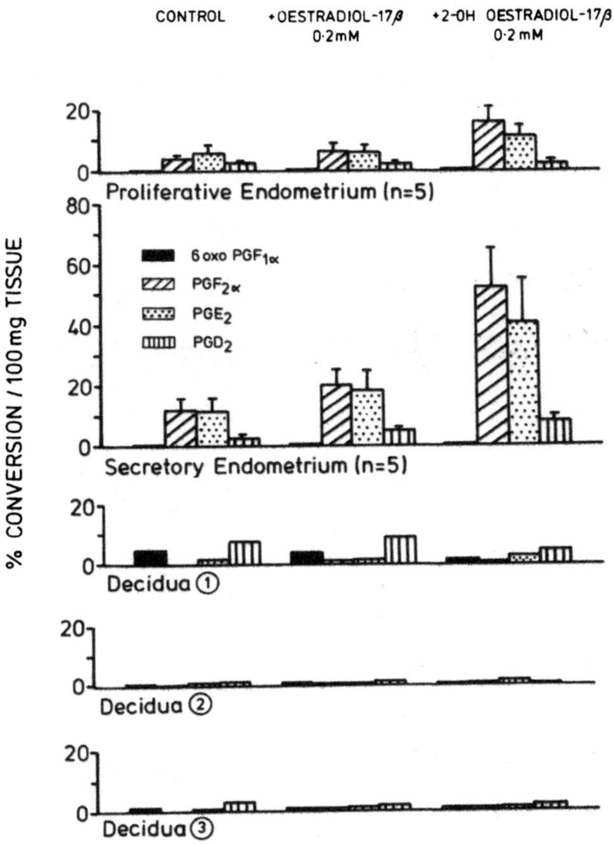

Figure 6. The conversion of ^{14}C-arachidonic acid to 6-oxo-$PGF_{1}\alpha$, $PGF_{2}\alpha$ and PGE_2 and PGD_2 by homogenates of proliferative endometrium, (10-14 days), secretory endometrium (20-26 days) and endometrium from three intrauterine pregnancies, 7.5, 12 and 10 weeks respectively. Results are expressed as percentage conversion of arachidonic/acid 100 mg tissue.

It remains possible that another pregnancy associated protein may be responsible for the inhibition of prostaglandin synthesis in the endometrium although hCG has no effect on endometrial prostaglandin production in vitro. (MH Abel, unpublished observations). An endogenous inhibitor of prostaglandin synthesis has been reported in the globulin fraction of human plasma (Saeed et al, 1977) and pregnancy specific α-2-glycoprotein has been localised in decidua in late pregnancy (Horne et al, 1976). In several of the incubations of endometrium from early pregnancy with ^{14}C-arachidonic acid a number of less polar products, not corresponding to known prostaglandins were seen (Figure 7). It is possible that these could represent products

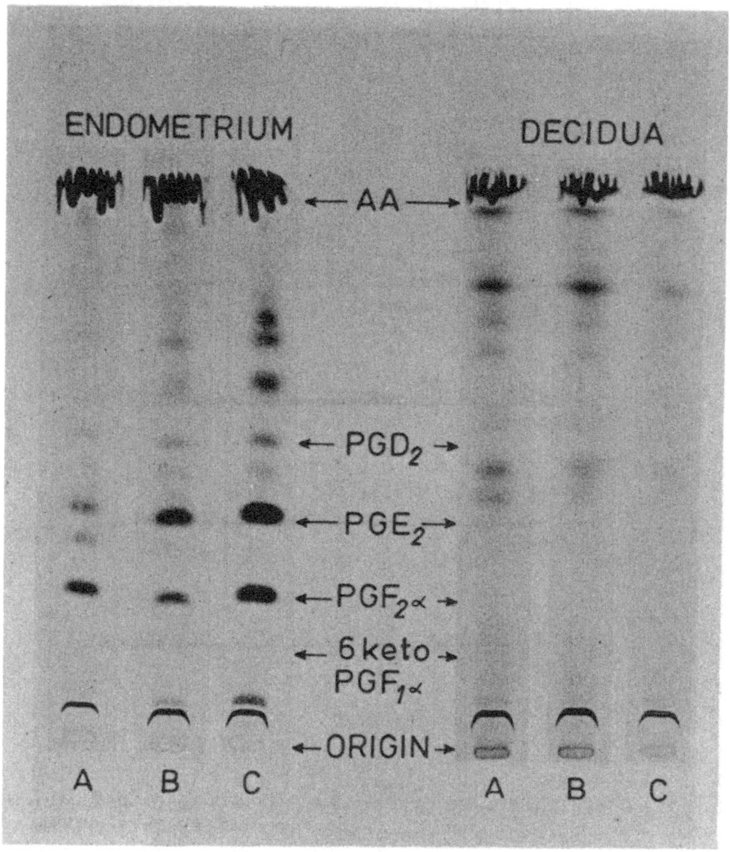

Figure 7. Autoradiographs of the products isolated after incubation of homogenates of secretory endometrium (day 22) and endometrium from a 12 week pregnancy with ^{14}C-arachidonic acid. The positions of authentic prostaglandins run in the same system are indicated.

formed by metabolism of arachidonic acid via a different pathway. This could result in the low concentration of $PGF_{2\alpha}$ and PGE_2 in endometrium during early pregnancy. This remains to be investigated.

In summary, a significant reduction in the concentration of both $PGF_{2\alpha}$ and PGE_2 is seen in the endometrium during early pregnancy in the human. This reduction appears to result from inhibition of prostaglandin synthesis within the endometrium. Inhibition or inactivation of the cyclooxygenase enzyme is probably the rate limiting step since endometrium is unable to metabolise exogenous arachidonic acid to prostaglandins.

It appears therefore, that the human conceptus, in addition to secreting a luteotrophic factor (hCG) responsible for maintaining progesterone output by the corpus luteum in early pregnancy, may also secrete a substance capable of inhibiting prostaglandin production in the maternal endometrium. Such a factor may act systemically, although a local action has not been ruled out. The nature of this substance is unknown.

ACKNOWLEDGEMENTS

Authentic prostaglandins were generously supplied by Dr. J Pike, The Upjohn Company, Kalamazoo. I gratefully acknowledge the collaboration of my colleagues Dr. RW Kelly and Dr. SK Smith in these studies. I should like to thank Professors RV Short and DT Baird and Dr. NL Poyser for helpful discussions. These studies were supported by the Royal Society Foulerton Gift Research Fellowship.

REFERENCES

Abel, MH and Baird, DT (1980). The effect of oestradiol-17β on prostaglandin production by human endometrium maintained in organ culture. Endocrinology (In press).

Abel, MH and Kelly, RW (1979). Differential production of prostaglandins within the human uterus. Prostaglandins (In press).

Abel, MH, Smith, SK and Baird, DT (1980). Suppression of endometrial prostaglandin concentration in early intrauterine and ectopic pregnancy in women. J Endocrinol (In press).

Baird, DT (1977). Local utero-ovarian relationships. In : Control of ovulation. Eds. DB Crighton and GE Lamming. Butterworths p 217-233.

Beling, CG, Marcus, SL and Markham, SM (1970). Functional activity of the corpus luteum following hysterectomy. J Clin Endocrinol 30: 30-39.

Bradbury, JT, Brown, WE and Gray, LA (1950). Maintenance of the corpus luteum and physiologic actions of progesterone. Rec Prog Horm Res 5: 151-190.

Downie, J, Poyser, NL and Wunderlich, M (1974). Levels of prostaglandins in human endometrium during the normal menstrual cycle. J Physiol 236: 465-472.

Eglinton, G, Raphael, RA, Smith, GN, Hall, WJ and Pickles, VR (1963). Isolation and identification of two smooth muscle stimulants from human menstrual fluid. Nature 200: 960 and 933-995.

Fenwick, L, Jones, RL, Naylor, B, Poyser, NL and Wilson, NH (1977). Production of prostaglandins by the pseudopregnant rat uterus in vitro, and the effect of tamoxifen with the identification of 6-keto-prostaglandin $F_{1}\alpha$ as a major product. Br J Pharmacol 59: 191-199.

Fraser, IS, Baird, DT, Hobson, BM, Michie, EA and Hunter, W (1973). Cyclical ovarian function in women with congenital absence of the uterus and vagina. J Clin Endocrinol Metab 36: 634-637.

Ham, EA, Cirillo, VJ, Zanetti, ME, and Kuehl, FA (1975). Estrogen directed synthesis of specific prostaglandins in the uterus. Proc Nat Acad Sci US 72: 1420-1424.

Horne, CHW, Bohn, H and Towler, GM (1976). Pregnancy-associated α-2-glycoprotein. In : Plasma hormone assays in evaluation of fetal well being. Ed., A Klopper. Churchill, Livingston, Edinburgh, p 147-173.

Horton, EW and Poyser, NL (1976). Uterine luteolytic hormone. A physiological role for prostaglandin F_2. Physiol Rev 56: 595-651.

Jones, RL, Poyser, NL and Wilson, NH (1977). Production of 6-oxo prostaglandin F_1 by rat, guinea pig and sheep uteri in vitro. Br J Pharmacol 59: 436-437P.

Kelly, RW and Abel, MH (1980). Catechol oestrogens stimulate uterine prostaglandin production. In : Advances in prostaglandin and thromboxane research, Vol. 8. Eds., B Samuelsson, PW Ramwell and R Paoletti, Raven Press, New York, p 1369-1370.

Kierse, MJNC, Williamson, JG and Turnbull, AC (1975). Metabolism of prostaglandin $F_{2}\alpha$ within the human uterus in early pregnancy. Br J Obstet Gynaecol 82: 142-145.

Kosasa, TS, Levesque, LA Foldstein, DP and Taymor, ML (1973). Early detection of implantation using a radioimmunoassay specific for human chorionic gonadotrophin. J Clin Endocrinol Metab 36: 622-624.

Krebhiel, RH (1937). Cytological studies of the decidual reaction in the rat during early pregnancy and in the production of deciduomata. Physiol Zool 10: 212-234.

Levitt, TM, Tobon, H and Josimovich, JB (1975). Prostaglandin content of human endometrium. Fertil and Steril 26: 296-300.

Lundstrom, V and Green, K (1978). Endogenous levels of prostaglandin $F_{2}\alpha$ and its main metabolites in plasma and endometrium of normal and dysmenorrhoeic women. Am J Obstet Gynecol 130: 540-646.

Maathuis, JB and Kelly, RW (1978). Concentrations of prostaglandins $F_{2}\alpha$ and E_2 in endometrium throughout the human menstrual cycle, after administration of clomiphene or an oestrogen-progesterone pill and in early pregnancy. J Endocrinol 77: 361-371.

Mapletoft, RJ, Del. Campo, MR and Ginther, OJ (1975). Unilateral luteotrophic effect of uterine venous effluent of a gravid uterine horn in sheep. Proc Soc Exp Biol Med 150: 129-133.

Markee, JE (1940). Menstruation in intra-ocular endometrial transplants in the Rhesus monkey. Contrib Embryol 177: 219-316.

Martin, NJ, Bydgeman, M and Eneroth, P (1978). The influence of locally administered prostaglandin E_2 and $F_{2}\alpha$ on uterine motility in the intact non-pregnant uterus. Acta Obstet Gynaecol Scand 57: 141-147.

Pickles, VR (1957). A plain muscle stimulant in the menstruum. Nature 180: 1198-1199.

Pickles, VR and Hall, WJ (1963). Some physiological properties of the "menstrual stimulant" substances A1 and A2. J Reprod Fertil 6: 315-317.

Pickles, VR, Hall, WJ, Best, FA and Smith, GN (1965). Prostaglandins in endometrium and menstrual fluid from normal and dysmenorrhoeic subjects. J Obstet Gynaecol Br Commonw 72: 185-192.

Poyser, NL and Maule-Walker, FM (1979). Anti-luteolytic effect of the embryo. In : Maternal recognition of pregnancy. Ciba Symposium, 64: Excerpta Medica, p 261-291.

Saeed, SA, McDonald-Gibson, WJ, Cuthbert, J, Copas, JL, Schneider, C, Gardiner, PJ, Butt, NM and Colher, HOJ (1977). Endogenous inhibitor of prostaglandin synthetase. Nature 270: 32-36.

Singh, EJ, Baccarini, IM and Zuspan, FP (1975). Levels of prostaglandin $F_{2}\alpha$ and E_2 in human endometrium during the menstrual cycle. Am J Obstet Gynecol 121: 1003-1006.

Sun, FF, Chapman, JP and McGuire, JE (1977). Metabolism of prostaglandin endoperoxides in animal tissue. Prostaglandins 14: 1055-1074.

Tulchinsky, D and Hobel, CJ (1973). Plasma human chorionic gonadotrophin, estradiol, estriol, progesterone and 17 hydroxy-progesterone in human pregnancy. III. Early normal pregnancy. Am J Obstet Gynaecol 117: 884-893.

Willman, EA and Collins, WP (1976). Distribution of prostaglandins E_2 and $F_{2}\alpha$ within the foetoplacental unit throughout human pregnancy. J Endocrinol 69: 413-419.

Willman, EA, Collins, WP and Clayton, SG (1976). Studies in the involvement of prostaglandins in uterine symptomatology and pathology. Br J Obstet Gynaecol 83: 337-341.

DISCUSSION

KATZENELLENBOGEN: Were you in fact using 0.2 mM 2-hydroxy-estradiol?

ABEL: Yes.

KATZENELLENBOGEN: Do you require such high concentrations of either estradiol or 2-hydroxy-estradiol?

ABEL: Yes. I am not suggesting that these levels of estrogen are physiological, however, this is a useful tool. Very high estradiol concentrations are required to increase PG production in this endometrial broken cell preparation. Therefore when we started using 2-hydroxy-estradiol, we used it at a similar concentration. You can, in fact, go to much lower concentrations with this catechol estrogen.

KATZENELLENBOGEN: In the dose-response studies, are you past the peak of stimulation with estradiol at the 0.2 mM concentration? Have you looked at lower concentrations?

ABEL: We have found very little effect of estradiol in this endometrial broken cell preparation.

GLASSER: I have two observations on embryo life or death and the maintenance of pregnancy that might be of interest. In the rat removal of all the fetuses but one will not precipitate the termination of pregnancy. Second, I've had the opportunity to work with patients whose fetus had died in utero. We have now examined the placentae in four women whose fetus had been dead since mid-pregnancy. In none of those cases did the death of the fetus precipitate the termination of the pregnancy. In considering a possible inhibitor of prostaglandin synthesis produced by the embryo, I offer this information only in terms of interest and information.

ABEL: I think that the nonembryonic or trophoblast tissue is the most likely site of production for this possible inhibitor. In ectopic pregnancies it was frequently very difficult to locate the gestational sac, but one could invariably identify trophoblastic tissue in quite large amounts. This is often a characteristic of ectopic development. Therefore, persistence of trophoblast tissue after fetal death may result in continued secretion of this PG synthesis inhibitor. In addition, there seems to be a prolonged effect of this inhibition so that you might not expect immediate stimulation of parturition mechanisms following death of the fetus.

GLASSER: If you place the site of synthesis of this putative inhibitor in the trophoblast, then I would have to say that our data would support the trophoblast as the site. In human fetal death the trophoblast tissue which is responsible for the synthesis of the peptide hormones which maintain pregnancy is maintained until term.

KENNEDY: Do you need an embryonic inhibitor? Is it not possible that the differentiation of stromal cells to decidual cells by itself brings about some change in cellular function such that prostaglandin biosynthesis is suppressed?

ABEL: Histological changes which occur during decidualization may reflect biochemical changes within these cells, such as a decreased ability to synthesize PGs. However, predecidual changes are apparent in the endometrium during the mid to late secretory phase of the menstrual cycle, when both the PG synthesizing capacity and endogenous concentrations of $PGF_{2\alpha}$ and PGE_2 are high.

In addition, in the nine women with an intact ectopic pregnancy we found a variable degree of endometrial decidualization which probably reflects variations in plasma progesterone concentration, despite consistently low levels of both $PGF_{2\alpha}$ and PGE. Therefore, I think that the histological appearance of the endometrium does not necessarily reflect its ability to synthesize PGs.

GERSCHENSON: What is the concentration of added arachidonic acid in your organ cultures?

ABEL: 2.5 μg/ml

GERSCHENSON: Do you have sera in your culture medium?

ABEL: Yes. The culture medium is Trowel's T_8 supplemented with 20% donor calf serum.

GERSCHENSON: What percentage of your arachidonic acid is metabolized to prostaglandins?

ABEL: Adding arachidonic acid to the cultures didn't increase the output of either $PGF_{2\alpha}$ or PGE_2 into the medium. Although arachidonic acid may be taken up by cells or tissue there is evidence that it may not be immediately available for prostaglandin synthesis. Simply increasing the arachidonic acid content of the medium does not necessarily increase the free arachidonic acid concentration within the cell.

GERSCHENSON: Our experience was years ago working with Drs. Mead and Haggerty at UCLA, before I was aware of the biological importance of prostaglandins. When either linoleic or arachidonic acid was added to the culture systems practically all the fatty acid was β-oxidized. Can you add enough other kinds of fatty acids so that the arachidonic may be available for prostaglandin synthesis? We also found there are certain concentrations of arachidonic acid at which there was tremendous generation of peroxides that were somehow inhibitory for the cells.

ABEL: Perhaps a better system for looking at arachidonic acid metabolism is the short-term incubation of a tissue homogenate with arachidonic acid, rather than a long-term culture system.

BIGGERS: A comment on this last question. Utilization of arachidonic acid by tissues can be quite variable and people that work, for example on renal tissue, find arachidonic acid cannot be metabolized directly to give the prostaglandin products, although arachidonic acid gets into the cellular phospholipids. The trick that's used is to cause release of arachidonic acid from the phospholipid stores by means of stimulating intracellular calcium release which activates phospholipase A_2. You can do this by use of a calcium ionophore. We've been using this technique on blastocysts. So, the fact that you don't get arachidonic acid utilized directly is the same experience other people have had with other tissues.

The question I wanted to ask was: If the lower concentrations of prostaglandins in the endometrium in pregnancy are the result of what is produced and what is destroyed, is it possible that these lower PG concentrations result from increased uterine metabolic activity which is eliminating it faster than the nonpregnant state?

ABLE: There is little evidence for metabolism of PGs by uterine tissue. Tissues of trophoblastic origin, chorion and placenta, have a much higher 15-PG dehydrogenase activity than either myometrium or decidua from both early (Kierse, et al, 1975) and late pregnancies (Kierse and Turnbull, 1975). After incubation of decidual tissue with $^3HPGF_{2\alpha}$ for 30 minutes, approximately 85% of the radioactivity was recovered as $PGF_{2\alpha}$.

In addition, in our incubations of homogenates of decidual tissue with ^{14}C-arachidonic acid, we have not found evidence of increased amounts of the 15-keto-13,14-dihydro-derivatives of $PGF_{2\alpha}$ or PGE_2 following TLC separation of the products when compared with incubations with nonpregnant tissue.

SHAPIRO: Seven or eight years ago Claude Villee's lab did similar culture experiments and reported perhaps three to five times as high a level of $PGF_{2\alpha}$ in their culture tissue. Could you contrast your work to Villee's to explain that difference?

ABEL: Cane and Villee (1975) used a 48 hour incubation to look at the effect of estradiol and progesterone on PGF production by human endometrium in vitro. Concentrations of PGF were measured in both tissue and medium at the end of the incubation period. Comparison of our results with those reported by Cane and Villee is difficult, first because different culture systems were used, second, because of the heterogeneous nature of the three samples used by these workers and third because we have expressed our results in a different manner. Thus the levels of PGF of approximately 100 ng/ml reported by Cane and Villee in control cultures appear considerably higher than levels reported here because they have not been corrected for tissue weight and represent production over a 48 hour period. In our study output of $PGF_{2\alpha}$ by proliferative tissue cultured in the absence of exogenous steroids was approximately 5.0 ng/mg/24 hour and for secretory endometrium approximatey 10.0 ng/mg/24 hour. The tissue weight in each case was in region of 5.0 mg. Therefore, if tissue weight, nature of tissue and time period are taken into account the apparent differences are reduced. However, since PG production can be readily stimulated by any form of trauma it is likely that one will always find differences between different workers and different systems with respect to PGs.

BAZER: I wanted to make one comment relative to what Stan Glasser brought up with the dead human fetuses. In domestic animals, if the embryo develops normally beyond a certain critical period you can then either flush it out of the uterus or kill it, and corpus luteum function continues. There seems to be a period of gestation in all these species beyond which you have to pass, after that, the corpus luteum is maintained through some mechanism which isn't understood.

References:

Cane, EM and Villee, CA (1975). The synthesis of prostaglandin F by human endometrium in organ culture. Prostaglandins 9:281-288.

Kierse, MJNC and Turnbull, AC (1975). Metabolism of prostaglandins within the pregnant uterus. Br J Obstet Gynaecol 82:887-893.

Kierse, MJNC, Williamson, JG and Turnbull, AC (1975). Metabolism of prostaglandin $F_{2\alpha}$ within the human uterus in early pregnancy. Br J Obstet Gynaecol 82:142-145.

The Endometrium

17

Prostaglandin I_2 and Increased Endometrial Vascular Permeability Preceding the Decidual Cell Reaction

T.G. Kennedy
G.J. Barbe
C.A. Evans

SUMMARY

The possibility that the increased endometrial vascular permeability which precedes the decidual cell reaction is mediated by prostaglandin I_2, rather than prostaglandin E_2, was investigated in rats. Immature rats were pretreated with hormones so that at the time of uterine stimulation they were sensitized for the decidual cell reaction. To determine if a deciduogenic stimulus resulted in increased uterine prostaglandin I_2, rats received a unilateral intrauterine injection of 50 µl phosphate buffered saline containing gelatin, and were killed at varying times thereafter. As determined by radioimmunoassay, the levels of 6-keto-prostaglandin $F_{1\alpha}$ were elevated in the injected uterine horns compared to the noninjected horns 30 min, 2 h and 8 h after injection, suggesting that uterine production of prostaglandin I_2 had been stimulated. Prostaglandin E levels were also elevated in the injected horns. To determine if prostaglandin I_2 was able to increase endometrial vascular permeability when given into the uterus, rats treated with indomethacin to inhibit endogenous prostaglandin synthesis received a unilateral intrauterine injection of either vehicle (50 µl 0.01M Tris, 0.145 M NaCl, pH 9.0), 50 µg prostaglandin I_2 or 50 µg prostaglandin E_2. The alkaline pH was used in an attempt to reduce the breakdown of prostaglandin I_2. Endometrial vascular permeability indices (ratios of the concentrations of radioactivity in the injected to noninjected uterine horns 15 min after an intravenous injection of ^{125}I-labelled bovine serum albumin) were determined 4 or 8 h later. Prostaglandin I_2 had no significant effect on the indices at either time of sacrifice, whereas prostaglandin E_2 significantly increased the indices. Prostaglandin I_2 did not interact significantly with prostaglandin E_2. The inability of prostaglandin I_2 to alter endometrial vascular permeability suggests that it does not mediate the increase in permeability which results from a deciduogenic stimulus. However, because of the instability of prostaglandin I_2 at neutral pH, this possible role for prostaglandin I_2 cannot be eliminated.

INTRODUCTION

The differentiation of endometrial cells into decidual cells in rodents occurs in response to either blastocysts or artificial stimuli and is always preceded by an increase in endometrial vascular permeability (Psychoyos, 1973). Although many different kinds of artificial stimuli are effective, decidualization can be obtained only during a limited period of pregnancy, pseudopregnancy, or when the uterus has been sensitized by giving the animals an appropriate regimen of hormone injections (Finn and Porter, 1975).

Recently, considerable evidence has been presented which suggests that prostaglandins mediate the changes in endometrial vascular permeability and subsequent decidualization in both the pregnant and non-pregnant animal. In pregnancy, indomethacin, an inhibitor of prostaglandin biosynthesis, not only delays or inhibits the appearance of increased vascular permeability in uterine areas surrounding the blastocysts (Kennedy, 1977; Evans and Kennedy, 1978; Hoffman _et al_., 1978), but also inhibits implantation (Lau _et al_., 1973; Gavin _et al_., 1974; Saksena _et al_., 1976). The concentrations of prostaglandins are elevated in the areas of increased endometrial vascular permeability (Kennedy, 1977; Evans and Kennedy, 1978; Kennedy and Zamecnik, 1978), and exogenous prostaglandins can at least partially reverse the effect of indomethacin on implantation (Saksena _et al_., 1976). In non-pregnant animals, artificially induced decidualization is reduced by indomethacin treatment (Castracane _et al_., 1974; Tobert, 1976; Sananes _et al_., 1976; Rankin _et al_., 1979a), as also are the changes in endometrial vascular permeability (Kennedy, 1979).

At present, there is uncertainty about which prostaglandins are involved in mediating the endometrial vascular permeability changes. Kennedy (1979), for several reasons, suggested that prostaglandin E_2 may be the mediator. First, E-series prostaglandins are elevated in the areas of increased endometrial vascular permeability, relative to the rest of the uterus, at implantation in rats (Kennedy, 1977) and hamsters (Evans and Kennedy, 1978). Secondly, artificial stimuli applied to uteri sensitized for the decidual cell reaction result in elevated uterine prostaglandin E levels prior to any demonstrable increase in permeability, suggesting that the prostaglandin levels are increased as a cause, rather than a consequence, of the change in permeability (Kennedy, 1979). Finally, intrauterine administration of prostaglandin E_2, but not prostaglandin $F_{2\alpha}$, to rats in which endogenous prostaglandin production has been inhibited by indomethacin, increases endometrial vascular permeability. However, as noted by Kennedy (1979), prostaglandin I_2 may also be of significance as a mediator since rat uterine homogenates produce large amounts of 6-keto-prostaglandin $F_{1\alpha}$, the stable product of prostaglandin I_2 (Fenwick _et al_., 1977) and, at implantation, the concentrations of 6-keto-prostaglandin $F_{1\alpha}$ are elevated within the uterus at the sites of increased endometrial vascular permeability (Kennedy and Zamecnik, 1978). In addition, there are suggestions that prostaglandin I_2 may be involved in mediating the changes in vascular permeability associated with the inflammatory response (Murota _et al_., 1978; Komoriya _et al_., 1978; Williams, 1979).

In this report, we examine the possibility that prostaglandin I_2 mediates the increase in endometrial vascular permeability induced by the application of an artificial deciduogenic stimulus to the sensitized rat uterus. Uterine prostaglandin I_2 production was estimated by measuring the uterine concentration of its stable break-down product, 6-keto-prostaglandin $F_{1\alpha}$.

MATERIALS AND METHODS

Animals

Female Sprague-Dawley rats, 26 or 27 days old, were obtained from Bio Breeding Laboratories of Canada, Ltd., Ottawa, Ontario and housed under temperature- and light-controlled conditions (lights on from 0500 to 1900 h) with free access to food and water.

All rats were pretreated so that at the time of intrauterine treatment, their uteri were sensitized for the decidual cell reaction. When 28 days old, the rats received a s.c. injection of 5 I.U. of pregnant mare serum gonadotropin (Equinex, Ayerst Laboratories) to induce ovulation. On the morning of the day after ovulation, the rats were ovariectomized under ether anesthesia and given 2 mg progesterone in 0.2 ml sesame oil s.c. For the next three days, the animals received daily s.c. injections of 0.5 μg estrone and 2 mg progesterone. All intrauterine injections were given between 1200 and 1500 h on the third day.

Treatments

Indomethacin, an inhibitor of prostaglandin biosynthesis (Vane, 1971; Flower, 1974), when administered, was given s.c. as 1 mg doses in 0.2 ml sesame oil at 1100 and 1700 h on the day of treatment.

The artificial stimulus given to the uterus was a unilateral intraluminal injection of 50 μl of phosphate buffered saline containing gelatin (PBS-G; 0.1 M phosphate in 0.154 M NaCl, 0.1% gelatin, pH 6.9). Saline introduced into the sensitized uterus of the rat will precipitate the decidual cell reaction (Finn and Porter, 1975).

At neutral pH, prostaglandin I_2 is chemically unstable at 37°C (Gryglewski et al., 1976). In an attempt to decrease the rate of hydrolysis of prostaglandin I_2 after intrauterine administration, prostaglandins in this study were dissolved in an alkaline Tris-saline buffer (0.01 M Tris, 0.145 M NaCl, pH 9.0). Control animals received an equivalent volume (50 μl) of the Tris-saline buffer.

All intrauterine injections were made into the uterine lumen of one uterine horn at the cervical end through a 30 gauge needle. Before withdrawing the needle, a tight ligature (5-0 silk) was tied just cranial to the site of injection to prevent loss of the injected material through the cervix (Kennedy, 1976) or the puncture wound. Care was taken to restrict mechanical trauma of the uterus to the site of injection.

Endometrial Vascular Permeability

Changes in endometrial vascular permeability were quantified by the use of [^{125}I]-labelled bovine serum albumin ([^{125}I]-BSA) (Psychoyos, 1961; Kennedy, 1979), prepared by the chloramine-T method of Greenwood et al. (1963). At the appropriate time after the intrauterine treatment, the rats were lightly anesthetized and given appropriately 2 μCi [^{125}I]-BSA/100 g body weight in 0.2 ml saline, via a tail vein. Fifteen min later, the animals were decapitated and trunk blood collected for subsequent determination of serum radioactivity levels. The uterus was removed and cleaned. The injected horn was cut approximately 0.5 cm cranial to the position of the ligature to avoid the area which had been traumatized mechanically at the time of intrauterine injection. The noninjected, contralateral horn was cut at an equivalent position. After gentle blotting, the uterine horns were weighed and placed in tubes for the determination of radioactivity.

Uterine Prostaglandin Levels

At various times after the intrauterine injections of PBS-G, rats were killed by cervical dislocation, their uteri removed and placed in ice-cold saline containing 20 μg/ml indomethacin. After at least 1 min in this solution, the uteri were cleaned of extraneous tissue and the injected horn cut approximately 0.5 cm cranial to the ligature; the contralateral horn was cut at the equivalent position. After blotting, freezing on dry ice and weighing, the tissue was placed in ice-cold ethanol and stored at -20°C. Before prostaglandin concentrations were determined, the samples were homogenized at 4°C in ethanol in Kontes all-glass Dual homogenizers and centrifuged. The supernatants were then utilized to estimate uterine prostaglandin levels by radioimmunoassays, conducted as described by Kennedy (1979) for prostaglandin E, and as described below for 6-keto-prostaglandin $F_{1\alpha}$.

Antisera against 6-keto-prostaglandin $F_{1\alpha}$ was generated in rabbits, essentially as described by Salmon (1978), except that crystalline 6-keto-prostaglandin $F_{1\alpha}$ (The Upjohn Company) was conjugated to BSA. The tracer for the assay was obtained by labelling histamine, coupled to 6-keto-prostaglandin $F_{1\alpha}$, with ^{125}I (Maclouf et al., 1976), using 10 μg chloramine T and 10 μg sodium metabisulphite in 10 μl phosphate buffer. For the assay, 0.1 ml diluted antiserum (1:1750) was incubated overnight at 4°C with tracer (approximately 15,000 cpm) and unknown sample or standard (7.8-1000 pg) in a final volume of 0.3 ml. This dilution of antiserum resulted in approximately 50% binding of the tracer in the absence of unlabelled 6-keto-prostaglandin $F_{1\alpha}$. To separate bound from free, 1 ml dextran-charcoal (25 mg Dextran T-70, 250 mg Norit A per 100 ml buffer) at 4°C was added to each tube. The tubes were then allowed to incubate for 1 h before being centrifuged at 4°C for 15 min at approximately 2000 x g. The supernatant was counted in a gamma spectrometer.

Sensitivity of the assay varied between 7.8 and 15.6 pg per tube. Specificity, as assessed by inhibition of binding of tracer to antiserum by a series of prostaglandins, is presented in Table 1. Accuracy of the assay was estimated by determining the content of 6-keto-prostaglandin $F_{1\alpha}$ before and after the addition of standard amounts of this compound

TABLE 1. Cross-reactivity of various prostaglandins and related compounds in the 6-keto-prostaglandin $F_{1\alpha}$ assay

Compound	Relative cross-reaction (%)*
6-Keto-prostaglandin $F_{1\alpha}$	100%
Prostaglandin E_2	2.1%
Prostaglandin $F_{2\alpha}$	4.0%
Prostaglandin D_2	< 1%
Prostaglandin A_2	< 1%
Thromboxane B_2	< 1%
13,14-Dihydro-15-keto-prostaglandin $F_{1\alpha}$	< 1%
13,14-Dihydro-15-keto-prostaglandin $F_{2\alpha}$	< 1%
13,14-Dihydro-15-keto-prostaglandin E_1	< 1%
15-Keto-prostaglandin $F_{1\alpha}$	< 1%

*Ratio of mass of compound to mass of 6-keto-prostaglandin $F_{1\alpha}$, expressed as a percentage, which caused 50% inhibition of binding of tracer 6-keto-prostaglandin $F_{1\alpha}$.

to rat uterine homogenates; when 100 pg 6-keto-prostaglandin $F_{1\alpha}$ was added, 107 ± 5 pg (mean ± SEM, n = 7) was recovered.

For rat uterine homogenates, prepared as described above, direct assay of the supernatant was compared with assay after purification on silicic acid columns, using the system described by Kennedy (1978). The 6% and 10% methanol in chloroform fraction was omitted; 6-keto-prostaglandin $F_{1\alpha}$ was eluted in 7 ml 20% methanol in chloroform. When allowances were made for column blanks and chromatographic losses (estimated by the recovery of $[^3H]$-6-keto-prostaglandin $F_{1\alpha}$), there was good agreement between the values obtained by the two procedures (correlation coefficient, r = 0.929, n = 6, $P < 0.01$). For the direct assay, different aliquot sizes (50, 100, 200 μl ethanolic extract) gave results which were parallel to the standard curve.

The intra- and inter-assay coefficients of variation were 5% and 13%, respectively.

Data Analysis

To assess changes in endometrial vascular permeability, the ratios of the concentrations of radioactivity in the injected to the non-injected uterine horns were calculated and referred to as the endometrial vascular permeability indices (Kennedy, 1979). An index of 1 is presumed to indicate that vascular permeability is identical in both horns; an index greater than 1 indicates that vascular permeability in the injected horn is greater than in the noninjected horn.

The significance of treatment effects was determined by analysis of variance. When heterogeneity of variance was present, as determined by Bartlett's test (Snedecor, 1956), the data were transformed logarithmically prior to statistical analysis.

RESULTS

Uterine Prostaglandins following Intrauterine Treatment

To determine if the application of an artificial stimulus resulted in increased uterine prostaglandin I_2 production, as estimated by uterine levels of 6-keto-prostaglandin $F_{1\alpha}$, rats with uteri sensitized for the decidual cell reaction were given a unilateral intrauterine injection of 50 µl PBS-G and killed 30 min, 2 h or 8 h later. As indicated by analysis of variance, the levels of 6-keto-prostaglandin $F_{1\alpha}$ (Fig. 1) were elevated ($\underline{P} < 0.001$) in the injected uterine horns, whereas the later times of autopsy were associated with lower

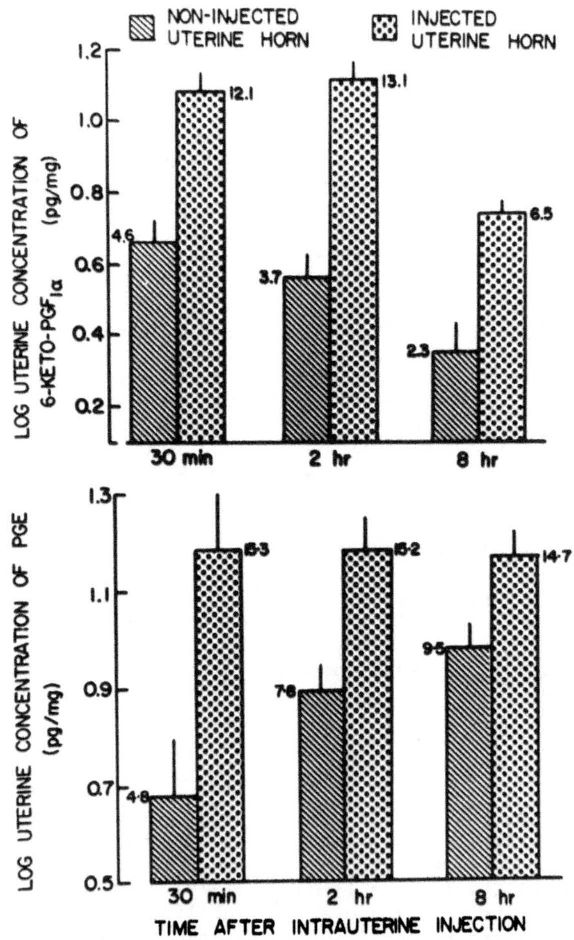

FIGURE 1. Uterine concentrations of 6-keto-prostaglandin $F_{1\alpha}$ and prostaglandin E at varying times after the unilateral, intrauterine injection of 50 µl PBS-G. Each bar represents the mean (± SEM) of the logarithmically transformed data of 7 rats. The geometric mean is given beside each bar.

(P < 0.001) levels. For prostaglandin E, time of autopsy had no significant effect on uterine concentrations, whereas intrauterine treatment was associated with elevated (P < 0.001) levels.

Effect of Prostaglandin I_2 and Prostaglandin E_2 on Endometrial Vascular Permeability

Rats which had been treated with indomethacin to inhibit endogenous prostaglandin biosynthesis were given a unilateral intrauterine injection of 50 µg prostaglandin I_2 or 50 µg prostaglandin E_2, and killed 4 or 8 h later, 15 min after an i.v. injection of [^{125}I]-BSA. As indicated by analysis of variance, prostaglandin E_2 increased (P < 0.005) the endometrial vascular permeability indices over those seen in controls (Fig. 2); prostaglandin I_2 was without effect. The indices tended (0.05 < P < 0.1) to be greater for autopsy at 8 h, compared to those at 4 h.

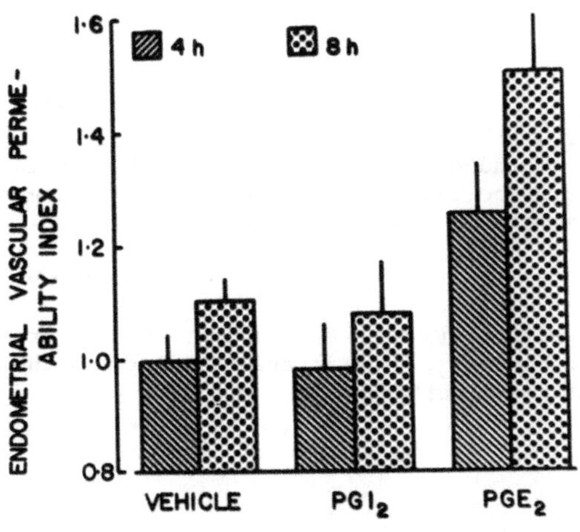

FIGURE 2. Effect of a unilateral, intrauterine injection of 50 µg prostaglandin I_2 or 50 µg prostaglandin E_2, given in 50 µl Tris-saline buffer to indomethacin-treated animals, on endometrial vascular permeability indices 4 or 8 h later. Each bar represents the mean (± SEM) of 7 rats.

Interaction between Prostaglandin E_2 and I_2

In a 2x2 factorial experiment, indomethacin-treated rats were given a unilateral intrauterine injection of 50 µl Tris-saline buffer with and without 50 µg prostaglandin E_2 and prostaglandin I_2. The animals were killed 8 h later, 15 min after an i.v. injection of [^{125}I]-BSA. Analysis of variance of the permeability indices (Fig. 3) indicated

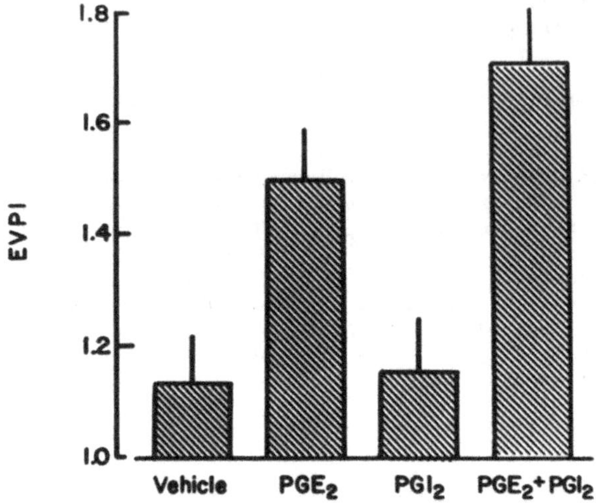

FIGURE 3. Effect of a unilateral, intrauterine injection of 50 µl Tris-saline buffer, with and without 50 µg prostaglandin E_2 and 50 µg prostaglandin I_2, on endometrial vascular permeability indices (EVPI) measured 8 h later. The rats were pretreated with indomethacin. Each bar represents the mean (± SEM) of 8-9 animals.

---

that they were significantly ($\underline{P} < 0.001$) increased by prostaglandin E_2 but not by prostaglandin I_2. The interaction between the two prostaglandins was not significant ($\underline{P} > 0.25$).

DISCUSSION

The application of an artificial deciduogenic stimulus to the uterus of rats sensitized for the decidual cell reaction resulted in increased concentrations of 6-keto-prostaglandin $F_{1\alpha}$ in the stimulated uterine horn. The levels of 6-keto-prostaglandin $F_{1\alpha}$ were elevated within 30 min, and remained higher than in the nonstimulated horns for at least 8 h. These changes in 6-keto-prostaglandin $F_{1\alpha}$ presumably reflect increased uterine prostaglandin I_2 synthesis and, since the levels are elevated prior to the increase in endometrial vascular permeability (Kennedy, 1979), are consistent with prostaglandin I_2 functioning as a mediator of the change in permeability. However, attempts to override the indomethacin-inhibition of the permeability response to artificial uterine stimulation (Kennedy, 1979) with prostaglandin I_2 were unsuccessful. When given into the uterine lumen of rats in which endogenous prostaglandin production had been inhibited by pretreatment of the animals with indomethacin, prostaglandin I_2 did not alter endometrial vascular permeability, as measured with [^{125}I]-BSA. However, because of the instability of prostaglandin I_2, particularly at neutral pH (Gryglewski et al., 1976), these negative results do not rule out the possibility that prostaglandin I_2 is a mediator of endometrial vascular permeability changes. In an attempt to circumvent this problem of instability, relatively large amounts of prostaglandin I_2 were administered to the uterine lumen in an alkaline buffer. Nevertheless, it is possible that the prostaglandin I_2 was hydrolysed to the relatively inactive 6-keto-prostaglandin $F_{1\alpha}$ before it could alter endometrial vascular permeability.

The suggestion that prostaglandin I_2 may be the mediator of decidualization has come from Rankin et al. (1979b), who found that tranylcypromine, a selective inhibitor of prostaglandin I_2 synthesis (Gryglewski et al., 1976) inhibits decidualization in mice. However, the selectivity of this inhibitory action of tranylcypromine on prostaglandin I_2 synthesis has been questioned (Rajtar and de Gaetano, 1979), and the inhibition has not been overridden with prostaglandin I_2.

At present, the available experimental evidence suggests that prostaglandin E_2 mediates the changes in endometrial vascular permeability. The levels of prostaglandin E were elevated within the uterus following the application of the artificial stimulus and, when given into the lumen of indomethacin-treated animals, prostaglandin E_2 increased vascular permeability. Larger amounts of this prostaglandin were administered in the present study than previously (Kennedy, 1979), because of its instability in alkaline solutions.

Thus, at present there is considerable evidence for, and none against, a role for prostaglandin E_2 as a mediator for changes in endometrial vascular permeability, whereas there is only suggestive evidence for prostaglandin I_2.

Despite the considerable evidence for the involvement of prostaglandins in mediating changes in endometrial vascular permeability, little is known about their mode of action. The effects of prostaglandins on vascular permeability have been most studied in the inflammatory response. Williams (1977) and Williams and Peck (1977) have recently emphasized that during this response, there is not only an increase in vascular permeability but also vasodilation, and that these two components of the response, both essential, may have separate chemical mediators. There is general agreement that prostaglandins, probably of the E or I series, mediate the vasodilation of the inflammatory response (Kuehl et al., 1977; Williams, 1977, 1979; Williams and Peck, 1977), but disagreement about the mediators of the changes in vascular permeability, with histamine and bradykinin being proposed by Williams and Peck (1977), and the endoperoxide, prostaglandin G_2, or some non-prostaglandin product of it, by Kuehl et al. (1977). The report of Bitton et al. (1965) that, in pseudopregnant rats, vasodilation accompanies increased endometrial vascular permeability suggests that the two mediator hypothesis may be applicable to this endometrial response. The vasodilation may be mediated by prostaglandins of the E or I series, with the experimental evidence at present favouring the former. The involvement of histamine in the endometrial vascular permeability response is suggested by the report of Brandon and Wallis

(1977) that histamine H_1- and H_2-receptor antagonists reduce the number and intensity of localised areas of increased endometrial vascular permeability at implantation.

ACKNOWLEDGEMENTS

Ms. L. A. Lukash provided excellent technical assistance during the course of the study. Drs. J. E. Pike and K. T. Kirton, The Upjohn Company, Kalamazoo, Michigan, generously provided the prostaglandins and the antiserum used in the prostaglandin E assay, respectively. The indomethacin was a gift from Dr. F. A. Kuehl, Jr., Merck Institute for Therapeutic Research, Rahway, New Jersey. The research was supported by a grant from the Medical Research Council (Canada). T.G.K. is a Scholar of the Medical Research Council.

REFERENCES

Bitton, V., Vassent, G. and Psychoyos, A. (1965). Réponse vasculaire de l'utérus au traumatisme, au cours de la pseudogestation chez la ratte. C. R. Acad. Sci. 261: 3474-3477.

Brandon, J.M. and Wallis, R.M. (1977). Effect of mepyramine, a histamine H_1-, and burimamide, a histamine H_2-receptor antagonist, on ovum implantation in the rat. J. Reprod. Fert. 50: 251-254.

Castracane, V.D., Saksena, S.K. and Shaikh, A.A. (1974). Effect of IUDs, prostaglandins and indomethacin on decidual cell reaction in the rat. Prostaglandins 6: 397-404.

Evans, C.A. and Kennedy, T.G. (1978). The importance of prostaglandin synthesis for the initiation of blastocyst implantation in the hamster. J. Reprod. Fert. 54: 255-261.

Fenwick, L., Jones, R.L., Naylor, B., Poyser, N.L. and Wilson, N.H. (1977). Production of prostaglandins by the pseudopregnant rat uterus, in vitro, and the effect of tamoxifen with the identification of 6-keto-prostaglandin $F_{1\alpha}$ as a major product. Br. J. Pharmacol. 59: 191-199.

Finn, C.A. and Porter, D.G. (1975). "The Uterus". Publishing Sciences Group, Acton.

Flower, R.J. (1974). Drugs which inhibit prostaglandin biosynthesis. Pharmacol. Rev. 26: 33-67.

Gavin, M.A., Dominguez Fernandez-Tejerina, J.C., Montañes de las Heras, M.F. and Vijil Maeso, E. (1974). Efectos de un inhibidor de la biosíntesis de las prostaglandinas (indometacina) sobre la implantación en la rata. Reproducción 1: 177-183.

Greenwood, F.C., Hunter, W.M. and Glover, J.S. (1963). The preparation of ^{131}I-labelled human growth hormone of high specific radioactivity. Biochem. J. 89: 114-123.

Gryglewski, R.J., Bunting, S., Moncada, S., Flower, R.J. and Vane, J.R. (1976). Arterial walls are protected against deposition of platelet thrombi by a substance (prostaglandin X) which they make from prostaglandin endoperoxides. Prostaglandins 12: 685-713.

Hoffman, L.H., DiPietro, D.L. and McKenna, T.J. (1978). Effects of indomethacin on uterine capillary permeability and blastocyst development in rabbits. Prostaglandins 15: 823-828.

Kennedy, T.G. (1976). Effects of analogues of prostaglandins E_2 and $F_{2\alpha}$ on uterine luminal fluid accumulation in the estrogen-treated ovariectomized rat: an indirect measure of cervical tone. Prostaglandins 12: 1061-1071.

Kennedy, T.G. (1977). Evidence for a role for prostaglandins in the initiation of blastocyst implantation in the rat. Biol. Reprod. 16: 286-291.

Kennedy, T.G. (1978). Effect of oxytocin on estrogen-induced uterine luminal fluid accumulation in ovariectomized rats and the role of prostaglandins. Can. J. Physiol. Pharmac. 56: 908-914.

Kennedy, T.G. (1979). Prostaglandins and increased endometrial vascular permeability resulting from the application of an artificial stimulus to the uterus of the rat sensitized for the decidual cell reaction. Biol. Reprod. 20: 560-566.

Kennedy, T.G. and Zamecnik, J. (1978). The concentration of 6-keto-prostaglandin $F_{1\alpha}$ is markedly elevated at the site of blastocyst implantation in the rat. Prostaglandins 16: 599-605.

Komoriya, K., Ohmori, H., Azuma, A., Kurozumi, S., Hashimoto, Y., Nicolaou, K.C., Barnette, W.E. and Magolda, R.L. (1978). Prostaglandin I_2 as a potentiator of acute inflammation in rats. Prostaglandins 15: 557-564.

Kuehl, F.A., Humes, J.L., Egan, R.W., Ham, E.A., Beveridge, G.C. and Van Arman, C.G. (1977). Role of prostaglandin endoperoxide PGG_2 in inflammatory processes. Nature 265: 170-173.

Lau, I.F., Saksena, S.K. and Chang, M.C. (1973). Pregnancy blockade by indomethacin, an inhibitor of prostaglandin synthesis: its reversal by prostaglandins and progesterone in mice. Prostaglandins 4: 795-803.

Maclouf, J., Pradel, M., Pradelles, P. and Dray, F. (1976). ^{125}I derivatives of prostaglandins. A novel approach in prostaglandin analysis by radioimmunoassay. Biochim. Biophys. Acta 431: 139-146.

Murota, S., Morita, I., Tsurufuji, S., Sato, H. and Sugio, K. (1978). Effect of prostaglandin I_2 and related compounds on vascular permeability response in granuloma tissues. Prostaglandins 15: 297-301.

Psychoyos, A. (1961). Perméabilité capillaire et décidualisation utérine. C.R. Acad. Sci. 252: 1515-1517.

Psychoyos, A. (1973). Endocrine control of egg implantation. In: Handbook of Physiology (R.O. Greep, E.B. Astwood and S.R. Geiger, eds.), Section 7, Volume II, Part 2. American Physiological Society, Washington, D.C., pp. 187-215.

Rajtar, G. and de Gaetano, G. (1979). Tranylcypromine is not a selective inhibitor of prostacyclin in rats. Thrombosis Res. 14: 245-248.

Rankin, J.C., Ledford, B.E., Jonsson, H.T. and Baggett, B. (1979a). Prostaglandins, indomethacin and the decidual cell reaction in the mouse uterus. Biol. Reprod. 20: 399-404.

Rankin, J.C., Ledford, B.E. and Baggett, B. (1979b). The effect of tranylcypromine on the artificially stimulated decidual cell reaction in the mouse uterus. Soc. Study Reprod., 12th Annual Meeting, Abstract No. 174.

Saksena, S.K., Lau, I.F. and Chang, M.C. (1976). Relationship between oestrogen, prostaglandin $F_{2\alpha}$ and histamine in delayed implantation in the mouse. Acta Endocr. 81: 801-807.

Salmon, J.A. (1978). A radioimmunoassay for 6-keto-prostaglandin $F_{1\alpha}$. Prostaglandins 15: 383-397.

Sananes, N., Baulieu, E.-E. and Le Goascogne, C. (1976). Prostaglandin(s) as inductive factor of decidualization in the rat uterus. Mol. Cell. Endocrinol. 6: 153-158.

Snedecor, G.W. (1956). "Statistical Methods". 5th ed. The Iowa State University Press, Ames.

Tobert, J.A. (1976). A study of the possible role of prostaglandins in decidualization using a non-surgical method for the instillation of fluids into the rat uterine lumen. J. Reprod. Fert. 47: 391-393.

Vane, J.R. (1971). Inhibition of prostaglandin synthesis as a mechanism of action of aspirin-like drugs. Nature (New Biol.) 231: 232-235.

Williams, T.J. (1977). Chemical mediators of vascular responses in inflammation: a two mediator hypothesis. Br. J. Pharmac. 61: 447P-448P.

Williams, T.J. (1979). Prostaglandin E_2, prostaglandin I_2 and the vascular changes of inflammation. Br. J. Pharmac. 65: 517-524.

Williams, T.J. and Peck, M.J. (1977). Role of prostaglandin-mediated vasodilatation in inflammation. Nature 270: 530-532.

DISCUSSION

ABEL: Prostacyclin, as measured by 6-keto-$PGF_1\alpha$ production, has been identified as the major prostaglandin produced by the uterus in the rat or sheep in studies using the whole uterus. One advantage in working with human uterine tissue is that endometrium and myometrium can be easily separated. Human endometrium produces predominantly PGF and PGE whereas human myometrium is relatively inactive, with 6-keto-$PGF_1\alpha$ the major PG identified. 6-Keto-$PGF_1\alpha$ is produced in significant amounts only when endometrium and myometrium are combined, possibly as a result of endoperoxide precursors being supplied to the myometrial prostacyclin synthetase. I wonder if the 6-keto-$PGF_1\alpha$ synthesized predominately in the myometrium is the causative agent in modifying vascular permeability within the endometrium. Have you looked at the endometrium and myometrium separately?

KENNEDY: No. What I presented were uterine concentrations of prostaglandins. We don't know whether the prostaglandins are in the endometrium or myometrium or in both.

BAULIEU: Two questions. Can you say anything about the prostacylin effects on the formation of deciduoma and on vascular permeability?

KENNEDY: The short answer is no, we have been looking much earlier, prior to the differentiation of the decidual cells. However, prostaglandin synthesis is probably required over a prolonged period if decidualization is to occur. Tolbert (1976) has reported that decidualization is inhibited when the administration of indomethacin is not initiated until 8 hrs after the application of a deciduogenic stimulus. By 8 hrs the changes in endometrial vascular permeability had presumably already occurred. This indicates that prostaglandins are not only involved in initiating the changes in permeability but also the subsequent differentiation of decidual cells. Which prostaglandins are involved in the differentiation and whether they are the same one which are involved in permeability changes are not known.

BAULIEU: The second question is, did you coadminister indomethacin with PGE_2? We find that the effect of $PGF_2\alpha$ on decidualization is antagonized by indomethacin. I believe your indomethacin treatment is by parenteral administration. Have you introduced indomethacin directly into the uterine horn?

KENNEDY: No. I am aware of those data from your laboratory which indicate that $PGF_2\alpha$ given into the uterine lumen will precipitate decidualization and am at a loss to explain the apparent difference between those results and ours. In our hands, $PGF_2\alpha$ inhibits the ability of PGE_2 to increase endometrial vascular permeability. Given the evidence that increased permeability is essential if decidualization is to occur, I would therefore expect $PGF_2\alpha$ to inhibit decidualization. However, Hoffman et al (1978) have shown that PGE_2 placed in the rabbit uterine lumen in silastic capsules is much more potent than $PGF_2\alpha$ in bringing about decidualization. I look forward to seeing your dose-response curves for the effect of $PGF_2\alpha$, as well as the effect of PGE_2, on decidualization.

BAULIEU: We work, as you know, in a slightly different model. Instead of having a uterus sensitized by estrogen as you have, we administer only progesterone and trauma. The prostaglandin effect starts from a lower baseline than in your animals, whether we use immature or castrated rats. So the different systems may explain the different results.

KENNEDY: As an alternative interpretation of your results, is it not possible that you were not giving the appropriate prostaglandin along with the indomethacin?

BAULIEU: Indomethacin blocks decidualization provoked by trauma or by arachidonic acid. This is easier to understand than the antagonism against $PGF_2\alpha$, a result which suggests that PGs do not always act directly, but may involve a loop somewhere in the arachidonic acid cascade.

BIGGERS: This is not a question, just a comment. Dr. Abel raised the issue of possible PGI_2 effects. El Tahir and Williams (1979) separated endometrium and myometrium and found a marked increase in PGI_2 in the myometrium in the area of the implantation sites. This may need to be taken into consideration.

References:

El Tahir, KEH and Williams, KI (1979). Myometrial prostacyclin synthesis - a new factor in pregnancy in the rat? J Physiology 296:86P.

Hoffman, LJ, DiPietro, DL and McKenna, TJ (1978). Effects of indomethacin on uterine capillary permeability and blastocyst development in rabbits. Prostaglandins 15:823-828.

Tolbert, JA (1976). A study of the possible role of prostaglandins in decidualization using a non-surgical method for the instillation of fluids into the rat uterine lumen. J Reprod Fert 47:391-393.

Index

GPSR Compliance

The European Union's (EU) General Product Safety Regulation (GPSR) is a set of rules that requires consumer products to be safe and our obligations to ensure this.

If you have any concerns about our products, you can contact us on ProductSafety@springernature.com

In case Publisher is established outside the EU, the EU authorized representative is:

Springer Nature Customer Service Center GmbH
Europaplatz 3
69115 Heidelberg, Germany

Batch number: 10607212

Printed by Printforce, the Netherlands